T0257776

Advanced Research in Quality Control

Edited by **Theresa Heen**

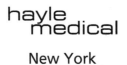

New York

Published by Hayle Medical,
30 West, 37th Street, Suite 612,
New York, NY 10018, USA
www.haylemedical.com

Advanced Research in Quality Control
Edited by Theresa Heen

© 2015 Hayle Medical

International Standard Book Number: 978-1-63241-014-6 (Hardback)

This book contains information obtained from authentic and highly regarded sources. Copyright for all individual chapters remain with the respective authors as indicated. A wide variety of references are listed. Permission and sources are indicated; for detailed attributions, please refer to the permissions page. Reasonable efforts have been made to publish reliable data and information, but the authors, editors and publisher cannot assume any responsibility for the validity of all materials or the consequences of their use.

The publisher's policy is to use permanent paper from mills that operate a sustainable forestry policy. Furthermore, the publisher ensures that the text paper and cover boards used have met acceptable environmental accreditation standards.

Trademark Notice: Registered trademark of products or corporate names are used only for explanation and identification without intent to infringe.

Printed in the United States of America.

Advanced Research in Quality Control

Edited by **Theresa Heen**

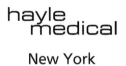

New York

Published by Hayle Medical,
30 West, 37th Street, Suite 612,
New York, NY 10018, USA
www.haylemedical.com

Advanced Research in Quality Control
Edited by Theresa Heen

© 2015 Hayle Medical

International Standard Book Number: 978-1-63241-014-6 (Hardback)

This book contains information obtained from authentic and highly regarded sources. Copyright for all individual chapters remain with the respective authors as indicated. A wide variety of references are listed. Permission and sources are indicated; for detailed attributions, please refer to the permissions page. Reasonable efforts have been made to publish reliable data and information, but the authors, editors and publisher cannot assume any responsibility for the validity of all materials or the consequences of their use.

The publisher's policy is to use permanent paper from mills that operate a sustainable forestry policy. Furthermore, the publisher ensures that the text paper and cover boards used have met acceptable environmental accreditation standards.

Trademark Notice: Registered trademark of products or corporate names are used only for explanation and identification without intent to infringe.

Printed in the United States of America.

Contents

Preface

Quality control is an important and growing aspect in every field of life. Quality control is a process that is used to ensure a certain level of quality in a product or service. It might encompass whatever actions a business seems necessary to provide for the control and verification of certain characteristics of a product or service. With the improvement of technology, we come across new and complicated devices and methods in different fields. Quality control is necessary in all of those new techniques. Our objective was to gather information about quality control in various fields. This book aims at disseminating useful and practical knowledge about quality control in several fields such as quality control in herbal medicine, food science, and in pharmaceutics.

This book is a result of research of several months to collate the most relevant data in the field.

When I was approached with the idea of this book and the proposal to edit it, I was overwhelmed. It gave me an opportunity to reach out to all those who share a common interest with me in this field. I had 3 main parameters for editing this text:

1. Accuracy – The data and information provided in this book should be up-to-date and valuable to the readers.
2. Structure – The data must be presented in a structured format for easy understanding and better grasping of the readers.
3. Universal Approach – This book not only targets students but also experts and innovators in the field, thus my aim was to present topics which are of use to all.

Thus, it took me a couple of months to finish the editing of this book.

I would like to make a special mention of my publisher who considered me worthy of this opportunity and also supported me throughout the editing process. I would also like to thank the editing team at the back-end who extended their help whenever required.

Editor

Quality Control of Herbal Medicine

Quality Control of *Rheum* and *Cassia* Species by Immunological Methods Using Monoclonal Antibodies Against Sennosides

Osamu Morinaga and Yukihiro Shoyama

Additional information is available at the end of the chapter

1. Introduction

Recently, medical usage of Japanese traditional medicine has been expanded by reaching aging society and increasing various chronic diseases. Therefore, the demand of crude drugs prescribed for Japanese traditional medicine has been increased. However, over 90% of crude drugs are imported in our country, and those over 70% are supplied by the collection of wild species. It is well known that the natural resources bring the difficulty of quality control depending on collection season, cultivation place, a variety of species and so on. The other problem, shortage of crude drug comes up. For these general environment, micropropagation and clonal propagation systems using tissue and cell culture were investigated in this laboratry.

Sennoside A (SA) and B (SB) have the strong catharsis activity and contained in rhubarb and senna (Figure 1) [1]. The concentration of sennosides in rhubarb and senna is variously dependent on the genetic heterogeneity of species, differences in soil condition and climate influence. Sennosides are metabolized by intestinal bacteria to rheinanthrone which acts in the intestines as a direct purgatives [2, 3] and functions as similar to a natural prodrug (Figure 2). Despite the rising availability of a number of synthetic cathartics, sennoside- containing prescriptions are still among the most widely used today, and their importance is increasing.

Rhubarb, the rhizome and root of *Rheum* spp. (Polygonaceae), is an important drug in traditional Japanese herbal medicine as well as in western medicine since ancient times. It was already recorded in *Chinese Materia Medica* 2000 years ago. It is used in many traditional Japanese herbal medicines prescribed with other herbal medicines for the syndrome of stasis of blood, as an anti-inflammatory, sedative agent and as a stomachic. Furthermore, it is widely used as cathartics in Japan. The main purgative principles of rhubarb have proved to be sennosides [1], identical with those isolated from senna leaves, and rheinosides, which were also isolated as purgatives of rhubarb, together with various kinds of phenolics, like tannins, stilbenes, naphthalenes and lindleyin. The quality of rhubarb is severely regulated by Japanese Pharmacopeia as rhubarb contains SA of over 0.25% dry weight in root [4].

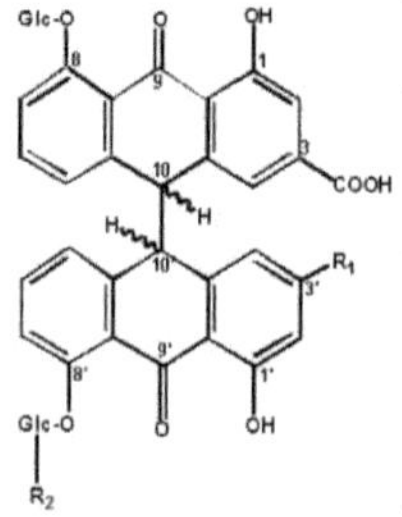

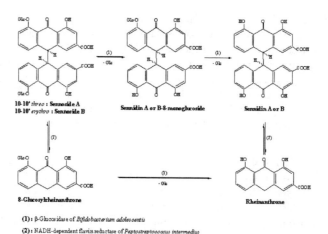

Compound	R_1	R_2	10-10'
Sennoside A	COOH	H	threo
Sennoside B	COOH	H	erythro
Sennoside C	CH₂OH	H	threo
Sennoside D	CH₂OH	H	erythro
Sennoside E	COOH	HOOC-CO	threo
Sennoside F	COOH	HOOC-CO	erythro

Figure 1. Structures of sennosides

10-10' *threo* : Sennoside A
10-10' *erythro* : Sennoside B

Sennidin A or B-8-monoglucoside

Sennidin A or B

8-Glucosylrheinanthrone

Rheinanthrone

(1) : β-Glucosidase of *Bifidobacterium adolescentis*

(2) : NADH-dependent flavin reductase of *Peptostreptococcus intermedius*

Figure 2. Metabolic pathways of sennosides by intestinal bacteria.

Senna, the leaf and pod of *Cassia* spp. (Leguminosae), is one of the most popular in herbal remedies and in health food industry. It has been widely used in cathartics for the relief of constipation prescribed with other health teas and dieter's teas in Japan, and often used as natural dietary supplements for enhancement of bloodflow and metabolism in USA, Europe and Australia. These pharmaceutical properties are due to sennosides, which are contained in *Cassia acutifolia* Delile and *Cassia angustifolia* Vahl. *C. angustifolia* listed in Japanese Pharmacopeia, and the quality is severely regulated as senna contains total sennosides (SA and SB) of over 1.0% dry weight in leaf [4].

In the breeding research on the plant, a lot of stages are required as follows : dedifferentiation, extension of mutation by the mutagen, redifferentiation, analysis of the redifferentiated plant, mass propagation of the higher yielding plant and transplanting to soil. Therefore, it is very important to study a large number of plant samples in the phytochemical field and a small sample size *in vitro* for the breeding of *Rheum* and *Cassia* species yielding high concentration of sennosides. Many analytical approaches have been investigated for the determination of sennosides in plant extracts. Among these methods, the use of high-performance liquid chromatography (HPLC) appears most frequently and widely today. However, when the assay of very low concentration of sennosides in the regenerated plantlets is needed, the HPLC method is not appropriate and efficient.

Recently, the immunological assay method is widely developed for the purpose of analysis for a small amount of constituent. In general immunological methodologies in particular enzyme-linked immunosorbent assay (ELISA) have promoted the development of higher sensitive assay system.

On the one hand, monoclonal antibodies (MAbs) have many potential uses in addition to immunological methods in plant sciences. MAbs are superior to polyclonal antibodies (PAbs) in the antigenic specificity and stability. Therefore, immunoassay using MAbs against pharmacologically active compound having small molecular weight has become an important tool for the studies on receptor binding analysis, enzyme assay and quantitative and/or qualitative analytical techniques in plants owing to its specific affinity, and possesses an extremely high possibility in the phytochemical analysis. Up to now, immunological approach for assaying quantities of sennosides in *C. angustifolia* using PAb against SB has been investigated by Atzorn *et al* [5]. However, since no success with MAbs against SA and SB has been reported, objectives of this work are shown as following.

1. Production of MAb against SA, its characterization and use for ELISA.

2. Production of MAbs against SB, their characterization and use for ELISA.

3. Establishments of a new eastern blotting, double staining and immunohistochemical staining using anti-SA and SB MAbs.

2. Production of MAb against SA, its characterization and use for ELISA

2.1. Preface

In the immunologically analytical methodology, there are two measuring methods using the antiserum (polyclonal antibody ; PAb) and MAb in general. PAb is a heterogeneous mixture of antibody molecules arising from a variety of constantly evolving B lymphocytes. Therefore, PAb can often show high affinity because different antibody populations react with the variety of epitopes that characterize the antigen. On the other hand, there are some problems of PAb that the extensive cross-reactivity occurs between the antibody and the multiple antigens which have the same antigenic determinant, and it is impossible to supply for identical antibody permanently. In the meantime, MAb is produced from a single B lymphocyte and can react with one antigenic determinant of the specific antigen. Besides MAb has identical specificity and affinity. There are some advantages that the complete purity of the immunized antigen is not required and the hybridoma cells can be preserved as freeze stock, and it is possible to get MAb depending on necessary respond.

There are several formats for ELISA like direct ELISA, competitive ELISA, sandwich ELISA and competitive ELISA according to the immune complexes formed during manipulation. Analysis of low molecular weight compound by immunoassay is still limited to competitive format.

Quality control of the Japanese herbal medicine is necessary because it is believed that approximately 70% of these crude drugs prescribed are collected from natural resource. Furthermore, since MAbs become necessary for the assay of concentrations of active constituents in our on-going plant biotechnological projects, we have already produced MAbs against natural compounds such as forskolin [6], solamargine [7], opium alkaloids [8], marihuana compounds [9], glycyrrhizin [10], crocin [11], ginsenoside Rb1 [12] and Rg1 [13], and developed individual competitive ELISAs. An immunological approach for assaying quantities of sennosides using a PAbs has been investigated by Atzorn et al.[5]. However, since no result of MAb related to sennosides has been reported yet, anti-SA MAb was produced as described [14].

2.2. Experimental

2.2.1. Chemicals and immunochemicals

SA was purchased from Wako Pure Chemical Ind., Ltd. (Osaka, Japan). 1-Ethyl-3-(3'-dimethylaminopropyl)-carbodiimide HCl (EDC) was purchased from Nacalai Tesque Inc. (Kyoto, Japan). BSA and HSA were provided by Pierce (Rockford, IL, USA). Peroxidase-labeled anti-mouse IgG was provided by Organon Teknika Cappel Products (West Chester, PA, USA). Enriched RPMI1640-Dulbecco's-Ham's F12 (eRDF) medium and RD-1 additives (containing 9 µg/mL insulin, 20 µg/mL transferrin, 20 µM ethanolamine, 25 µM sodium selenite) were purchased from Kyokuto Pharmaceutical Industrial Co., Ltd. (Tokyo, Japan). Hypoxanthine-aminopterin-thymidine (HAT) additives were obtained from Sigma Chemical Company (St. Louis, MO, USA). Fetal calf serum (FCS) was purchased from Cambrex Corporation (Walkersville, MA, USA). All other chemicals were standard commercial products of analytical grade. Samples of various rhubarb roots were purchased from the Tochimototenkaido Corporation (Osaka, Japan).

2.2.2. Extraction of various rhubarb samples

Dried samples (30 mg) of various rhubarb roots were powdered, and then extracted five times with MeOH containing 0.1% (w/v) NH_4OH (0.5 mL) with sonication, filtered using a Cosmonice Filter W (0.45 μm Filter Unit, Nacalai Tesque Inc., Kyoto, Japan), and the combined extracts were diluted with 10 mM $NaHCO_3$ to prepare a solution suitable for the ELISA.

2.2.3. Synthesis of antigen conjugates

To SA (6 mg) dissolved in 1 mL of tetrahydrofuran-20 mM phosphate buffer of pH 5.5 (7:3), 0.3 mL of 20 mM phosphate buffer (pH 5.5) containing 6 mg of EDC was added. Then, 0.3 mL of 20 mM phosphate buffer (pH 5.5) containing 6 mg of BSA was added, with stirring at room temperature for 14 hr. The reaction mixture was dialyzed five times against H_2O, and then lyophilized to give 5.8 mg of SA conjugate (SA-BSA). SA-HSA conjugate was also synthesized in the same manner.

2.2.4. Determination of hapten density in SA-carrier protein conjugate by matrix-assisted laser desorption/ionization (MALDI)-time of flight (TOF) mass spectrometry

The hapten number in the SA-carrier protein conjugate was determined by MALDI-TOF mass spectrometry as previously described [15]. A small amount (1-10 pmol) of antigen conjugate was mixed with a 10^3-fold molar excess of sinapinic acid in an aqueous solution containing 0.15% trifluoroacetic acid (TFA). The mixture was subjected to a JEOL Mass Spectrometers (JMS) time-of-flight (TOF) mass monitor (model Voyager Elite, PerSeptive Biosystems Inc., Framingham, MA, USA) and irradiated with a N_2 laser (337 nm, 150 ns pulse). The ions formed by each pulse were accelerated by a 20 kV potential into a 2.0 m evacuated tube and detected using a compatible computer as previously reported [15].

2.2.5. Competitive ELISA for SA

SA-HSA (five molecules of SA per molecule of HSA) (100 μL, 1 μg/mL) dissolved in 50 mM carbonate buffer (pH 9.6) was adsorbed to the wells of a 96-well immunoplate then treated with 300 μL S-PBS for 1 hr to reduce non-specific adsorption. Fifty μL of various concentrations of SA or samples dissolved in 10 mM $NaHCO_3$ solution were incubated with 50 μL of MAb solution (0.218 μg/mL) for 1 hr. The plate was washed three times with T-PBS, and then incubated with 100 μL of a 1:1000 dilution of POD-labeled anti-mouse IgG for 1 hr. After washing the plate three times with T-PBS, 100 μL of substrate solution [0.1 M citrate buffer (pH 4) containing 0.003% H_2O_2 and 0.3 mg/mL of ABTS] was added to each well and incubated for 15 min. The absorbance was measured by a micro plate reader at 405 nm and 490 nm.

The cross-reactivities (CR) of sennosides and related compounds were determined as following.

$$CR(\%) = \frac{\mu g/mL \text{ of SA yielding } A/A_0 = 50\%}{\mu g/mL \text{ of compound under investigation yielding } A/A_0 = 50\%} \times 100$$

where A is the absorbance in the presence of the test compound and A_0 is the absorbance in the absence of the test compound.

2.3. Results and discussion

2.3.1. Direct determination of SA-carrier protein conjugate by MALDI-TOF mass spectrometry

In general, the low molecular weight compounds (hapten) like plant secondary metabolite have no immunogenicity. Therefore, it should be conjugated with some high molecular compound like protein resulting in immunogenic. The specificity of immunoassay method is dependent on the site of linkage between hapten and carrier protein moiety, and enumeration of hapten in immunogen conjugate. SA-BSA and SA-HSA conjugates were synthesized as immunogen and the immobilization antigen for ELISA, respectively. Figure 3 shows the typical synthetic pathway of SA-BSA conjugate. The commonly used methods to link carboxyl group and amino group in a hapten or carrier involve activation by carbodiimides, isobutylchloroformate or carbonyldiimidazole. Carbodiimides react with carboxyl groups to form an unstable O-acetylisourea intermediate, which reacts with amines to form amide bonds. EDC can be used commonly as a carbodiimide. In this case, carrier protein combined directly to antigen as indicated in Figure 3.

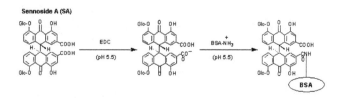

Figure 3. Typical synthetic pathway of SA-BSA. Carboxyl group of SA was activated by EDC and subsequently combined to amino residues of lysine and/or arginine on the protein to form amide bond.

Figure 4 shows the MALDI-TOF mass spectrum of the antigen, SA-BSA conjugate. A broad peak coinciding with the conjugate of SA and BSA appeared from m/z 68,500 to 73,500 centering at around m/z 70,600. Using experimental results and a molecular weight of 66,433 for BSA, the calculated values of SA component (MW 862) are 4,218 resulting in the range of two to eight molecules of SA (five on average) conjugated with BSA. In general eight to twenty five molecules of hapten conjugated with carrier protein in the conjugate were sufficient for immunization. Therefore, the hapten number was estimated to be sufficient for immunization because an antigen conjugate having a similar hapten number was sufficient for immunization in a previous study [10]. The number of SA contained in the SA-HSA conjugate was also determined to be around five molecules by its spectrum.

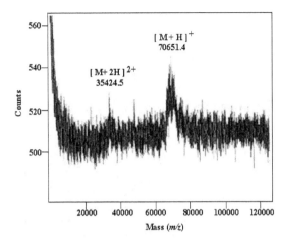

Figure 4. Direct determination of SA-BSA by MALDI-TOF MS. [M+H]+, [M+2H]²+ are single and double protonated molecules of SA-BSA, respectively.

2.3.2. Production and characteristic of MAb against SA

After the cell fusion and HAT selection, hybridoma producing MAb reactive to SA was obtained, and classfied into IgG$_1$ which had k light chains. Refined MAb was confirmed to be IgG compared to the MALDI-TOF MS measurement. The molecular weight of MAb was 151,396 calculated [16]. The reactivity of IgG type MAb 6G8 was tested for varying the antibody concentration and for performing a dilution curve in direct ELISA. The antibody concentration of 0.218 µg/mL showed the absorbance at 0.8 in direct ELISA, therefore it was selected for the competitive ELISA.

2.3.3. Assay sensitivity and assay specificity

The free MAb 6G8, following incubation with competing antigen, was bound to the polystyrene microtitre plates precoated with SA-HSA. Under these conditions, the full measuring range of the assay extended from 20 to 200 ng/mL as indicated in Figure 5.

SA is a unique anthraquinone having individual double of carboxylic acid-, hydroxyl-, carbonyl- and O-glucosyl-groups at C-3, C-1, C-9 and C-8 positions in a molecule, respectively. Moreover, SA possessed a *threo-* configuration between C-10 and C-10' positions as indicated in Figure 6. Therefore, a MAb should detect all these functions, and also the stereochemical recognition is needed for this complicated compound. Since the newly established ELISA against SA is expected to be applied for phytochemical investigations involving crude plant extracts, the assay specificity was checked by determining the cross-reactivities of MAb with various related compounds. The cross-reactivities of the MAb was examined by competitive ELISA.

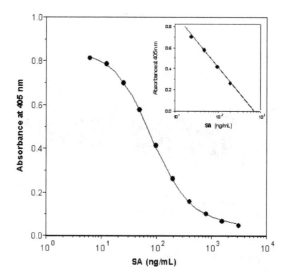

Figure 5. Calibration curve for SA.

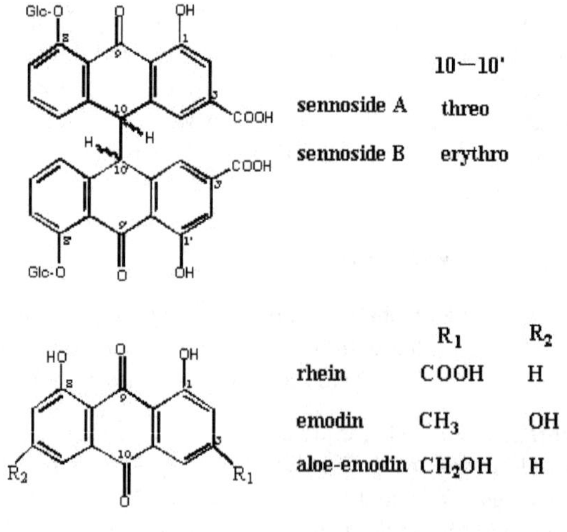

Figure 6. Chemical structures of SA, SB and its structurally related compounds.

Table 1 indicates the cross-reactivities of anti-SA MAb against related anthraquinone, anthrone and phenol carboxylic acid. MAb 6G8 cross-reacted with rhein and SB weakly; 0.28 and 0.35%, respectively. However, the other related anthraquinone and anthrone did not have appreciable cross-reactivities. From these results it is suggested that a basal structure of rhein and sugar moiety caused immunization. In addition the most important property of MAb 6G8 is an ability of stereochemical recognition because the differences of structure between SA and SB are only the stereochemical configuration at the C-10 and C-10' positions. Therefore, it is suggested that *threo*-configurational structure of bisanthrone is indispensable as an immunodominant molecule for reactivity of MAb 6G8.

Compound	Cross-reactivities (%)
Anthraquinone and anthrone	
sennoside A	100
sennoside B	0.28
rhein	0.35
emodin	< 0.04
aloe-emodin	< 0.04
barbaloin	< 0.04
1,4-dihydroxy-anthraquinone	< 0.04
Stilbene	
rhaponticin	< 0.04
Phenol carboxylic acid	
gallic acid	< 0.04
vanillic acid	< 0.04
caffeic acid	< 0.04
homogentisic acid	< 0.04

Table 1. Cross-reactivities (%) of MAb-6G8 against sennosides and other compounds.

2.3.4. Correlation of results of SA determination in crude extracts of rhubarb roots between HPLC and ELISA using MAb 6G8

The ELISA was utilized to measure the concentrations of SA in various rhubarb (Table 2). Oshio and Kawamura determined sennoside concentrations in various crude rhubarbs by HPLC [17]. More recently Seto *et al.* reported the comparative concentrations of sennosides determined by HPLC in various commercial rhubarbs [18]. They required a lager sample size compared to the newly established ELISA due to some pretreatments because the crude materials contained several kinds of phenolics such as tannins, stilbens, naphthalen derivatives and lindleyin as previously indicated.

Table 2 shows the SA concentrations in various rhubarbs. Shinshu Daio bred by crossing *R. palmatum* and *R. coreanum* in order to increase the concentration of SA in Japan, contained the highest SA; 13.69±0.69 μg/mg dry wt. Ga-wo which was estimated to be high grade, contained 6.62±0.42 μg/mg dry wt. The other three species showed almost the same concentrations of SA, around 3.3 μg/mg dry wt. These results are in good agreement with the previous reports [18]. The correlation between results from ELISA and HPLC is reasonable except for Kinmon Daio. The concentration analyzed by HPLC was very low compared to the others. The reason is still obscure although individual peaks separated by HPLC were analyzed by ELISA.

Sample	Concentration (μg/mg dry wt. powder)	
	ELISA	HPLC
Shinshu Daio	13.69±0.69	12.28±0.41
Ga-wo	6.62±0.42	6.93±0.02
Kinmon Daio	3.34±0.02	0.85±0.04
Itto-Ga-wo (powder)	3.27±0.20	3.69±0.32
Itto-Ga-wo (refuse)	3.43±0.16	3.69±0.28

Table 2. SA concentrations in various rhubarb samples. Data are the means of triplicate assays.

3. Production of MAbs against SB, their characterization and use for ELISA

3.1. Preface

SB is a very important natural bioactive component of rhubarb and senna as well as SA. Total sennoside (SA and SB) concentrations are important, when rhubarb and senna are used as a raw material of medical supply and traditional Japanese herbal medicine for the purgative effect.

A number of methods for the quantification of SB have been published, most of which have been performed by HPLC [17]. Immunological approaches for assaying quantities of sennosides and SA using PAb and MAb have been investigated by Atzorn et al. [5] and by us [14], respectively. However, no success with MAb against SB has been reported. In here, production of anti-SB MAb and the competitive ELISA using anti-SA and SB MAbs for the direct determination of SA and SB in various samples are described [19].

3.2. Experimental

3.2.1. Plant materials

Samples of various rhubarb roots were purchased from the Tochimototenkaido Corporation (Osaka, Japan). Samples of leaves of *Cassia* plants were collected in Thailand. Traditional Japanese prescriptions were procured from Tsumura & Co. (Tokyo, Japan). Dietary supplements (health teas and dieter's teas) were purchased from drug and department stores.

3.2.2. Sample preparation

Dried samples (30 mg) of various rhubarb roots, *Cassia* plant leaves, traditional Japanese prescriptions and dietary supplements were powdered, and then extracted five times with MeOH containing 0.1% (w/v) NH_4OH (0.5 mL) with sonication, filtered using a Cosmonice Filter W (0.45 μm Filter Unit, Nacalai Tesque Inc., Kyoto, Japan), and the combined extracts were diluted with 10 mM $NaHCO_3$ to prepare a solution suitable for the ELISA.

3.2.3. Synthesisi of antigen conjugates

To SB (6 mg) dissolved in 1 mL of tetrahydrofuran-20 mM phosphate buffer of pH 5.5 (7:3), 0.3 mL of 20 mM phosphate buffer (pH 5.5) containing 6 mg of EDC was added. Then, 0.3 mL of 20 mM phosphate buffer (pH 5.5) containing 6 mg of BSA was added, with stirring at room temperature for 14 hr. The reaction mixture was dialyzed five times against H_2O, and then lyophilized to give 5.5 mg of SB-BSA conjugate. SB-HSA conjugate was also synthesized in the same manner.

3.2.4. Determination of hapten density in SB-carrier protein conjugate by MALDI-TOF mass spectrometry

The hapten number in the SB-carrier protein conjugate was determined by MALDI-TOF mass spectrometry as previously described [15].

3.2.5. Competitive ELISA for SB

SB-HSA (four molecules of SB per molecule of HSA) (100 μL, 1 μg/mL) dissolved in 50 mM carbonate buffer (pH 9.6) was adsorbed to the wells of a 96-well immunoplate then treated with 300 μL S-PBS for 1 hr to reduce non-specific adsorption. Fifty μL of various concentrations of SB or samples dissolved in 10 mM $NaHCO_3$ solution were incubated with 50 μL of MAb solution (0.121 μg/mL) for 1 hr. The plate was washed three times with T-PBS, and then incubated with 100 μL of a 1:1000 dilution of POD-labeled anti-mouse IgG for 1 hr. After washing the plate three times with T-PBS, 100 μL of substrate solution [0.1 M citrate buffer (pH 4) containing 0.003% H_2O_2 and 0.3 mg/mL of ABTS] was added to each well and incubated for 15 min. The absorbance was measured by a micro plate reader at 405 nm and 490 nm.

3.3. Results and discussion

3.3.1. Direct determination of SB-carrier protein conjugate by MALDI-TOF mass spectrometry

It is well known that hapten number in an antigen conjugate is important for immunization against low molecular weight compounds. Figure 7 shows the MALDI-TOF mass spectrum of the antigen, SB-BSA conjugate. A broad peak coinciding with the conjugate of SB and BSA appeared from *m/z* 67,300 to 70,700 centering at around *m/z* 68,900. Using experimental results and a molecular weight of 66,433 for BSA, the calculated values of SB component

(MW 862) are 2,500 resulting in the range of one to five molecules of SB (three on average) conjugated with BSA. This conjugate, although having a relatively low hapten number, proved sufficiently immunogenic in agreement with our previous results [10]. The number of SB contained in the SB-HSA conjugate was also determined to be around four molecules by its spectrum.

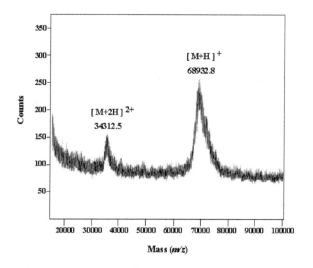

Figure 7. Direct determination of SB-BSA by MALDI-TOF MS.

3.3.2. Production and characteristics of Mabs against SB

The immunized BALB/c mice yielded splenocytes which were fused with P3-X63-Ag8-653 myeloma cells by the routinely established procedure in this laboratory [6]. Hybridoma producing MAbs reactive to SB were obtained, and classified as IgG1 (5G6, 7H12) and IgG2b (5C7) which had k light chains. The reactivity of IgG type MAb 7H12 was tested by varying the antibody concentration and by performing a dilution curve in direct ELISA. The antibody concentration (0.121 µg/mL) at which the absorbance was about 1.0 in direct ELISA was selected for competitive ELISA.

3.3.3. Assay sensitivity and assay specificity

The free MAb 7H12 following competition was bound to the polystyrene microtitre plates precoated with SB-HSA. Under these conditions, the full measuring range of the assay extends from 0.5 ng/mL to 15 ng/mL as indicated in Figure 8 and the ELISA using a MAb 7H12 is more sensitive than those using MAb 5C7 and 5G6.

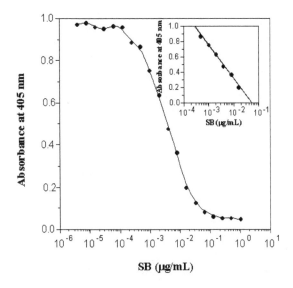

Figure 8. Calibration curve for SB.

SB is a unique anthraquinone having individual double-carboxylic acid-, hydroxyl-, carbon-yl- and *O*-glucosyl-groups at C-3, C-1, C-9 and C-8 positions in the molecule, respectively. Moreover, SB possesses an *erythro*-configuration between C-10 and C-10' positions. There-fore, MAbs should distinguish all these functional groups, and also recognize the stereo-chemistry of this complicated compound. Since the newly established ELISA against SB is expected to be used for phytochemical investigations involving crude plant extracts, the as-say specificity was checked by determining the cross-reactivities of the MAbs with various related compounds. The cross-reactivities of MAbs were examined by the competitive ELI-SA. Table 3 indicates the cross-reactivities of anti-SB MAbs against related anthraquinone, anthrone and phenol carboxylic acid. MAb 7H12 has weak cross-reactivities with SA (2.45%) and rhein (0.012%). However, the other related anthraquinone and anthrone did not have appreciable cross-reactivities. From these results it is suggested that the epitope consists of a basal structure of rhein and sugar moiety. In addition the most important property of MAb 7H12 is its ability to distinguish between SB and SA, which differ only in the stereochemical configuration at the C-10 and C-10' positions. Therefore, it is suggested that *erythro*-configu-rational structure of bisanthrone is indispensable as an immunodominant molecule for the reactivity of MAb 7H12. So the ELISA using a MAb 7H12 possesses apparently high sensi-tivity and specificity for SB. Because we have also prepared an anti-SA MAb having a weak cross-reactivity with SB (0.28%) as already discussed, these two MAbs make it possible to investigate stereochemical recognition precisely.

Compound	Cross-reactivities (%)		
	7H12	5G6	5C7
Anthraquinone and anthrone			
sennoside B	100	100	100
sennoside A	2.45	2.30	8.53
rhein	0.012	0.030	0.007
emodin	< 0.004	< 0.023	< 0.006
aloe-emodin	< 0.040	< 0.023	< 0.006
barbaloin	< 0.004	< 0.023	< 0.006
1,4-dihydroxy-anthraquinone	< 0.004	< 0.023	< 0.006
Stilbene			
rhaponticin	< 0.004	< 0.023	< 0.006
Phenol carboxylic acid			
gallic acid	< 0.004	< 0.023	< 0.006
vanillic acid	< 0.004	< 0.023	< 0.006
caffeic acid	< 0.004	< 0.023	< 0.006
homogentisic acid	< 0.004	< 0.023	< 0.006

Table 3. Cross-reactivities of anti-SB MAbs against various compounds.

3.3.4. Correlation of results of SB determination in crude extracts of rhubarb roots between HPLC and ELISA using MAb 7H12

The concentrations of SB in various rhubarb samples were determined by ELISA (Table 4). Shinshu Daio, bred by crossing *R. palmatum* and *R. coreanum* in order to increase the level of SB concentration in Japan, contained the highest SB level of 6.01±0.18 µg/mg dry wt. Ga-wo, estimated to be high grade in the traditional Japanese medicine, contained SB level of 3.14±0.27 µg/mg dry wt. These results are in good agreement with previous reports [18]. The correlation between results from ELISA and HPLC is also good.

Sample	Concentration (µg/mg dry wt. powder)	
	ELISA	HPLC
Shinshu Daio	6.01±0.18	6.15±0.59
Ga-wo	3.14±0.27	3.80±0.16
Kinmon Daio	0.35±0.01	0.38±0.02
Itto-Ga-wo (powder)	1.44±0.12	1.52±0.18
Itto-Ga-wo (refuse)	1.42±0.07	1.40±0.11

Table 4. SB concentrations in various rhubarb samples. Data are the means of triplicate assays.

3.3.5. Determination of concentrations of SA and SB in various Cassia species

The concentrations of SA and SB in leaves of various *Cassia* species were determined by ELISA using anti-SA and SB MAbs (Table 5). The results indicate that *C. angustifolia* contains 4.56±0.25 µg/mg dry wt. powder of SA and 5.10±0.15 µg/mg dry wt. powder of SB indicating higher amounts of SA and SB compared to the other species. *C. alata* contains 1.19±0.12 µg/mg dry wt. powder of SA and 1.16±0.15 µg/mg dry wt. powder of SB. *C. fistula* (A)~(D) contain 0.10-2.04 µg/mg dry wt. powder of SA and 0.13-2.05 µg/mg dry wt. powder of SB, respectively.

Sample	Concentration (µg/mg dry wt. powder)		
	Sennoside A	Sennoside B	Total sennosides
Cassia angustifolia	4.56±0.25	5.10±0.15	9.66±0.40
C. alata	1.19±0.12	1.16±0.15	2.35±0.27
C. bakeriana	0.40±0.03	0.44±0.02	0.84±0.05
C. fistula (A)	1.14±0.08	0.75±0.08	1.89±0.16
C. fistula (B)	2.04±0.32	1.52±0.12	3.56±0.44
C. fistula (C)	1.90±0.16	2.05±0.24	3.95±0.40
C. fistula (D)	0.10±0.01	0.13±0.00	0.23±0.01
C. mimosoides	$(1.30\pm0.24)\times10^{-2}$	$(1.88\pm0.29)\times10^{-4}$	$(1.32\pm0.24)\times10^{-2}$
C. floribunda	$(2.78\pm0.11)\times10^{-3}$	$(1.04\pm0.03)\times10^{-4}$	$(2.88\pm0.11)\times10^{-3}$
C. surattensis	$(1.15\pm0.18)\times10^{-2}$	$(2.44\pm0.17)\times10^{-4}$	$(1.17\pm0.18)\times10^{-2}$
C. tora	$(2.13\pm0.21)\times10^{-3}$	$(3.64\pm0.21)\times10^{-5}$	$(2.17\pm0.23)\times10^{-3}$
C. siamea	$(4.45\pm0.14)\times10^{-3}$	$(1.87\pm0.13)\times10^{-3}$	$(6.32\pm0.27)\times10^{-3}$

Table 5. Total sennoside concentrations in leaves of various *Cassia* species. Data are the means of triplicate assays.

4. Establishments of a new eastern blotting, double staining and immunohistochemical staining using anti-SA and SB MAbs

4.1. Preface

Thin-layer chromatography (TLC) is most widely used for detection, separation and monitoring of small molecular compounds like sennosides. If the direct TLC immunostaining with MAb can be done, this procedure must be contributive to the development of structural analysis of small molecular compounds. However, this procedure cannot be used for the direct detection of small molecular compounds on a TLC plate because the silica gel is sloughed off from the plate and the compounds on the plate are easily washed out without fixing during treatment. If the compounds are transferred from the TLC plate to a plastic membrane with hydrophobic properties and immobilized on the membrane, these difficulties can be solved. Therefore, I examined the transfer of sennosides from a TLC plate to a plastic membrane. Towbin *et al.* first reported the transfer of glycosphingolipids using nitrocellulose membranes [20]. However, since its transfer efficiency was poor and reproducible results were not obtained, I tested various plastic membranes and transfer conditions resulting in a polyvinylidene difluoride (PVDF) membrane to be the best [21]. The membrane is very stable against heating and various organic solvents in addition to retaining sennosides with high efficiency. I named this new method as eastern blotting (EB), because theoretically same methodology compared to previous EB except the way of sennoside-BSA conjugation for fixing sennosides on the membrane [22]. I communicate here the EB procedure for sennosides and its application for analytical survey of sennosides [23].

4.2. Experimental

4.2.1. Chemicals and immunochemicals

Polyvinylidene difluoride (PVDF) membranes (Immobilon-N) were purchased from Millipore Corporation (Bedford, MA, USA). Glass microfiber filter sheets (GF/A) were purchased from Whatman International Ltd. (Maidstone, England). All other chemicals were standard commercial products of analytical grade.

4.2.2. EB and Double staining

Sennosides were applied to a TLC plate and developed with 1-propanol-ethyl acetate-water-acetic acid (40:40:30:1, by volume). The developed TLC plate was dried and then sprayed with a blotting solution mixture of isopropanol-methanol-water (1:4:16, by volume). It was placed on a stainless steel plate and then covered with a PVDF membrane sheet. After covering with a glass microfiber filter sheet, the whole assembly was pressed evenly for 70 s with a 120 °C hot plate as previously described with some modifications [24, 25]. The PVDF membrane was separated from the TLC plate and dried.

The blotted PVDF membrane was dipped in 20 mM carbonate buffer solution (pH 9.6) containing BSA (1%) and EDC (20 mg/mL), and stirred at room temperature for 14 hr. After washing the PVDF membrane twice with T-PBS for 5 min and then treated with S-PBS for 3 hr to reduce non-specific adsorption. The PVDF membrane was washed with T-PBS twice for 5 min, and then immersed in anti-SA MAb (6G8) and stirred at room temperature for 3 hr. After washing the PVDF membrane twice with T-PBS for 5 min, a 1:1000 dilution of POD-labeled goat anti-mouse IgG in PBS cotaining 0.2% of gelatin (G-PBS) was added and stirred at room temperature for 1 hr. The PVDF membrane was washed twice with T-PBS and water, then exposed to 1 mg/mL 4-chloro-1-naphtol-0.03% H_2O_2 in PBS solution which was freshly prepared before use for 10 min at room temperature. The protocol of the EB technique is shown in Figure 9.

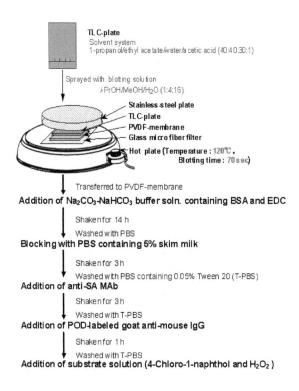

Figure 9. Eastern blotting protocol.

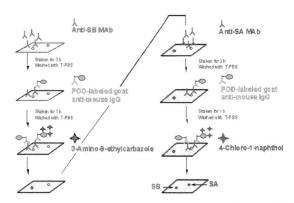

Figure 10. Double staining protocol.

For successive staining by anti-SB MAb (7H12), the PVDF membrane stained by anti-SA MAb was treated in the same way as anti-SA MAb (6G8) except that it was exposed to 2 mg/10 mL 3-amino-9-ethylcarbazole-0.03% H_2O_2 in acetate buffer (0.05 M, pH 5.0) containing 0.5 mL of N,N-dimethyl formamide. The protocol of double staining is shown in Figure 10.

4.2.3. EB for immunohistochemical staining of SA

A piece of PVDF membrane was placed on a glass microfiber filter sheet. A sliced fresh rhubarb root was placed on the PVDF membrane, and they were pressed together evenly for 1 hr. The blotted PVDF membrane was stained using the same procedure described for the EB method.

4.3. Results and discussion

4.3.1. EB of SA using anti-SA MAb

Previously we established a new immunostaining method named as eastern blotting for several glycosides like solasodine glycosides [21], ginsenosides [26, 27] and glycyrrhizin [22, 28] by using individual MAbs. In this methodology we separated the sugar moiety in a molecule into two functions, the epitope part and fixation ability part on a membrane after blotted to a PVDF membrane from a TLC plate, since small molecular compounds can not be fixed on the membrane. Although I followed the previous methodology for SA, unfortunately staining was not succeeded. Therefore, a new blotting method onto a PVDF membrane from the developed TLC plate is required. SA was transferred to the PVDF membrane by the same way as previously described, and treated with EDC solution followed by the addition of BSA as indicated in Figure 9. This reaction enhanced the fixation of SA via SA-BSA conjugate on the PVDF membrane and the pathway was indicated diagrammatically in Figure 11. When the blotted PVDF membrane was incubated in the absence of EDC, it was essentially free of immunostaining (data not shown).

Figure 12 shows the EB of sennosides and other structurally related compounds using anti-SA MAb (A) and the H_2SO_4 staining (B). The EB indicated only limited staining of SA as shown in Figure 12A, lane 7. Moreover, the EB method was considerably more sensitive than that of H_2SO_4 staining. Since anti-SA MAb cross-reacts against SB and rhein as 0.28 and 0.35%, respectively, they can be stained very weakly by anti-SA MAb, as described in the previous section. Previously Fukuda et al. succeeded the EB of ginsenoside Rb1 by using anti-ginsenoside Rb1 MAb resulting in staining together with ginsenoside Rc, Rd, Re and Rg1 [26, 27]. The difference between the newly established EB and the previous methodology is combine system of sugar moiety to PVDF membrane. The sugar moiety in ginsenosides was oxidatively cleavaged to release aldehyde groups which were conjugated with a protein to fix on a PVDF membrane. Since it was evident that a part of sugar moiety in ginsenoside Rb1 was immunized, the cleavage of sugar moiety by $NaIO_4$ expanded its cross-reactivity against other ginsenosides resulting in possibility of staining for ginsenoside Rc, Rd, Re and Rg1, though their cross reactivities are weak. On the other hand, the newly established EB in here does not hinder around sugar moiety in SA. Therefore, strength of staining for SA, SB and rhein was proportional to their cross-reactivities as described in ELISA.

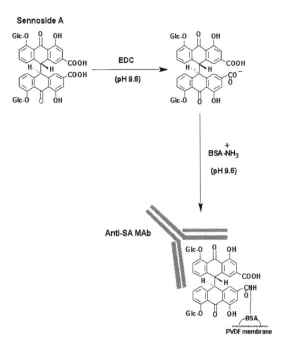

Figure 11. Schematic diagram illustrating the eastern blotting of SA onto the PVDF membrane and the detection using anti-SA MAb.

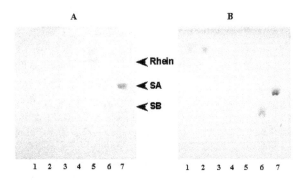

Figure 12. Eastern blotting of sennosides and related compounds stained by anti-SA MAb (A). B shows a TLC plate stained by 10% H_2SO_4. Lanes 1, 2, 3, 4, 5, 6 and 7 indicate rhaponticin, barbaloin, aloe-emodin, emodin, rhein, SB and SA (3 µg), respectively.

4.3.2. Double staining of sennosides using anti-SA and SB MAbs

Previously, I used 4-chloro-1-naphthol for staining of SB. However, since it could not function well for SB, the combination of 4-chloro-1-naphthol and 3-amino-9-ethylcarbazole was selected to improve double staining of sennosides as indicated in Figure 10. SA and SB were stained clearly by the purple and red color, respectively (Figure 13). From this result both antibodies can distinguish stereochemical configurations, *threo* and *erythro* between C-10 and C-10′ positions in a molecule on PVDF membrane stained as double coloring, respectively.

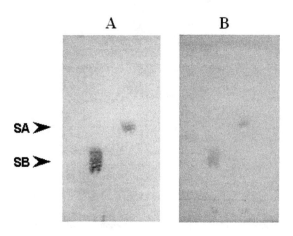

Figure 13. Double staining of sennosides using eastern blotting technique (A). B shows a result of H_2SO_4 staining. Red and purple colors were stained by anti-SB and SA MAb, respectively.

4.3.3. Detection of SA and SB in various Cassia species using double staining with a new EB technique

The crude extracts of various *Cassia* species were analyzed by the newly developed double staining system and TLC stained with H_2SO_4 as shown in Figure 14. Although H_2SO_4 staining (Figure 14B) detected many spots including probably sugars and different types of anthraquinone glycosides in various *Cassia* species, double staining (Figure 14A) detected clearly SA and SB, and very weakly other sennosides except appearance of chlorophylls around top. Band 1 indicated a purple color that means a *threo*-configuration between C-10 and C-10′ positions detected by EB using anti-SA MAb as shown in Figure 14A. Moreover, its Rf value indicated that band 1 has one sugar moiety and a CH_2OH group instead of COOH group in a molecule. I surveyed the previous papers regarding sennosides in senna [1]. Judging from these evidences, I suggested that band 1 is sennoside C (SC) having *threo*-configuration as indicated previously [1]. Band 2 was easily suggested to be *erythro*-configuration from its red color. The *Rf* value clearly showed that band 2 includes one sugar moiety having a HOOC-CO group. From these results I supposed that band 2 is sennoside F (SF) that has *erythro*-configuration as indicated previously [1]. The double staining by EB indicates that *C. angustifolia, C. alata, C. bakeriana* and *C. fistula* contain a higher concentration of sennosides compared to the other species. This result has a good agreement with that of ELISA. The limit of detection by the double staining method was confirmed to be 48 μg/mL of both SA and SB.

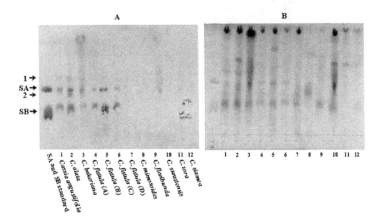

Figure 14. Double staining of SA and SB in various *Cassia* species (A). B shows a result of H₂SO₄ staining. Lefthand lane indicates SA (4 μg)and SB (3 μg). Lanes 1~12 indicate various *Cassia* species (3 μL).

4.3.4. Validation of EB for immunohistochemical staining of SA

As an other application of the EB method, the immunohistochemical staining of SA in rhubarb root, was investigated. A sliced fresh rhubarb root was placed on the PVDF membrane, and they were pressed together evenly for 1 hr. The blotted PVDF membrane was stained using the same procedure described for the EB method. Figure 15II illustrates the immunohistochemical staining of SA in fresh Hokkai Daio root. The phloem and cambium contained a higher concentration of SA compared to other tissues, pith and bud. To confirm this result, I analyzed these tissues individually by ELISA and HPLC. The concentrations of SA were determined by ELISA to determine 64.4±4.5, 48.1±8.2, 15.0±1.6 and 1.8±0.3 ng/mg fresh wt. in phloem, cambium, pith and bud, respectively. This result was a good agreement with those of HPLC resulting in 58.4±2.6, 49.0±3.9 and 13.3±0.5 ng/mg fresh wt. in phloem, cambium and pith, respectively.

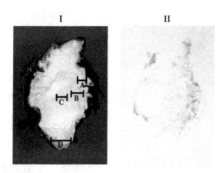

Figure 15. Immunohistochemical staining of SA using anti-SA MAb in rhubarb root. I, cross section of Hokkai Daio. root; II, direct eastern blotting on PVDF membrane of a cross section of Hokkai Daio root. A, Phloem; B, Cambium; C, Pith; D, Bud, respectively.

5. Conclusion

The recent developments of molecular biosciences and their biotechnological applications have opened up many new avenues of pharmaceutical areas. MAbs have many potential uses in addition to immunological methods to plant sciences. Therefore, immunoassay system using MAbs against pharmacologically active natural products having low molecular weight have become an important tool for the studies on receptor binding analysis, enzyme assay, and quantitative and/or qualitative analytical techniques in plants owing to their specific affinity.

In order to analyze the stereochemical isomers, SA and SB in plants, medicaments, prescriptions, health foods and patients'sera, I have produced MAbs against them. These MAbs have the most important ability to distinguish between SA and SB, which differ only in the stereochemical configuration at the C-10 and C-10′ positions, respectively. Moreover, they have no detectable cross-reaction with the other related anthraquinone and anthrone.

Analytical systems of SA and SB by competitive ELISA using anti-SA and SB MAbs were established. These ELISA systems are capable of measuring SA and SB in complex matrics without any pretreatments. Furthermore, these ELISA methods are approximately 2,000 times for SA and 10,000 times for SB more sensitive than that of HPLC method.

The newly developed EB methodology can be theoretically expanded for all compounds having carboxylic acid such as phenol carboxylic acids, glucuronides, furthermore compounds having only a carboxylic group in a molecule. A new double staining with EB method for sennosides using anti-SA and SB MAbs was established. SA and SB were stained purple and red color, respectively. This system visualized sennosides on a PVDF membrane. In fact, SA and SB in the crude extracts of various *Cassia* species were distinguished by their coloring and Rf values. Moreover, it could make it possible to survey the natural resources of sennosides and quickly determine their structures. Furthermore, EB also can be used for the survey of distribution of SA and/or SB in the *Rheum* specimen by immunohistochemical staining.

Acknowledgements

We thank Dr. Hiroyuki Tanaka (Faculty of Pharmaceutical Sciences, Kyushu University) for useful suggestions in this work. This research was supported in part by Japan Science and Technology Agency, Grant-in-Aid from the Ministry of Education, Culture, Sports, Science and Technology of Japan, the research grant from Takeda Science Foundation.

Author details

Osamu Morinaga and Yukihiro Shoyama*

*Address all correspondence to: shoyama@niu.ac.jp

Department of Pharmacognosy, Faculty of Pharmaceutical Sciences, Nagasaki International University, Sasebo, Japan

References

[1] Oshio, H., Naruse, Y., & Tsukui, M. (1978). Quantilative analysis of the purgative components of rhubarb and senna. *Chemical Pharmaceutical Bulletin*, 26, 2458-2464.

[2] Yang, L., Akao, T., Kobashi, K., & Hattori, M. (1996). A sennoside-hydrolyzing β-glucosidase from Bifidobacterium sp.strain SEN is inducible. *Biological Pharmaceutical Bulletin*, 19, 701-704.

[3] Yang, L., Akao, T., Kobashi, K., & Hattori, M. (1996). Purification and characterization of a novel sennoside-hydrolyzing β-glucosidase from Bifidobacterium sp. strain SEN, a human intestinal anaerobe. *Biological Pharmaceutical Bulletin*, 19, 705-709.

[4] Japanese Pharmacopoeia (2011). The Japanese Pharmacopoeia, 16. th ed.; Jiho

[5] Atzorn, R., Weiler, E. W., & Zenk, M. H. (1981). Formation and distribution of sennosides in Cassia angustifolia, as determined by a sensitive and specific radioimmunoassay. *Planta Medica*, 41, 1-14.

[6] Sakata, R., Shoyama, Y., & Murakami, H. (1994). Production of monoclonal antibodies and enzyme immunoassay for typical adenylate cyclase activator, forskolin. *Cytotechnology*, 16, 101-108.

[7] Ishiyama, M., Shoyama, Y., Murakami, H., & Shinohara, H. (1995). Production of monoclonal antibodies and development of an ELISA for solamargine. *Cytotechnology*, 18, 153-158.

[8] Shoyama, Y., Fukada, T., & Murakami, H. (1995). Production of monoclonal antibodies and ELISA for thebaine and codeine. *Cytotechnology*, 19, 55-61.

[9] Tanaka, H., Goto, Y., & Shoyama, Y. (1996). Monoclonal antibody based enzyme immunoassay for marihuana (cannabinoid) compounds. *Journal of Immunoassay*, 17, 321-342.

[10] Tanaka, H., & Shoyama, Y. (1998). Formation of a monoclonal antibody against glycyrrhizin and development of an ELISA. *Biological Pharmaceutical Bulletin*, 21, 1391-1393.

[11] Xuan, L., Tanaka, H., Xu, Y., & Shoyama, Y. (1999). Preparation of monoclonal antibody against crocin and its characterization. *Cytotechnology*, 29, 65-70.

[12] Tanaka, H., Fukuda, N., & Shoyama, Y. (1999). Formation of monoclonal antibody against a major ginseng component, ginsenoside Rb1 and its characterization. *Cytotechnology*, 29, 115-120.

[13] Fukuda, N., Tanaka, H., & Shoyama, Y. (2000). Formation of monoclonal antibody against a major ginseng component, ginsenoside Rg1 and its characterization. Monoclonal antibody for a ginseng saponin. *Cytotechnology*, 34, 197-204.

[14] Morinaga, O., Tanaka, H., & Shoyama, Y. (2000). Production of monoclonal antibody against a major purgative component, sennoside A, its characterization and ELISA. *Analyst*, 125, 1109-1113.

[15] Shoyama, Y., Sakata, R., Isobe, R., & Murakami, H. (1993). Direct determination of forskolin-bovine serum albumin conjugate by matrix-assisted laser desorption ionization mass spectrometry. *Organic Mass Spectrometry*, 28, 987-988.

[16] Langone, J. J. (1980). A simple procedure to use whole serum as a source of either IgG- or IgM-specific antibody. *Journal of Immunol Methods*, 32, 51-58.

[17] Oshio, H., & Kawamura, N. (1985). Determination of the laxative compounds in rhubarb by high performance liquid chromatography. *Shoyakugaku Zasshi*, 39, 131-38.

[18] Seto, T., Yasuda, I., Hamano, T., Takano, I., Kiyono, S., Nishijima, M., & Akiyama, K. (1996). Determination method of sennoside A, sennoside B, rhein and rhein 8-glucoside in kampo or crude drug preparations and the comparison of these components in processed rhubarb. *Natural Medicines*, 50, 138-144.

[19] Morinaga, O., Nakajima, S., Tanaka, H., & Shoyama, Y. (2001). Production of monoclonal antibodies against a major purgative component, sennoside B, their characterization and use in ELISA. *Analyst*, 126, 1372-1376.

[20] Towbin, H., Schoenenberger, C., Ball, R., Braun, D. G., & Rosenfelder, G. (1984). Glycosphingolipid-blotting: an immunological detection procedure after separation by thin layer chromatography. *Journal of Immunological Methods*, 72, 471-479.

[21] Tanaka, H., Putalun, W., Tsuzaki, C., & Shoyama, Y. (1997). A simple determination of steroidal alkaloid glycosides by thin-layer chromatography immunostaining using monoclonal antibody against solamargine. *FEBS Letters*, 404, 279-82.

[22] Shan, S. J., Tanaka, H., & Shoyama, Y. (2001). Enzyme-linked immunosorbent assay for glycyrrhizin using anti-glycyrrhizin monoclonal antibody and an eastern blotting technique for glucuronides of glycyrrhetic acid. *Analytical Chemistry*, 73, 5784-5790.

[23] Morinaga, O., Uto, T., Sakamoto, S., Putalun, W., Lhieochaiphant, S., Tanaka, H., & Shoyama, Y. (2009). Development of eastern blotting technique for sennoside A and sennoside B using anti-sennoside A and anti-sennoside B monoclonal antibodies. *Phytochemical Analysis*, 20, 154-158.

[24] Towbin, H., Staehelin, T., & Gordon, J. (1979). Electrophoretic transfer of proteins from polyacrylamide gels to nitrocellulose sheets: procedure and some applications. *Proceedings of the National Academy of Sciences of the United States of America*, 76, 4350-4.

[25] Taki, K., Kasama, T., Handa, S., & Ishikawa, D. (1994). A simple and quantitative purification of glycosphingolipids and phospholipids by thin-layer chromatography blotting. *Analytical Biochemistry*, 223, 232-8.

[26] Fukuda, N., Tanaka, H., & Shoyama, Y. (1999). Western blotting for ginseng saponins, ginsenosides using anti-ginsenoside Rb1 monoclonal antibody. *Biological Pharmaceutical Bulletin*, 22, 219-20.

[27] Fukuda, N., Tanaka, H., & Shoyama, Y. (2001). Double staining of ginsenosides by Western blotting using anti-ginsenoside Rb1 and Rg1 monoclonal antibodies. *Biological Pharmaceutical Bulletin*, 24, 1157-1160.

[28] Shan, S. J., Tanaka, H., & Shoyama, Y. (1999). Western blotting method for the immunostaining detection of glucuronides of glycyrrhetic acid using anti-glycyrrhizin monoclonal antibody. *Biological Pharmaceutical Bulletin*, 22, 221-223.

Chapter 2

Microbial Quality of Medicinal Plant Materials

Marcelo Gonzaga de Freitas Araújo and
Taís Maria Bauab

Additional information is available at the end of the chapter

1. Introduction

The use of medicinal plants is continually expanding worldwide. The increasing search for therapeutic agents derived from plant species is justified by the emergence of diseases, yet without proper treatment, and the growth of scientific knowledge about the herbal medicines as important treatment alternatives. Therefore, the quality and safety of herbal preparations are also of great concern [1]. The reference [2] explained that quality is the basis of reproducible efficacy and safety of herbal drugs, and to ensure the standard of research on herbal medicines, the quality of the plant materials or preparations is of utmost importance. With the ever increasing use of herbal medicines and the global expansion of the herbal medicines market, safety has become a concern for both health authorities and the public in many countries. This is because many contaminants and residues that may cause harm to the consumers have been reported [3].

The microbial load of plants is the result of a series of influences (Figure 1). By their origin, herbal drugs are subject to contamination by microorganisms from soil, air and water may be present potentially pathogenic microorganisms to man. Microbial contamination of medicinal herbal can be influenced by environmental factors such as temperature, humidity and extent of rainfall during pre-harvesting and post-harvesting periods, handling practices and the storage conditions of crude and processed medicinal-plant materials. In order to improve the purity and safety of the products, observation of basic hygiene during preparation, standardization of some physical characteristic such as moisture content, pH and microbiological contamination levels are desirable [1,4,5].

The presence of microbial contaminant in non sterile pharmaceutical products can reduce or even inactivate the therapeutic activity of the products and has the potential to adversely affect patients taking the medicines. As herbal medicinal products are complex mixtures which originate from biological sources, great efforts are necessary to guarantee a constant and adequate quality. Manipulation and processing factors largely determine the microbiological quality of the final products [6]. Previous studies have confirmed the presence of potential contaminants in herbal preparations [7-10]. Thus, manufacturers should ensure the lowest possible level of microorganisms in the raw material, finished dosage forms and the packaging components to maintain appropriate quality, safety and efficacy of the natural products [9].

This review intends to contribute to knowledge regarding the microbial contamination of medicinal plants by considering the influence of different commonly used pharmaceutical preparation techniques on the microbiological status of the products. Finally, quality standards will be discussed, considering the main guidelines of microbial quality control and through quality assurance measures such as good manufacturing practices (GMP) for herbal medicines.

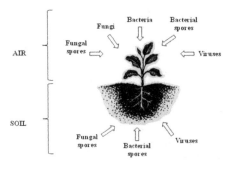

Figure 1. Influence of environmental factors and possible pathways of microbial contamination of medicinal herbs (adapted from [4]).

2. Common microbial contaminants associated with medicinal plants

The growing, harvesting and manipulation methods usually applied cannot avoid microbial contamination of the plant material which therefore reflects the environmental conditions as well as the specific hygiene during the diverse treatments [4]. Biological contamination refers to impurities in medicinal herbs and their preparations and products, and may involve living microbes such as bacteria and their spores, yeasts and moulds, viruses, protozoa, insects (their eggs and larvae), and other organisms. However, products of microbial metabolism such as toxic, low-molecular-weight metabolites from moulds are important chemical contaminants [11]. The main microbial contamination of plant materials, in general, are attributed to total aerobic mesophilic, enterobacterial, yeast and mould [4].

The presence of higher numbers of spores bacteria could be explained by the fact that some of these organisms (e.g. *Bacillus* and *Clostridium* spp.) produce spores which are resistant to harsh processing, elevated heat and dry conditions. Therefore, they can survive for a long time on the product in a dormant state. *Bacillus cereus* and *Clostridium perfringens* are recognized as having potential pathogenicity and have been incriminated in food poisoning [12]. Although bacterial endospores and fungal spores can be regarded as the two dominating groups of contaminants associated with medicinal plants, a broad diversity of bacterial, fungal cells and viruses can be found either in or on the plant material [4]. *B. cereus* and *C. perfrigens* were isolated from chamomile and other herbs by [13].

Although enterobacteria can be found in nature, this family possesses some indicative value towards faecal contamination. The presence of enterobacteria and *E. coli* reflect the situation regarding faecal contamination [7]. Together with the group of coliforms, it can be taken as an indicator for undesirable hygiene conditions, although this conclusion has to be related to the magnitude of viable count measured [4]. *Staphylococcus aureus* is not common contaminant of this type of plant material and relatively rarely found. However, contamination could provide amount of enterotoxin produced by *S. aureus*, depending on the specific nature of the individual [11].

Herbal medications are likely to be contaminated with a wide variety of others potentially pathogenic bacteria. In a study whose was evaluated the bacterial contamination of powdered herbal medicinal preparations sourced from identified herbal retail outlets in different parts of Kaduna, Nigeria, the results showed that a number of herbal remedies were contaminated with *Salmonella typhi* and *Shigella* spp., besides *E. coli* and *S. aureus* [1]. In addiction, the presence of pathogenic bacteria like *B. cereus*, *Aeromonas hydrophila*, *Shigella* spp., *Enterobacter agglomerans*, *E. cloacae*, *Vibrio fluvialis*, *Pasteurella multocida*, *S. epidermidis*, *Acinetobacter iwoffii*, *Klebsiella* spp., *B. subtilis* and *Pseudomonas aeruginosa*, and fungi *Rhizopus stolonifer* also were observed to be present in plant samples analyzed recently [14,15].

Because they are widespread in the atmosphere, moulds are common natural contaminants of medicinal herbs. It is known that, under favourable conditions, some fungi can synthesize toxical metabolites – mycotoxins. Among the known mycotoxins, the most toxic one is aflatoxin synthesised by species of *A. flavus* and *A. parasiticus*, and a minor number of other fungi [10]. Contamination by *A. flavus*, the most famous aflatoxin producer, is common in medicinal plant and herbal tea [16]. *A. flavus* colonization does not necessarily reduce yield, but causes economic losses by contaminating with aflatoxin [17]. In a study of 91 medicinal herb samples in Brazil [18], were found that 50 % of aerial part samples were contaminated with fungi. Samples of medicinal plants were evaluated by [5] for the fungal contamination, and results indicated that predominant mycoflora (89.9% of the isolates) corresponded to genera *Aspergillus* and *Penicillium*, which are extremely important from the mycotoxicological standpoint. The fungal contamination of powdered herbal medicinal preparations sourced from some herbal retail outlets in some parts of Nigeria was evaluated by [19] and the results showed that all of the herbal preparations had the presence of fungal contaminants with predominance of *Aspergillus* spp. and *Penicillium* spp., but *Mucor* spp., *Candida* spp., *Trichosporium* spp., also were found. The fungal deterioration adversely affects the chemical composition of the raw materials and thereby decreases the medicinal potency of herbal drugs [20].

The risk of the presence of microorganisms in a plant product depends on this finality of the use, its nature and its potential damage that may be caused to the consumers. Considering natural flora, current production conditions and the need to warrant the quality and the safety of these products, monographs establish a maximum fungal contamination limit for products that contain raw material of natural origin [5]. Although high fungal loads may be accepted due to the natural origin of those products, they indicate the potential for spoilage and mycotoxigenesis.

3. Influence of different preparation techniques on the microbiological quality

The production of an herbal medicine generally involves the steps in which a vegetable is subjected to unfavorable conditions to survival of microorganisms. Next, we introduce some of these processes and their influence on the microbial load.

3.1. Drying process

Drying is basically defined as the decreasing of plant moisture content, aimed at preventing enzymatic and microbial activity, and consequently preserving the product for extend shelf life [21]. Drying is the most common and fundamental method for post-harvest preservation of medicinal plants because it allows for the quick conservation of the medicinal qualities of the plant material in an uncomplicated manner. This process may also contribute to facilitate the marketing of plants, because drying results in reduction of the weight and volume of the plant with positive consequences for transport and storage [21,22].

The optimization of the drying process contributes to physical, chemical and microbiological stability of the medicinal herbs. The choice of drying conditions depend on the moisture content of tissue at harvest, the plant parts used, and the temperature best suited for preservation of the requested ingredients. For this reason, adequate dryers are needed, using temperature, velocity and humidity values for drying air that provides a rapid reduction in the moisture content without affecting the quality of the active ingredients of medicinal plants [21].

Medicinal plants can be dried in a number of ways: in the open air (shaded from direct sunlight); placed in thin layers on drying frames, wire-screened rooms or buildings; by direct sunlight, if appropriate; in drying ovens/rooms and solar dryers; by indirect fire; baking;

lyophilization; microwave; or infrared devices. When possible, temperature and humidity should be controlled to avoid damage to the active chemical constituents. In the case of natural drying in the open air, efforts should be made to achieve uniform drying of medicinal plant materials and so avoid mould formation [23].

Spray drying technique has been widely used to obtain dried extracts presenting better technological characteristics and greater concentration of biological active constituents. This method is widely used in the pharmaceutical industry, despite the high temperature drying (100°C to 200°C), the contact time between the material to be dry and hot air is extremely fast, less than 1 minute, theoretically is not enough to remove the microorganisms [24]. Comparative microbiological analysis of drug pulverized, extraction in liquid phase and the the spray drying extraction, using *Phyllanthus niruri* L., revealed that there is a significant reduction in microbial load, caused by the extraction in liquid process, while the spray dryer, despite the high temperature, did not affect the microbial load [25].

Drying at high temperature decreases the total aerobic microbial count in herbs. Water is a significant component of biological materials. Drying methods can lower the water activity to the level required for preventing growth of *Aspergillus* species and also for ensuring quality of medicinal herbs which may get destroyed upon over drying [10]. Exposure of herbs to microwaves and warm-air ovens can be efficient to reduce the microbial load, but they are not recommend to medicinal herbs containing volatile oils. The reference [26] evaluated both method of drying of plant, and reduction the microbial load present on the plants was observed but the effect on the volatile oil profile was profound by microwave drying, and warm drying air revealed that at temperatures >60°C, most of the volatile constituents were lost.

Other methods such as freeze-drying, oven drying and tray drying have been previously used to preserve medicinal herbs but to date there is little information in the literature on the effect of these drying conditions on the decrease of microbial loads [27].

Once drying is complete, plants are packaged in preparation for shipping or other further processing.

3.2. Extraction methods

Water is almost universally the solvent used to extract activity. At home, dried plants can be ingested as teas (plants steeped in hot water) or, rarely, tinctures (plants in alcoholic solutions) or inhaled via steam from boiling suspensions of the parts. Dried plant parts can be added to oils or petroleum jelly and applied externally. Poultices can also be made from concentrated teas or tinctures [28]. These kinds of preparations are usually called medicinal teas and are prepared using natural plants collected, dried and packaged without an effective hygienic and sanitary control. In addition, there can be microbiological contamination and controlling microbial contamination can be difficult in aqueous extracts [13].

Environmental dust settled on different parts of the plant and other contaminations can carry very significant amounts of bacterial and moulds spores [13]. However, those drugs which are subjected to cold water extraction (herbal maceration) may host a considerable amount of microbes, and the extraction procedure carried out at ambient temperature usually enables microbial multiplication [4]. The application of hot water extraction usually compensates for microbiological contaminations, since it can be expected that boiling water markedly reduces the viable counts by several log units and also inactivates possible pathogens [4]. However, bacterial spores of the Bacillaceae family are resistant to thermal treatment usually applied in infusion preparation, and this thermal shock may stimulate spore germination. Some of these bacteria like *B. cereus* and *C. perfringens* are recognized as having potential pathogenicity and have been incriminated in food poisoning [12]. Thus, in extractions using only water, hot or cold, as extractor liquid, the stability of the extract becomes compromised and the risk of microbiological contamination increases significantly. This contamination can compromise the quality and integrity of the plant material itself, as well as products arising from its use [29-30].

In addition to extraction temperature, the choice of extraction solvent is another important factor to prevent microbial contamination. The aim of an extraction process should be, of course, to provide for the maximum yield of substances and of the highest quality (concentration of target compounds and pharmacological power of the extracts). For extraction of active phytochemicals, the most commonly used solvents are methanol, ethanol, hexane, chloroform and diethyl ether [31]. Herbal extraction which made by ethanol or methanol extraction should, in general, provide good hygiene conditions, but the result depends on the alcoholic concentration applied [4].

3.3. pH influence

The pH value is one of the main factors influencing the quality of medicine. It always controls many chemical and microbiological reactions [32]. When the pH value is low (presence of acidic substances), the bacterial count could be low, but at neutral or higher pH the level of contamination of the herbal preparations could observed to be higher. This suggests that a neutral or alkaline pH favoured high contamination levels of the herbal preparations. This agrees with the observation that bacterial growth is optimal at more or less neutral pH, around pH 5-8.5 [1].

3.4. Storage

Most pre-storage processing of plant material, such as that involving drying, heat, cooling and packaging, can prevent the degradation of plant material during storage [33]. Storage of medicinal herbs is an important part in the process production. During storage, due the factors in the outside world and their own physical and chemical properties of the interaction, gradually occurring physical, chemical and biological changes. Prolonged storage in poorly ventilated storehouse usually increases sample moisture content in the bulk due to heat exchange capacity, rendering herbs more susceptible to molds growth and toxin production. Fungi are the predominant contaminants of herbs, but most such microbial populations are probably regarded as commensal residents on the plant that survived drying and storage. Most fungi are present on plants, which develop after harvest if relative humidity is not controlled during storage [34-35].

Moulds are responsible for biodeterioration of a number of substrates including raw materials of some medicinal plants. These moulds reduce raw herbal drugs shelf life and market value. The fungal deterioration adversely affects the chemical composition of the raw materials and thereby decreases the medicinal potency of herbal drugs [20]. Samples of herbal parts stored for sale in markets located in Ibadan, Nigeria were analysed for mycoflora associated with their storage and twenty eight fungal species were isolated, showing that herbal drug plant pieces are hazardous for human health [36]. Some samples of herbal raw materials have been reported to contain aflatoxin. The reference [37] determined the incidence of toxigenic fungi and their mycotoxins on 152 dried medicinal and aromatic herbs from Argentina, which are used as raw material for drugs. A. flavus and A. parasiticus were the predominant species isolated, and high aflatoxin concentrations were detected. There is a potential risk for mycotoxins contamination, especially during prolonged storage in poorly conditions without temperature and moisture control that usually render medicinal plants more susceptible to moulds growth and mycotoxins production [5,10,20].

The reduction of plant enzyme activity and inactivation of microorganisms is achieved by drying. Dried plant materials tend to be hygroscopic (readily absorbing moisture) and must be stored under controlled humidity. Rehydration can lead to the decomposition of the bioactive metabolites by enzymes from microorganisms or the plant itself. Significant contamination by bacteria and fungi suggest inadequate storage facilities and poor hygienic practice during preparation of these medicinal plants. The storage processes of such products are stages during which it is important to avoid even further contamination [38].

Studies on long-term stability of dried herbal teas and preparations are rare. In a study of [20] was examined the deterioration of herbal drug samples which were stored for 6-9 months by traders after collection. Some of the contaminated materials were found to be deteriorated by toxigenic strains of A. flavus and contain aflatoxin B1 which was above the permissible limit. In a study of [38], dried P. lanceolata leaves were exposed to atmospheres of different relative humidity (75, 45 and 0%) for 24 weeks and was evaluated the chemical changes of the compounds of interest. It was shown that exposure to water results in loss of bioactive molecules of P. lanceolata dried leaves, and that colonising fungi are the key contributors to this loss. The fungal deterioration adversely affects the chemical composition of the raw materials and thereby decreases the medicinal potency of herbal drugs. Biodeterioration of herbal products samples by associated fungi during storage has drawn attention regarding quality maintenance of these products [35,38-40].

It is common practice for herbalists to prepare herbal medicines and store them in a refrigerator. However, in previous study the effect of microbial contaminants on active compounds of African plant extracts was assessed and indicated that after 25 days of storage in low temperature there may be little or no active compounds due to spontaneous biodegradation by naturally-occurring microbes [41]. The World Health Organization (WHO) recommends that whenever required and when possible, fresh medicinal plant materials should be stored at appropriate low temperatures, ideally at 2-8°C; frozen products should be stored at less than -20°C.

Processed medicinal plant materials should be packaged as quickly as possible to prevent deterioration of the product and to protect against unnecessary exposure to potential pest attacks and other sources of contamination.

4. Decontamination of plant materials

Attempts have always been made to decontaminate and preserve these medicinal plants so as to get more safe, natural and potent medicines. The number of methods has been tried for decontamination such as heat treatment, UV irradiation and fumigation. However, volatility and heat sensitivity of the delicate flavor and aroma components of the medicinal plants do not permit the use of heat treatment [42].

Low penetration power of UV radiations makes this irradiation method unsuitable [42]. Fumigation with gaseous ethylene oxide brings down the microbial burden but this method is now prohibited or restricted in many countries due to the carcinogenic nature of one of its residue in treated medicinal plants [43,44]. Various disinfectant technologies have been suggested which include electromagnetic radiations, photodynamic pulsing, ultrahigh pressure and CO_2 treatment [42].

Gamma irradiation is now getting recognition throughout the world as a phytosanitary treatment of herbal materials. It improves the hygienic quality of various herbal materials and reduces the losses due to microbial contamination and insect damage [45]. Besides, it is a fast, safe, convenient, eco-friendly method which reduces the reliance on chemical fumigants and preservatives currently used by industries. The chances of recontamination are also reduced, as it can be done after packaging [46]. Some studies showed that the exposition of plant samples to different doses of gamma radiation can result in reduction in total bacterial counts and also indicated that the microbial load could be decreased by increasing the radiation-absorbed dose. These studies indicate that gamma irradiation is an effective treatment for microbial decontamination of medicinal plants [42,47,48].

Certain plants contain natural barriers and antimicrobial substances which exert typical inhibitory effects on microbial growth and stability. It has been estimated that around 1400 herbs and spices may possess antimicrobial agents of different chemical nature as oils, peptides, liquid and organic extracts [4]. Some medicinal herbs contain essential oils which act as natural antimicrobials and may inhibit mould development and mycotoxin production [11]. Different studies have demonstrated the effectiveness of antimicrobials and their effective compounds to control or inhibit the growth of pathogenic and spoilage microorganisms [49-51].

5. Microbial quality parameters

The most widely accepted and used technique is that recommended by WHO for total count of microorganisms in plant materials. According to the methodology of the WHO, 10 g of sample should be suspended in 90 ml of buffer sodium chloride-peptone, adjusting the pH to 7.0. To count total aerobic bacteria, sample should be plated in duplicate, using the official technique of sowing depth on casein-soybean digest agar, and then incubated at 30-35°C for 48h. To count yeast and mold, the technique employed is the sowing depth in Sabouraud-dextrose plus a solution of 10% tartaric acid to obtain pH 3.0 to 3.5. The dilution is plated in duplicate and incubated at 20-25°C for 5 days [52]. Analysis of specific pathogens, Enterobacteriaceae and other Gram negative bacteria (*E. coli*, *Salmonella* sp., *P. aeruginosa* and *S. aureus*) consists of specific methods of cultivation and through biochemical and serological tests. The specification of WHO for total aerobic microorganisms is not more than 10^7 CFU/g for the plant material for use as teas and infusions and at most 10^5 CFU/g for internal use. The specification of WHO for yeasts and molds are at most 10^4 CFU/g for the plant material for use as teas and infusions and at most 10^3 UFC/g for internal use. High counts of fungi are a risk because of the possibility to produce mycotoxin, such as aflatoxin, which is a carcinogen toxin. The WHO also recommends a test to detect the possible presence of aflatoxins, which are highly dangerous contaminants in any material of plant origin.

In Brazil, despite the large consumption of products derived from plants, products sold and consumed were not subject to any kind of quality control. In 1995, the Ministry of Health instituted the ordinance MS/SNVS No. 6, January 31, 1995 [53] that regulated the registration of herbal products for commercial purposes. Then came the Resolution RDC No. 17 [54] and, more recently, the RDC No. 48 [55] which confirms definitely that are herbal medicines and thereby rescues the need for the existence of safety studies, efficacy and quality, prior to the registration of these products. The Resolution RDC No. 48 of March 16 of 2004 [55] recommends that the contamination analysis on herbal medicines must be in accordance with pharmacopoeial specifications.

Both the Brazilian Pharmacopeia [56], as the United States Pharmacopeia [57] draw the following specifications for products for oral use: 104 aerobic bacteria/g or mL, 10^2 fungi/g and absence of *Salmonella* spp, *E. coli* and *S. aureus*. However, the Brazilian Pharmacopeia also indicates the detection of other indicators of increased risk for oral administration, such as *P. aeruginosa*, *B. cereus*, *Enterobacter* spp, *C. albicans*, *A. flavus* and *A. parasiticus*. High microbial loads are indicative of the possibility of potentially pathogenic microorganisms.

In Europe the evaluation of microbial contamination of medicinal plants has increasingly become an integral part of Good Agricultural Practice (GAP) and Hazard Analysis and Critical Control Point (HACCP) concepts [33]. The limits of microbial contamination given in European Pharmacopoeia [58] for herbal medicinal products to which boiling water is added before use are: total aerobic bacteria (10^7 CFU/g), fungi (10^5 CFU/g); for herbal medicinal products to which boiling water is not added before use are: total aerobic bacteria (10^5

CFU/g), fungi (10^4 CFU/g); Enterobacteria and other Gram-negative organisms (10^3 CFU/g); *E. coli* and *Salmonella* sp. should be absent. In general, the tests used to verify the presence of microorganisms in plant drugs and microbial limits show no significant variation and follow the recommendations used for non-sterile pharmaceutical products (Table 1).

	United States Pharmacopoeia[a]	European Pharmacopoeia[b]	WHO[c]	Brazilian Pharmacopoeia[d]
Aerobic bacteria	10^5 / 10^4 / 10^2	10^7 / 10^5	* / 10^7 / 10^5	10^7 / 10^5 / 10^4
Mold and yeast	10^3 / 10^2 / 10	10^5 / 10^4	10^5 / 10^4 / 10^3	10^4 / 10^3 / 10^2
Enterobacteria and other Gram negative bacteria	10^3 / * / *	* / 10^3	* / 10^4 / 10^3	10^4 / 10^3 / 10^2
E. coli	absent	10^3 / absent	10^4 / 10^2 / 10	absent
Salmonella	absent	* / absent	* / absent /absent	absent

[a] United States Pharmacopoeia: The first value represents dried or powdered botanicals and botanicals to be treated with boiling water before use; The second value represents tinctures, powdered botanicals extracts, fluid extracts and nutritional supplements with botanicals; The third value represents infusions/decoctions. [b] European Pharmacopoeia: Herbal medicinal products consisting solely of one or more herbal drugs (whole, reduced or powdered): the first value represents herbal medicinal products to which boiling water is added before use; The second value represents herbal medicinal products to which boiling water is not added before use. [c] WHO: The first value represents contamination of "crude" plant material intended for further processing; The second value represents for plant materials that have been pretreated (e.g. with boiling water as used for herbal teas and infusions) or that are used as topical dosage forms; The third value represents For other plant materials for internal use: [d] Brazilian Pharmacopoeia: The first value represents herbal drugs to which boiling water is added before use; The second value represents herbal drugs to which the extractive process made in cold temperature; The third value represents final products for oral use. * Limits are not specified.

Table 1. Recommended microbial limits for herbal drugs (values in CFU/g).

6. Conclusion

Microbial contamination can lead to impaired performance of the product due to disruption of the stability of the formulation, modification of physical characteristics and appearance and lead to inactivation of the active ingredients and excipients in the formulation and also cause loss of confidence in the company. Herbalists should be trained to apply Good Manufacturing Practices, good harvesting practices and the safe handling and storage of herbal medicinal products. Further studies are recommended for herbal products to establish other contaminants and ways in which the contaminants can be reduced to recommended levels. The microbial loads should be established and the contaminants isolated and identified. In addition, alternative methods such as treatment with ethylene oxide or radiation with ionic rays lead to decontamination effects. These methods can be seen as a compromise between ensuring the microbiological safety of the product and avoiding consumer's risk and special legal permissions are required in many countries. It is evident that more detailed studies of plant species popularly used are needed in order to ensure the quality, an important concept for providing the wished security and reliability for its use.

Author details

Marcelo Gonzaga de Freitas Araújo* and Taís Maria Bauab

*Address all correspondence to: mgfaraujo@yahoo.com.br

Biological Sciences Department, Faculty of Pharmaceutical Sciences, São Paulo State University – UNESP, Araraquara, Brazil

References

[1] Abba, D., Inabo, H. I., Yakubu, S. E., & Olonitola, O. S. (2009). Contamination of herbal medicinal products marketed in Kaduna Metropolis with selected pathogenic bacteria. *African Journal of Traditional, Complementary and Alternative Medicines, 6,* 70-77.

[2] Zhang, X. (1998). Regulatory situation of herbal medicines: a worldwide review. 2003: World Health Organization. Available at:, http://apps.who.int/medicinedocs/en/d/Jwhozip57e/, (accessed 8 June 2012).

[3] Kunle, O. F., Egharevba, H. O., & Ahmadu, P. O. (2012). Standardization of herbal medicines- A review. *International Journal of Biodiversity and Conservation, 4,* 101-112.

[4] Kneifel, W., Czech, E., & Kopp, B. (2002). Microbial contamination of medicinal plants- A review. *Planta Medica,* 5-15, 68.

[5] Bugno, A., Almodovar, A. A. B., Pereira, T. C., Pinto, T. J. A., & Sabino, M. (2006). Occurrence of toxigenic fungi in herbal drugs. *Brazilian Journal of Microbiology, 37,* 47-51.

[6] Busse, W. (2000). The significance of quality for efficacy and safety of herbal medicinal products. *Drug Information Journal, 34,* 15-23.

[7] Czech, E., Kneifel, W., & Kopp, B. (2001). Microbiological status of commercially available medicinal herbal drugs- A screening study. *Planta Medica, 67,* 263-269.

[8] Tassaneeyakul, W., Razzazi-Fazeli, E., Porasuphatana, S., & Bohm, J. (2004). Contamination of aflatoxins in herbal medicinal products in Thailand. *Mycopathologia, 158,* 239-244.

[9] Okunlola, A., Adewoyin, B. A., & Odeku, A. O. (2007). Evaluation of pharmaceutical and microbial qualities of some herbal medicinal products in South Western Nigeria. *Tropical Journal of Pharmaceutical Research*, 6, 661-670.

[10] Kulshrestha, R., Gupta, C. P., Shukla, G., Kundu, M. G., Bhatnagar, S. P., & Katiyar, C. K. (2008). The effect of water activity and storage temperature on the growth of *Aspergillus flavus* in medicinal herbs. *Planta Medica*, 74, 1308-1315.

[11] Kosalec, I., Cvek, J., & Tomic, S. (2009). Contaminants of medicinal herbs and herbal products. *Archives of Industrial Hygiene and Toxicology*, 60, 485-501.

[12] Kunene, N. F., Hastings, J. W., & von Holy, A. (1999). Bacterial populations associated with a sorghum-based fermented weaning cereal. *International Journal of Food Microbiology*, 49, 75-83.

[13] Martins, H. M., Martins, M. L., Dias, M. I., & Bernardo, F. (2001). Evaluation of microbiological quality of medicinal plants used in natural infusions. *International Journal of Food Microbiology*, 68, 149-153.

[14] Alwakeel, S. S. (2008). Microbial and heavy metals contamination of herbal medicines. *Research Journal of Microbiology*, 3(12), 683-691.

[15] Idu, M., Erhabor, J. O., & Idele, S. O. (2011). Microbial load of some medicinal plants sold in local markets of Benin City, Nigeria. *International Journal of Medicinal and Aromatic Plants*, 1(3), 272-277.

[16] Halt, M. (1998). Moulds and mycotoxins in herb tea and medicinal plants. *European Journal of Epidemiology*, 14, 269-274.

[17] Amaike, S., & Keller, N. P. (2011). *Aspergillus flavus* . *Annual Review of Phytopathology*, 49, 107-133.

[18] Bugno, A., Buzzo, A. A., Nakamura, C. T., Pereira, T. C., Matos, D., & Pinto, T. J. A. (2005). Avaliação da contaminação microbiana em drogas vegetais. *Revista Brasileira de Ciências Farmacêuticas*, 41(4), 491-497.

[19] Anyanwu, C. U. (2010). Fungal contaminants of powdered herbal drugs sold in parts of Enugu State, Southeast, Nigeria. *Plant Product Research Journal*, 14, 46-50.

[20] Kumar, A., Shukla, R., Singh, P., & Dubey, N. K. (2009). Biodeterioration of some herbal raw materials by storage fungi and aflatoxin and assessment of *Cymbopogon flexuosus* essential oil and its components as antifungal. *International Biodeterioration & Biodegradation*, 63, 712-716.

[21] Rocha, R. P., Melo, E. C., & Radünz, L. L. (2011). Influence of drying process on the quality of medicinal plants: A review. Journal of Medicinal Plants Research, 5(33), 7076-7084.

[22] Müller, J., & Heindl, A. (2006). Drying of medicinal plants. In: Bogers RJ, Craker LE, Lange D. (eds.), *Medicinal and Aromatic Plants*, Dordrecht: Springer, 237-252.

[23] World Health Organization (WHO). (2003). WHO guidelines on good agricultural and collection practices [GACP] for medicinal plants. Geneva, World Health Organization.

[24] Oliveira, O. W., & Petrovick, P. R. (2010). Secagem por aspersão (spray drying) de extratos vegetais: bases e aplicações. *Revista Brasileira de Farmacognosia, 20,* 641-650.

[25] Souza, T. P., Lionzo, M. I. Z., & Petrovick, P. R. (2006). Avaliação da redução da carga microbiana de droga vegetal através do processamento tecnológico: decocção e secagem por aspersão. *Revista Brasileira de Farmacognosia, 16,* 94-98.

[26] Deans, S. G., Svoboda, K. P., & Bartlett, M. C. (1991). Effect of microwave oven and warm-air drying on the microflora and volatile oil profile of culinary herbs. *Journal of Essential Oil Research, 3,* 341-347.

[27] Harbourne, N., Marete, E., Jacquier, J.C., & O'Riordan, D. (2009). Effect of drying methods on the phenolic constituents of meadowsweet (Filipendula ulmaria) and willow (Salix alba). *Food Science and Technology, 42,* 1468-1473.

[28] Cowan, M. M. (1999). Plant products as antimicrobial agents. Clinical Microbiology Reviews, 12, 564-582.

[29] Migliato, K. F., Moreira, R. R. D., & Mello, J. C. P. (2007). Sacramento LVS, Correa MA, Salgado HRN. Controle de qualidade do fruto de Syzygium cumini (L.) Skells. *Revista Brasileira de Farmacognosia, 17,* 94-101.

[30] Araújo, M. G. F., Galeane, M. C., Castro, A. D., Salgado, H. R. N., Almeida, A. E., Cunha, W. R., Veneziani, R. C. S., & Moreira, R. R. D. (2010). Pharmacognostical evaluation of fruits of Solanum lycocarpum A. St.-Hill. (Solanaceae). *Pharmacognosy Journal,* 2(9), 248-253.

[31] Castillo, F., Hernández, D., Gallegos, G., Mendez, M., Rodríguez, R., Reyes, A., & Aguilar, C. N. (2010). In vitro antifungal activity of plant extracts obtained with alternative organic solvents against Rhizoctonia solani Kühn. *Industrial Crops and Products, 32,* 324-328.

[32] Liu, X., Qiu, Z., Wang, L., & Chen, Y. (2011). Quality evaluation of Panax notoginseng extract dried by different drying methods. *Food and Bioproducts Processing, 89,* 10-14.

[33] Fennel, C. W., Light, M. E., Sparg, S. G., Stafford, G. I., & van Staden, J. (2004). Assessing African medicinal plants for efficacy and safety: agricultural and storage practices. *Journal of Ethnopharmacology, 95,* 113-121.

[34] Aziz, N. H., Youssef, Y. A., El -Fouly, M. Z., & Moussa, L. A. (1998). Contamination of some common medicinal plant samples and spices by fungi and their mycotoxins. *Botanical Bulletin of Academia Sinica, 39,* 279-285.

[35] Mandeel, Q. A. (2005). Fungal contamination of some imported spices. *Mycopathologia, 159,* 291-298.

[36] Efunyoye, M. O. (1996). Fungi associated with herbal drug plants during storage. *Mycopathologia*, 136, 115-118.

[37] Rizzo, I., Vedoya, G., Maurutto, S., Haidukowski, M., & Varsavsky, E. (2004). Assessment of toxigenic fungi on Argentinean medicinal herbs. *Microbiological Research*, 159, 113-120.

[38] Gonda, S., Tóth, L., Gyémánt, G., Braun, M., Emrid, T., & Vasas, G. (2012). Effect of high relative humidity on dried *Plantago lanceolata* L. leaves during long-term storage: Effects on chemical composition, colour and microbiological quality. *Phytochemical Analysis*, 23, 88-93.

[39] Singh, P., Srivastava, B., Kumar, A., & Dubey, N. K. (2008). Fungal contamination of raw materials of some herbal drugs and recommendation of Cinnamomum camphora oil as herbal fungitoxicant. *Microbial Ecology*, 56, 555-560.

[40] Shukla, R., Kumar, A., Prasad, C. S., Srivastava, B., & Dubey, N. K. (2008). Antimycotic and antiaflatoxigenic potency of Adenocalymma alliaceum Miers. on fungi causing biodeterioration of food commodities and raw herbal drugs. *International Biodeterioration & Biodegradation*, 62, 348-351.

[41] Du Plessis-Stoman, D., Downing, T. G., van de Venter, M., & Govender, S. (2009). Traditional herbal medicines: potential degradation of sterols and sterolins by microbial contaminants. *South African Journal of Science*, 105, 147-150.

[42] Gupta, P. C., Garg, N., & Joshi, P. (2011). Effect of gamma irradiation on the extraction yield and microbial contamination of medicinal plants. *Internet Journal of Food Safety*, 13, 351-354.

[43] Kim, M. J., Yook, H. S., & Byun, M. W. (2000). Effects of gamma irradiation on microbial contamination and extraction yields of Korean medicinal herbs. [2]. *Radiation Physics and Chemistry*, 57, 55-58.

[44] Satomi, L. C., Soriani, R. R., & Pinto, T. J. A. (2005). Descontaminação de drogas vegetais empregando irradiação gama e óxido de etileno: aspectos microbianos e químicos. Revista Brasileira de Ciências Farmacêuticas, 41(4), 445-450.

[45] Farkas, J. (1998). Irradiation as a method for decontaminating food: A review. International Journal of Food Microbiology, 44, 189-204.

[46] Khattak, K. F., Simpson, T. J., & Ihasnullah, . (2009). Effect of gamma irradiation on the microbial load, nutrient composition and free radical scavenging activity of *Nelumbo nucifera* rhizome. *Radiation Physics and Chemistry*, 78, 206-212.

[47] Khattak, K. F. (2012). Evaluation of microbial loads, physical characteristics, chemical constituents and biological properties of radiation processed Fagonia arabica. *Radiation Physics and Chemistry*, 81, 679-685.

[48] Aquino, S., Gonçales, E., Rossi, M. H., Nogueira, J. H. C., Reis, T. A., & Corrêa, B. (2010). Evaluation of fungal burden and aflatoxin presence in packed medicinal plants treated by gamma radiation. *Journal of Food Protection*, 73(5), 932-937.

[49] Tiwari, B. K., Valdramidi, V. P., O'Donnell, C. P., Muthukumarappan, K., Bourke, P., & Cullen, P. J. (2009). Application of natural antimicrobials for food preservation. *Journal of Agricultural and Food Chemistry*, 57, 5987-6000.

[50] Wang, Y., Lu, Z., Wu, H., & Lv, F. (2009). Study on the antibiotic activity of microcapsule curcumin against foodborne pathogens. *International Journal of Food Microbiology*, 30, 71-74.

[51] Negi, P. S. (2012). Plant extracts for the control of bacterial growth: Efficacy, stability and safety issues for food application. *International Journal of Food Microbiology*, 156, 7-17.

[52] World Health Organization (WHO). (1998). Quality control methods for medicinal plant materials. Geneva, World Health Organization.

[53] Brasil, Ministério da Saúde, Secretaria Nacional de Vigilância Sanitária. (1995). Portaria nº 6., *Diário Oficial da Repúplica Federativa do Brasil*, 31 jan. Institui e normaliza o registro de produtos fitoterápicos.

[54] Brasil, Ministério da Saúde, Agência Nacional de Vigilância Sanitária. (2000). RDC nº 17., *Diário Oficial da República Federativa do Brasil*, 24 abr. Aprova regulamento técnico, normatizando o registro de medicamentos fitoterápicos junto ao Sistema de Vigilância Sanitária.

[55] Brasil. Resolução RDC nº 48. (2004). de 16 de março de 2004. Dispõe sobre o registro de medicamentos fitoterápicos. Diário Oficial [da] República Federativa do Brasil, Brasília, DF, 18 mar. 2004. Disponível em:, http://www.anvisa.gov.br/legis/resol/2004/48_04rdc.htm, Acesso em: 8 june 2012.

[56] Farmacopéia Brasileira. (1988). 4. ed. São Paulo: Atheneu, Parte 1. pV.5.1.6.-1- V. 5.1.7.-6.

[57] The United States Pharmacopeia. (2005). 28 ed. Rockville: United States Pharmacopeial Convention, 3013.

[58] European Pharmacopoeia. (2007). Microbiological quality of pharmaceutical preparations. Chapter 5.1.4, 6. ed. Strasbourg: EDQM., 4451.

Chapter 3

Applications of Anti-natural Compound Immunoaffinity Purification on Quality Control

Takuhiro Uto, Nguyen Huu Tung, Hiroyuki Tanaka
and Yukihiro Shoyama

Additional information is available at the end of the chapter

1. Introduction

Worldwide demand of herbal medicines has increased in recent years owing to rising inter-est in the health benefits. Among with this, the quality control of plant extracts and plant-derived medicines is growing in importance to ensure their efficacy and safety. Effective quality control of the traditional Chinese medicines (TCM) and plant crude extracts requires the rapid and sensitive methods for separation and quantification of bioactive compounds. Various methods have been employed for the separation and quantification of certain con-stituents in medicinal plants or herbal medicines. However, the current methods in use are not necessarily optimal approaches. For example, separation and quantification of glycyrrhi-zin (GC), the main active constituent in licorice (*Glycyrrhiza* spp.), have been used gas chro-matography, high performance liquid chromatography (HPLC) and micellar trokinetic chromatography and so on [1,2]. Commercial purification of GC typically progressed through several steps, including crystallization, column chromatography, and liquid parti-tioning. These current methods are not sufficiently approaches because of insufficient sensi-tivity and reproducibility, large consumption of organic solvent for extraction and analysis, and long analysis time.

Immunoassay systems using monoclonal antibody (MAb) against drugs and small molecu-lar weight bioactive compounds have become an important tool for studies on receptor binding assays, enzyme assays, and quantitative and qualitative analytical techniques both *in vivo* and *in vitro* studies. Although immunoaffinity purification against higher molecule analyte such as peptides and proteins are widely used in the research and commercial ways, there are too few cases of immunoaffinity purification targeting a small molecule com-pound such as natural compounds. Our laboratory has prepared many kinds of MAbs against naturally occurring bioactive compounds such as terpenoids [3-5], alkaloids [6,7], saponins [8-12], and phenolics [13-16], and developed several applications. One of the applications by using MAbs is immunoaffinity column conjugated with anti-natural compound-specific MAbs and work by specifically binding and removing the target compounds. We have been establishing several affinity columns against a kind of terpenoid, forskolin [17], solasodine glycosides [18], ginsenosides Rb_1 [19], and GC [20]. Application of an immunoaffinity column to isolate and concentrate a natural compound may decrease the amount of solvent consumption and the number of purification steps, shorten analysis time, and simplify sample analysis compared to traditional cleanup techniques.

In this chapter, we focus on the immunoaffinity purification to separate and concentrate the target bioactive compounds from the crude extract. Our approaches effectively succeeded one-step purification of target compounds by MAb-conjugated immunoaffinity column, which leads to high-sensitivity detection and isolation of target compounds. In addition, the immunoaffinity column can prepare the knockout (KO) extract which contains all components except an antigen molecule, and KO extract will be useful for the pharmacological investigation to reveal the real effects of bioactive compound in the crude extract.The information in this chapter may provide new insight into quality control of plant-derived medicines.

2. Preparation of anti-ginsenoside Rb_1 immunoaffinity column and its application

Ginseng, the root of *Panax ginseng*, has been an important component in traditional medicines for more than 1000 years in Eastern Asia. It is now one of the most extensively used alternative medicines all over the world and appears in the pharmacopoeias of several countries. The biological and pharmacological activities of ginseng have been reported to have anti-aging, anti-cancer, anti-inflammation, anti-diabetics, anti-stress, maintenance of homeostasis, and to affect on central nervous system and immune function [21]. The bioactive components responsible for ginseng actions are ginsenosides, which are triterpenes saponins that possess a dammarane skeleton with sugar moieties [22]. Up to now more than 60 kinds of ginsenosides have been isolated from *Panax* genus [23]. It is well-known that the concentrations of ginsenosides vary in the ginseng root or the root extracts depending on the method of extraction, subsequent treatment, or even the season of its collection [24,25]. Due to the importance of ginseng, a number of researches has been carried out to develop the methods for the identification, quantification and quality control of ginsenosides in raw plants materials, extracts and commercial products. Currently, analytical and preparative HPLC are commonly used to quantify and purify the individual ginsenosides from ginseng [26]. However, isolation of ginsenosides by HPLC requires the repeated purification steps, including cumbersome handling and lengthy analysis times, and may result in the decrease of the final yield.Thus, the developed approaches are required for quality control of ginseng in the field of TCM.

Ginsenoside Rb_1 (G-Rb_1) is one of the main ginsenosides responsible for many pharmaceutical actions of ginseng [27]. G-Rb_1 has various biological activities, including facilitating acquisition and retrieval of memory [28], scavenging free radicals [29], inhibition of calcium over-influx into neurons [30], and preserving the structural integrity of the neurons [31].

In order to develop efficient quality control of ginseng, we have prepared anti-G-Rb$_1$ MAb, set up of enzyme-linked immunosorbent assay (ELISA), and a new immunostaining method named Eastern blotting [8,32]. Furthermore, we established an immunoaffinity column against G-Rb$_1$ and its application for one-step isolation from crude extract of ginseng root [19, 32]. Herein we describe the preparation of anti-G-Rb$_1$ immunoaffinity column and it applications for identification and concentration of G-Rb$_1$.

2.1. Preparation of MAb and immunoaffinity column against G-Rb$_1$

2.1.1. Analytical methodology for determination of hapten number in antigen, hapten-carrier protein conjugate

The first step for the MAb production is the synthesis of a hapten-carrier protein conjugate. Bovine serum albumin (BSA) conjugated with G-Rb$_1$ was produced for the preparation of specific MAb in mouse [8]. There had been no direct and appropriate methods for the determination of haptens conjugated carrier proteins without differential UV analysis, radiochemical or chemical methods. Therefore, immunization by the injection of hapten-carrier protein conjugate was unreliable. Wengatez *et al.* determined the hapten density of immuno-conjugates by matrix-assisted UV laser desorption/ionization (MALDI) mass spectrometry [33]. We also reported the direct analytical method of hapten and carrier protein conjugates by a MALDI tof mass spectrometry using internal standard [3-16]. Figure 1 shows the MALDI tof mass spectra of G-Rb$_1$-BSA conjugate. A broad peak coinciding with the conjugate of G-Rb$_1$ and BSA appeared from *m/z* 70,000 to 90,000 centering at around *m/z* 79,469. Using experimental results and a molecular weight of 66,433 for BSA, the calculated values of G-Rb$_1$component (MW1,109) are from 3,327 to 23,289 resulting in the range of 3 to 21 (12 in average) molecules of G-Rb$_1$ conjugated with BSA [8]. This method is suitable for characterization of conjugates between small molecule natural compound and carrier protein conjugates.

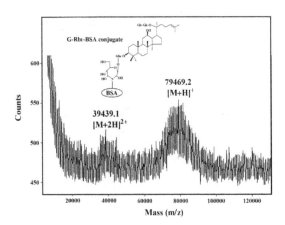

Figure 1. Direct detection of G-Rb$_1$-BSA conjugate by MALDI tof mass spectrometry. [M+H]$^+$, [M+2H]$^{2+}$ are single and double protonated molecules of G-Rb$_1$-BSA, respectively.

2.1.2. Preparation of anti-G-Rb₁ MAb and ELISA as an assay system

A hybridoma-producing MAb reactive to G-Rb$_1$ was obtained by general procedure and classified into IgG2b which had κ light chains [8]. The reactivity of IgG type MAb, 9G7 was tested by varying antibody concentration and by performing a dilution curve. The antibody concentration was selected for competitive ELISA. The free MAb following competition is bound to polystyrene microtiter plates precoated with G-Rb$_1$-human serum albumin (HSA). Under these conditions, the full measurement range of the assay extends from 20 to 400 ng/mL. The cross-reactivity against G-Rc and G-Rd, which possess a diglucose moiety attached to the C-3 hydroxy group, were weak compared with G-Rb$_1$ (0.024 and 0.020 %, respectively). G-Re and G-Rg$_1$ showed no cross-reactivity (less than 0.005 %). It is evident that the MAb reacted only with a small number of structurally related G-Rb$_1$ molecules, and very weakly and did not react with other steroidal compounds.

2.1.3. Preparation of anti-G-Rb₁ immunoaffinity column and appropriate buffer systems for separation of G-Rb₁

The purified IgG (10 mg) was treated by NaIO$_4$ to give dialdehyde group in sugar moiety which was coupled to Affi-Gel Hz hydrazide gel resulting in a hydrozone-type immunoaffinity gel [32]. The immunoaffinity gel was packed into plastic mini-column (Figure 2). Due to examine the optimal conditions of adsorption and elution, 400 μg of G-Rb$_1$ was dissolved in phosphate buffered saline (PBS) and loaded on anti-G-Rb$_1$ affinity column. After washing with washing buffer (20 mM PB containing 0.5 M NaCl), various buffer solutions for elution were loaded on the column, and then the recovery efficiency was determined by ELISA. The G-Rb$_1$ concentration was somewhat increased by eluting with a 20 mM phosphate buffer containing 0.5 M KSCN and 10 % MeOH. When the 20 mM phosphate buffer was changed to 100 mM AcOH buffer (pH 4), the elution ability reached the optimal level. Although 20 % MeOH could enhance the elution of G-Rb$_1$, higher MeOH concentration of over 20 % was ineffective. Thus, 100 mM AcOH buffer containing 0.5 M KSCN and 20 % MeOH could be used as an elution buffer in the immunoaffinity chromatography.

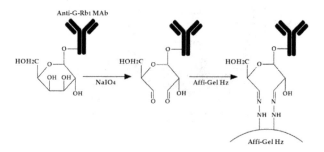

Figure 2. Preparation of anti-G-Rb₁ immunoaffinity column

2.2. Purification of G-Rb₁ by immunoaffinity column

2.2.1. One-step purification of G-Rb₁ from crude extract of P. ginseng roots by anti-G-Rb₁ immunoaffinity column

A crude extract (3.8 mg) of *P. ginseng* roots was loaded onto anti-G-Rb₁ immunoaffinity column. The column was washed with the washing buffer (fractions 1-20), and then eluted with elution buffer (fractions 21-40). As shown in Figure 3, the fractions 1-8 contained the overloaded G-Rb₁, which determined by ELISA. The other ginsenosides such as G-Rg₁, Rc, Re and Rd were also detected in these fractions by Eastern blotting procedure. After washing, a sharp peak was observed around fractions 21-24 of elution buffer, which contained G-Rb₁. However, these eluted fractions were still contaminated by a small amount of malonyl-G-Rb₁ as detected by Eastern blotting. The malonyl-G-Rb₁ has almost the same cross-reactivity with G-Rb₁ [32]. Therefore, the eluted fractions were treated with a mild alkaline solution (0.1 % KOH in MeOH) at room temperature to give pure G-Rb₁ [19]. Overcharged G-Rb₁ in washing solution (fractions 1-8) was repeatedly loaded and finally isolated in pure form. The anti-G-Rb₁ MAb was stable during all procedures, and the immunoaffinity column showed almost no decrease in capacity (20 μg of G-Rb₁/ml gel) after repeated use more than 10 times under same conditions, as reported for a one-step purification of forskolin from a crude extract of *Coleus forslohlii* root [17].

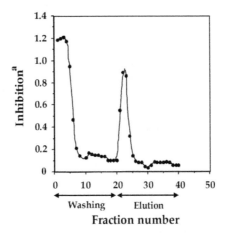

Figure 3. Elution profile of *P. ginseng* crude extract separated by anti-G-Rb₁ immunoaffinity column. The concentration of G-Rb₁ in each fraction was monitoring by ELISA using anti-G-Rb₁ MAb. Individual fraction (2 mL) were assayed by ELISA. [a]Inhibition = $(A_0-A)/A_0$;A_0 is the absorbance in the absence of the test compounds. A is the absence in the presence the test compounds.

This methodology is effective for the rapid and simple purification of G-Rb₁ and may open up a wide field of comparable studies with other families of saponins for which an acceptable method for one-step separation has not yet been developed. Furthermore, to separate the total ginseng saponins, a wide cross-reactive MAb against ginsenoside, like anti G-Re MAb which showed wide cross-reactivity, could be designed [34]. A combination of immunoaffinity column, Eastern blotting and ELISA could be used to survey low concentrations of ginsenoside Rb_1 of plant origin and/or in experimental animals and human. In fact we have succeeded in the isolation of $G-Rb_1$ from a different plant, *Kalopanax pictus* Nakai, which was not known previously to contain ginsenosides, using this combination of methods [35].

2.2.2. Isolation and determination of unknown compounds related to $G-Rb_1$ by anti-$G-Rb_1$ immunoaffinity column

Several species of ginseng are known to exist and contain different amount and kinds of ginsenosides. *P. japonicus* is distributed in Japan and China and it is morphologically different from the other *Panax* species. Yahara *et al.* indicated that $G-Rb_1$ was not detected in *P. japonicus*, and isolated oleanane-type saponins called chikusetsusaponins and determined their structures [36]. Morita *et al.* reported the varieties of saponins in *P. japonicus* by chemical analysis. These results suggested that the concentration of $G-Rb_1$ might be trace level in *P. japonicas* [37]. We previously analyzed the $G-Rb_1$ concentration in several ginseng roots by ELISA using anti-$G-Rb_1$ MAb and HPLC after pre-treatment under mildly alkaline condition [32]. As shown in Table 1, $G-Rb_1$ concentrationsof *P. ginseng, P. notoginseng* and *P. quinquefolius* were correlated between ELISA and HPLC. However, the $G-Rb_1$ of *P. japonicus* was higher concentrations compared with HPLC and previous reports [37]. This data suggest that anti-$G-Rb_1$ MAb using ELISA has the cross-reactivity with some unknown compounds contained in *P. japonicus*.

Sample		G-Rb₁ concentration (µg/mg dry weight powder)	
		ELISA	HPLC
P. ginseng	White ginseng	5.49 ±0.75	4.96 ± 0.05
	Red ginseng	3.57 ± 0.62	3.93 ± 0.34
	Fibrous ginseng	64.44 ± 3.64	69.75± 1.45
P. notoginseng		47.08 ± 3.34	42.39 ± 1.39
P. quinquefolium		48.51 ± 1.79	47.96 ± 1.04
P. japonicus		1.37 ± 0.34	0.63 ± 0.06

Table 1. G-Rb₁ concentration in various ginseng samples

To clarify the unknown compounds bound to anti-$G-Rb_1$ MAb, the crude extract of *P. japonicus* was concentrated by immunoaffinity column using anti-$G-Rb_1$ MAb. The crude root extract was loaded on the column and washed with the washing Buffer, followed by the elution buffer as already indicated. Figure 4 shows the H_2SO_4 staining (A) and the Eastern blotting (B) profiles of the washing fractions 1-4 and eluted fraction 5. Fraction 1 is first eluted fraction by the washing buffer, and showed many spots, indicating chikusetsusaponins, similar to the original extract of *P. japonicus*. After washing, the column was eluted by elution buffer (fraction 5), and then one spot was detected. As shown in Figure 4B, Eastern blotting indicated two different spots in washing fraction (Compound 1) and eluted fraction (Compound 2). These compounds bound with anti-G-Rb$_1$ MAb have a dammarane saponin having protopanaxadiol as a framework.

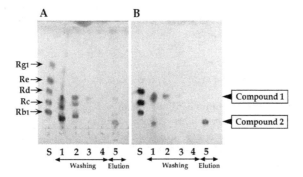

Figure 4. Purification and determination of ginsenosides of *P. japonicus* by the anti-G-Rb$_1$ immunoaffinity column. TLC (A) and Eastern blotting (B) profiles of the separated fractions from *P. japonicus* crude extract by the anti-G-Rb$_1$ immunoaffinity column. Lane S indicates the standard of ginsenosides (G-Rd, G-Rc, G-Rb$_1$, G-Rg$_1$, and G-Re). Lane 1-4 and Lane 5 were the washing fractions and the eluted fraction, respectively.

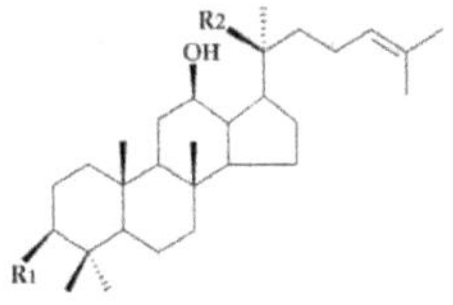

Compound	R$_1$	R$_2$
G-Rb1	-O-Glc-$\overset{2}{}$Glc	-O-Glc-$\overset{6}{}$Glc
Chikusetsusaponin III	-O-Glc-$\overset{6}{}$Xyl $\overset{2}{\searrow}$Glc	-OH
Chikusetsusaponin VI	-O-Glc-$\overset{6}{}$Xyl $\overset{2}{\searrow}$Glc	-O-Glc-$\overset{6}{}$Glc

Figure 5. Chemical structures of G-Rb$_1$ and chikusetsusaponins purified from *P. japonicus* by the anti-G-Rb$_1$ immunoaffinity column.

Compound 1 has three sugar moieties in a molecule because that the R_F value closes to that of G-Rd, indicating that this compound is chikusetsusaponin III (Figure 5). Finally, we identified that this compound as chikusetsusaponin III in a direct comparison with authentic sample [32]. Another unknown spot, compound 2 appeared in fraction 5 of the eluted fraction. Thus, compound 2 has a similar molecular structure and high cross-reactivity with G-Rb$_1$, and seems to be related ginseng saponin having protopanaxadiol as an aglycone. Moreover, compound 2 might have the same sugar fragments and possess five sugar moiety compared with G-Rb$_1$, as indicated by their R_F value. From these evidences compound 2 might be chikusetsusaponin III-20-O-gentiobiose, chikusetsusaponin VI (Figure 5), which has 5 sugars in a molecule in good agreement with the R_F value previously reported [38] and we confirmed that compound 2 is chikusetsusaponin VI by the direct comparison with authentic sample.

These data suggested that the anti-G-Rb$_1$ immunoaffinity column could isolate some unknown structurally resemble compounds having cross-reactivity against anti-G-Rb$_1$MAb. Therefore, this purification system will be applied to survey new compounds related to target compound of MAb. In our previous studies, we demonstrated the immunoaffinity purification against all solasodine glycosides from crude extract by one-step purification. In this case, all solasodine glycoside have almost same cross-reactivity against anti-solamargine MAb [12].

2.2.3. Preparation of G-Rb$_1$ knockout extract by anti-G-Rb$_1$ immunoaffinity column

The capacity of this anti-G-Rb$_1$immunoaffinity column is 20 µg of G-Rb$_1$/ml gel [32]. By loading the samples not to exceed the binding capacity against G-Rb$_1$, this immunoaffinity column becomes possible to remove all G-Rb$_1$ from crude ginseng extract. Figure 6 showed H_2SO_4 staining of TLC of the purification steps by the immunoaffinity column. Lane 1 and 2 were spotted the standard of ginsenosides (G-Rd, G-Rc, G-Rb$_1$, G-Rg$_1$, and G-Re). Lane A, B, and C were the crude extract, the washing fraction, and the eluted fraction, respectively. In the crude extract (lane A), all spots of ginsenosides were clearly detected. On the other hand, the washing fraction (lane B) contained all of the ginsenosides in the crude extract except G-Rb$_1$. Furthermore, the spot of G-Rb$_1$ was detected in the eluted fractions (lane C). These data strongly indicated that G-Rb$_1$ molecule in the ginseng extract can be eliminated by an anti-G-Rb$_1$ immunoaffinity column and the washing fractions was knockout only by the antigen molecule, G-Rb$_1$. Thus, we named the washing fractions a knockout (KO) extract [39,40]. This KO extract may be useful for the determination of real pharmacologically active principle in the TCMs.

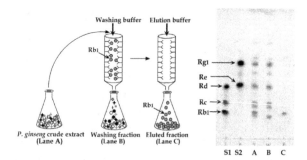

Figure 6. Preparation of G-Rb$_1$-KO extract from *P. ginseng* crude extract using anti-G-Rb$_1$ immunoaffinity column. Lane S1 and S2 indicate the standard of ginsenosides (G-Rd, G-Rc, G-Rb$_1$, G-Rg$_1$ and G-Re). Lane A, B, and C were the crude extract, the washing fraction, and the eluted fraction, respectively.

3. Glycyrrhizin-knockout extract and its application for *in vitro* assay

Licorice (*Glycyrrhiza* spp.) is also important crude drug used in over 70 % of the TCMs and Japanese Kampo medicines. It is prescribed with other herbal medicines as a demulcent in the treatment of sore throats, an expectorant for coughs and bronchial catarrh, an antitussive, a taste-modifying agent for relieving pain, an anti-inflammatory agent for anti-allergic reactions, rheumatism and arthritis, a prophylactic for liver disease and tuberculosis and adrenocorticoid insufficiency [41-43]. Accumulated evidence indicated that GC, a main saponin component of licorice, is one of the biologically active compounds. It has been reported that GC exhibits numerous pharmacological effects such as anti-inflammation, anti-ulcer, anti-tumor, anti-allergy, and hepatoprotective activities [44,45]. Clinically, GC has been used to treat patients with chronic hepatitis [46,47]. Although GC is supposed to be a major active principle in licorice crude extract, a number of studies by HPLC profiles suggested that licorice has many other bioactive components, including flavonoids, isoflavonoids and chalcones [43,48]. Biological studies showed that various flavonoid glycosides and their aglycones of licorice exhibit anti-inflammatory, anti-oxidative, anti-microbial, superoxide scavenging, and anti-carcinogenic activities [43,48]. In order to confirm the role of GC in TCM, we previously purified GC from TCM using an immunoaffinity column conjugated with anti-GC MAb [20]. In this section, we describe the preparation of GC-KO extract and its application for functional analysis of GC in licorice crude extract.

3.1. Preparation of GC-KO extract by anti-GC immunoaffinity column and the characterization of GC-KO extract

Our previous study demonstrated the preparation of anti-GC MAb [11]. The cross-reactivities of the anti-GC MAb against glycyrrhetic acid-3-O-glucuronide and glycyrrhetic acid were 0.585 % and 1.865 %, respectively. The other related compounds (deoxycholic acid, ursolic acid, and oleanolic acid) were all less than 0.005 %. Moreover, we established competitive ELISA and Eastern blotting method using anti-GC MAb [11,49].

The immunoaffinity column against GC was prepared by coupling the purified 60 mg of the anti-GC MAb to 25 ml of an Affi-Gel Hz gel [11]. To eliminate GC from licorice extract, 12 mg of licorice crude extract (GC content: 1275.0 µg) in loading buffer (5 % MeOH) was applied on the anti-GC MAb immunoaffinity column, and then the loading buffer was continuously circulated through the column to enhance the binding efficiency. After overnight circulation at 4 °C, the unbound fraction was separated. The column was washed with washing buffer (5 % MeOH) and then eluted with elution buffer (20 mM phosphate buffer containing 30 % MeOH). After separation, each fraction was deionized and the solvent was lyophilized. Figure 7 showed the recovery ratio of GC checked by ELISA. In the unbound fraction, 3.50 µg of GC (0.27% of the applied GC) was detected. On the other hand, 1269.26 µg of GC (99.55% of the applied GC) was obtained in the bound fraction. These data indicate that the anti-GC column could eliminate 99.55 % of the loading GC. Thus, we named this unbound fraction "GC-knockout (GC-KO) extract" [50].

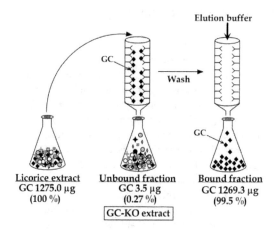

Figure 7. Preparation of GC-KO extract from licorice extract by anti-GC immunoaffinity column.

To further characterize GC-KO extract, the TLC analysis and Eastern blotting were performed [50]. As shown in Figure 8A, several spots including GC were detected in licorice extract (Lane B). However, the spot of GC was completely disappeared in GC-KO extract, although all other spots were clearly detected (lane C). Eastern blotting by anti-GC MAb indicated that GC was detected in licorice extract (Figure 8B, lane B), but the spot of GC was disappeared in GC-KO extract (Figure 8B, lane C). Therefore, these data suggest that GC was specifically eliminated from licorice extract by anti-GC MAb immunoaffinity column.

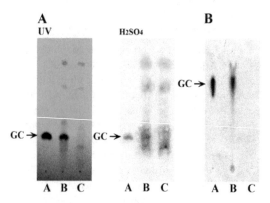

Figure 8. TLC profiles (A) and Eastern blotting by anti-GC MAb (B). Lane A, B, and C indicate GC, licorice extract, and GC-KO extract, respectively.

3.2. *in vitro* Assay by GC-KO extract prepared by anti-GC immunoaffinity column

Nitric oxide (NO), synthesized by NO synthase (NOS) from L-arginine, is an important reg-ulatory/modulatory mediator for several physiological processes [51]. However, during in-flammatory process, a large amount of NO is produced by inducible NOS (iNOS) stimulated by bacterial lipopolysaccharide (LPS) and inflammatory cytokines participates in the patho-genesis of inflammatory diseases [52]. Overproduced NO synthesized by iNOS triggers a variety of inflammatory diseases including sepsis, psoriasis, arthritis, multiple sclerosis, and systemic lupus *erythematosus* [53]. Therefore, inhibiting NO production by blocking iNOS expression may be useful strategy to treat a variety of inflammatory diseases.

In LPS-treated mouse RAW264 macrophages, licorice extract inhibited NO production and iNOS expression. At 100 μg/mL of licorice extract, iNOS protein and mRNA were complete-ly suppressed [50].

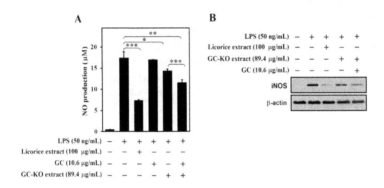

Figure 9. Effect of GC-KO extract and the combination of GC-KO extract and GC on NO production (A) and iNOS pro-tein expression (B) in LPS-treated RAW264 cells.Each bar indicates the mean S.D. of four individual experiments. *$P<0.05$, **$P<0.01$, ***$P<0.001$ indicate significant differences from the LPS alone

We next examined the inhibitory effect of GC alone, GC-KO extract and the combined treat-ment with GC and GC-KO extract on NO production [50]. Since 100 μg of licorice extract contains 10.6 ±0.618 μg of GC,the cells were pre-treated with licorice extract (100 μg/ml), GC-KO extract (89.4 μg/ml), or the combination of GC-KO extract (89.4 μg/ml) and GC (10.6 μg/ml). Figure9A indicated that the treatment of licorice extract led to a marked suppression of NO production as compared to LPS treatment [inhibition ratio (IR) 57.7%]. Interestingly, the inhibitory effect of GC-KO extract was lower (IR 17.8%) compared with licorice extract although GC alone could not block NO production as indicated above. On the other hand, the combined treatment with GC-KO extract and GC significantly improved the inhibitory ability (IR 33.5%). To determine whether the combinational effect of GC-KO extract and GC was related to iNOS expression, we performed Western blotting. As shown in Figure 9B, the treatment of GC-KO extract diminished the inhibitory ability of LE on iNOS expression, and addition of GC to GC-KO extract could improve it. These data suggest that GC alone cannot suppress iNOS expression, but combinational inhibition of iNOS expression may occur when GC coexists with the other constituents contained in licorice extract. The *in vitro* and in *vivo* analysis by using KO extract prepared by immunoaffinity column is a useful approach for determination of potential function of natural compound on *in vitro* and in *vivo* assays.

4. Conclusion

In this chapter, we introduce the unique strategy of one-step purification of target compounds from crude extract by anti-natural compound specific MAb-conjugated immunoaffinity column. The immunoaffinity column conjugated with anti-G-Rb$_1$ MAb could purify the G-Rb$_1$ from *P. ginseng* extract, and the washing fraction contained all compounds expect only G-Rb$_1$, which was named G-Rb$_1$-KO extract. By the use of the cross-reactivity of MAb, the anti-G-Rb$_1$ immunoaffinity column can identify new unknown compounds related to target compound of MAb and determine their structures. Furthermore, our data suggest that the combination of the immunoaffinity column and ELISA by using MAb provided a reliable and high sensitivity analysis for target compound in various TCMs and crude extract. We also demonstrated the in vitro assay by using GC-KO extract prepared by anti-GC immunoaffinity column from licorice extract. The KO extract may be able to support the pharmacological investigation for finding out a really active compound in a TCM and crude drug.

Acknowledgements

This work was funded by the Asahi Beer Science Promoting Foundation and Takeda Science Foundation. The research in this paper was also supported in part by Sasakawa Scientific Research Grant from Japan Science Society and "Science and Technology Research Partnership for Sustainable Development (SATREPS)" supported by the Japan Science and Technology Agency (JST) and the Japan International Cooperation Agency (JICA).

Author details

Takuhiro Uto[1], Nguyen Huu Tung[1], Hiroyuki Tanaka[2] and Yukihiro Shoyama[1*]

*Address all correspondence to: shoyama@niu.ac.jp

1 Faculty of Pharmaceutical Sciences, Nagasaki International University,, Japan

2 Faculty of Pharmaceutical Sciences, Kyushu University,, Japan

References

[1] Ong, E. S. (2002). Chemical assay of glycyrrhizin in medicinal plants by pressurized liquid extraction (PLE) with capillary zone electrophoresis (CZE). *J Sep Sci*, 25(13), 825-831.

[2] Tan, T. W., Huo, Q., & Ling, Q. (2002). Purification of glycyrrhizin from glycyrrhiza uralensis fisch with ethanol/phosphate aqueous two phase system. *Biochem Lett*, 24(17), 1417-1420.

[3] Sakata, R., Shoyama, Y., & Murakami, H. (1994). Production of monoclonal antibodies and enzyme immunoassay for typical adenylate cyclase activator, Forskolin. *Cytotechnology*, 16(2), 101-108.

[4] Xuan, L., Tanaka, H., Xu, Y., & Shoyama, Y. (1999). Preparation of monoclonal antibody against crocin and its characterization. *Cytotechnology*, 29(1), 65-70.

[5] Lu, Z., Morinaga, O., Tanaka, H., & Shoyama, Y. (2003). A quantitative ELISA using monoclonal antibody to survey paeoniflorin and albiflorin in crude drugs and traditional Chinese herbal medicines. *Biol Pharm Bull*, 26(6), 862-866.

[6] Shoyama, Y., Fukada, T., & Murakami, H. (1996). Production of monoclonal antibodies and ELISA for thebaine and codeine. *Cytotechnology*, 19(1), 55-61.

[7] Kim, J. S., Tanaka, H., & Shoyama, Y. (2004). Immunoquantitative analysis for berberine and its related compounds using monoclonal antibodies in herbal medicines. *Analyst*, 129(1), 87-91.

[8] Tanaka, H., Fukuda, N., & Shoyama, Y. (1999). Formation of monoclonal antibody against a major ginseng component, ginsenoside Rb_1 and its characterization. *Cytotechnology;* , 29(1), 115-120.

[9] Fukuda, N., Tanaka, H., & Shoyama, Y. (2000). Formation of monoclonal antibody against a major ginseng component, ginsenoside Rg_1 and its characterization Monoclonal antibody for a ginseng saponin. *Cytotechnology*, 34(3), 197-204.

[10] Zhu, S., Shimokawa, S., Tanaka, H., & Shoyama, Y. (2004). Development of an assay system for saikosaponin a using anti-saikosaponin a monoclonal antibodies. *Biol Pharm Bull*, 27(1), 66-71.

[11] Shan, S. J., Tanaka, H., & Shoyama, Y. (2001). Enzyme-linked immunosorbent assay for glycyrrhizin using anti-glycyrrhizin monoclonal antibody and an eastern blotting technique for glucuronides of glycyrrhetic acid. *Anal Chem*, 73(24), 5784-5790.

[12] Ishiyama, M., Shoyama, Y., Murakami, H., & Shinohara, H. (1996). Production of monoclonal antibodies and development of an ELISA for solamargine. *Cytotechnology*, 18(3), 153-158.

[13] Morinaga, O., Tanaka, H., & Shoyama, Y. (2000). Production of monoclonal antibody against a major purgative component, sennoside A, its characterization and ELISA. *Analyst*, 125(8), 1109-1113.

[14] Morinaga, O., Nakajima, S., Tanaka, H., & Shoyama, Y. (2001). Production of monoclonal antibodies against a major purgative component, sennoside B, their characterization and use in ELISA. *Analyst*, 126(8), 1372-1376.

[15] Tanaka, H., Goto, Y., & Shoyama, Y. (1996). Monoclonal antibody based enzyme immunoassay for marihuana (cannabinoid) compounds. *Immunoassay*, 17(4), 321-342.

[16] Loungratana, P., Tanaka, H., & Shoyama, Y. (2004). Production of monoclonal antibody against ginkgolic acids in Ginkgo biloba Linn. *Am J Chin Med*, 32(2), 33-48.

[17] Yanagihara, H., Sakata, R., Minami, H., Shoyama, Y., & Murakami, H. (1996). Immunoaffinity column chromatography against forskolin using an anti-forskolin monoclonal antibody and its application. *Anal Chim Acta*, 335(1-2), 63 -70.

[18] Putalun, W., Tanaka, H., & Yukihira, S. (1999). Rapid separation of solasodine glycosides by an immunoaffinity column using anti-solamargine monoclonal antibody. *Cytotechnology*, 31(1-2), 151-156.

[19] Fukuda, N., Tanaka, H., & Shoyama, H. (2000). Isolation of the pharmacologically active saponin ginsenoside Rb_1 from ginseng by immunoaffinity column chromatography. *J Nat Prod*, 63(2), 283-285.

[20] Xu, J., Tanaka, H., & Shoyama, Y. (2007). One-step immunochromatographic separation and ELISA quantification of glycyrrhizin from traditional Chinese medicines. *J Chromatog B*, 850(1-2), 53-58.

[21] Gillis, C. N. (1997). Panax ginseng pharmacology: a nitric oxide link? *Biochem Pharmacol*, 54(1), 1-8.

[22] Liu, C. X., & Xiao, P. G. (1992). Recent advances on ginseng research in China. *J. ethnopharmacol*, 36(1), 27-38.

[23] Yu, H., Zhang, C., Lu, M., Sun, F., Fu, Y., & Jin, F. (2007). Purification and characterization of new special ginsenosidase hydrolyzing multi-glycisides of protopanaxadiolginsenosides, ginsenosidase type I. *Chem Pharm Bull (Tokyo)*, 55(2), 231-235.

[24] Kitagawa, I., Taniyama, T., Yoshikawa, M., Ikenishi, Y., & Nakagawa, Y. (1989). Chemical studies on crude drug processing. IV. Chemical structures of malonyl-ginsenosides Rb_1, Rb_2, Re and Rd isolated from the root of Panax Ginseng C.A. Meyer. *Chem Pharm Bull*, 37(11), 2961-2970.

[25] Tanaka, O. (1989). Saponin-composition of Panax species. In: Shibata S, Ohtsuka Y, Saito H. (eds.) Recentadvances in ginseng studies. Tokyo, Hirokawa Publishing, 43-47.

[26] Fuzzati, N. (2004). Analysis methods of ginsenosides. *J Chromatogr B Analyt Technol Biomed Life Sci*, 812(1-2), 119 -33 .

[27] Washida, D., & Kitanaka, S. (2003). Determination of polyacetylenes and ginseno-sides in Panax species using high performance liquid chromatography. *Chem Pharm Bull*, 51(11), 1314-1317.

[28] Mook-Jung, I., Hong, H. S., Boo, J. H., Lee, K. H., Yun, S. H., Cheong, M. Y., Joo, I., Huh, K., & Jung, M. W. (2001). Ginsenoside Rb_1 and Rg_1 improve spatial learning and increase hippocampal synaptophysin level in mice. *J Neurosci Res*, 63(6), 509-515.

[29] Lim, J. H., Wen, T. C., Matsuda, S., Tanaka, J., Maeda, N., Peng, H., Aburaya, J., Ishihara, K., & Sakanaka, M. (1997). Protection of ischemic hippocampal neurons by gin-senoside Rb_1, a main ingredient of ginseng root. *Neurosci Res*, 28(3), 191-200.

[30] Liu, M., & Zhang, J. (1995). Effects of ginsenoside Rb_1 and Rg_1 on synaptosomal free calcium level, ATPase and calmodulin in rat hippocampus. *Chin Med J (Engl)*, 108(7), 544-547.

[31] Jiang, K. Y., & Qian, Z. N. (1995). Effects of Panax notoginseng saponins on posthy-poxic cell damage of neurons in vitro. *Zhongguo Yao Li Xue Bao*, 16(5), 399-402.

[32] Fukuda, N., Tanaka, H., & Shoyama, Y. (2000). Applications of ELISA, western blotting and immunoaffinity concentration for survey of ginsenosides in crude drugs of Panax species and traditional Chinese herbal medicines. *Analyst*, 125(8), 1425-1429.

[33] Wengatz, I., Schmid, R. D., Kreißig, S., Wittmann, C., Hock, B., Ingendoh, A., & Hillenkamp, F. (1992). Determination of the hapten density of immuno-conjugates by matrix-assisted UV laser desorption/ionization mass spectrometry. *Anal Lett*, 25(11), 1983-1997.

[34] Morinaga, O., Tanaka, H., & Shoyama, Y. (2006). Detection and quantification of gin-senoside Re in ginseng samples by a chromatographic immunostaining method using monoclonal antibody against ginsenoside Re. *J Chromatography B*, 830(1), 100-104.

[35] Tanaka, H., Fukuda, N., Yahara, S., Isoda, S., Yuan, C. S., & Shoyama, Y. (2005). Isolation of ginsenoside Rb_1 from Kalopanax pictus by eastern blotting using anti-ginse-noside Rb_1 monoclonal antibody. *Phytother Res*, 19(3), 255-258.

[36] Yahara, S., Kasai, R., & Tanaka, O. (1977). New dammarane type saponins of leaves of Panax japonicus C.A. Meyer. (1). Chikusetsusaponins L_5, L_{9a} and L_{10}. *Chem Pharm Bull*, 25(8), 2041-2047.

[37] Morita, T., Tanaka, O., & Kohda, H. (1985). Saponin composition of rhizomes of Pan-ax japonicus collected in South Kyushu, Japan, and its significance in oriental tradi-tional medicine. *Chem Pharm Bull*, 33(9), 3852-3858.

[38] Kohda, H., Tanaka, S., Yamaoka, Y., & Ohhara, Y. (1991). Saponins from Amaranthus hypochondriacus. *Chem Pharm Bull*, 39(10), 2609-2612.

[39] Tanaka, H., Fukuda, N., & Shoyama, Y. (2007). Eastern blotting and immunoaffinity concentration using monoclonal antibody for ginseng saponins in the field of tradi-tional chinese medicines. *J Agric Food Chem*, 55(10), 3783-3787.

[40] Wang, C. A., & Shoyama, Y. (2006). Herbal medicine: identification, analysis, and evaluationstrategies. In: Yuan CS, Bieber EJ, Bauer BA (eds) Textbook of complementary and alternative medicine, second edition. United Kingdom Informa Healthcare , 51-70.

[41] Kim, S. C., Byun, S. H., Yang, C. H., Kim, C. Y., Kim, J. W., & Kim, S. G. (2004). Cytoprotective effects of Glycyrrhizae radix extract and its active component liquiritigenin against cadmium-induced toxicity (effects on bad translocation and cytochrome c-mediated PARP cleavage). *Toxicology*, 197(3), 239-251.

[42] Fuchikami, J., Isohama, Y., Sakaguchi, M., Matsuda, M., Kucota, T., Akie, Y,k., Fujino, A., & Miyata, T. (2004). Effect of glycyrrhizin on late asthmatic responses induced by antigen inhalation in guinea pigs. *J Pharmacol Sci*, 94(Suppl.1), 251.

[43] Asl, M. N., & Hosseinzadeh, H. (2008). Review of pharmacological effects of Glycyrrhiza sp. and its bioactive compounds. *Phytother Res*, 22(6), 709-724.

[44] Jakkula, M., Boucher, T. A., Beyendorff, U., Conn, S. M., Johnson, J. E., Nolan, C. J., Peine, C. J., & Albrecht, J. H. (2004). A randomized trial of Chinese herbal medicines for the treatment of symptomatic hepatitis C. *Arch Intern Med*, 164(12), 1341-1346.

[45] Yanagawa, Y., Ogura, M., & Fujimoto, E. (2004). Effects and cost of glycyrrhizin in the treatment of upper respiratory tract infections in members of the Japanese maritime self-defense force: Preliminary report of a prospective, randomized, double-blind, controlled, parallel-group, alternate-day treatment assignment clinical trial. *Curr Ther Res Clin Exot*, 65(1), 26-33.

[46] Schalm, S. W., Brouwer, J. T., Bekkering, F. C., & van Rossum, T. G. (1999). New treatment strategies in non-responder patients with chronic hepatitis C. *J Hepatol*, 31(Suppl.1), 1184 -1188.

[47] Coon, J. T., & Ernst, E. (2004). Complementary and alternative therapies in the treatment of chronic hepatitis C: a systematic review. *J Hepatol*, 40(3), 491-500.

[48] Chin, Y. W., Jung, H. A., Liu, Y., Su, B. N., Castoro, J. A., Keller, W. J., Pereira, M. A., & Kinghorn, A. D. (2007). Anti-oxidant constituents of the roots and stolons of licorice (Glycyrrhiza glabra). *J Agric Food Chem*, 55(12), 4691-4697.

[49] Morinaga, O., Fujino, A., Tanaka, H., & Shoyama, Y. (2005). An on-membrane quantitative analysis system for glycyrrhizin in licorice roots and traditional Chinese medicines. *Anal Bioanal Chem*, 383(4), 668-672.

[50] Uto, T., Morinaga, O., Tanaka, H., & Shoyama, Y. (2012). Analysis of the synergistic effect of glycyrrhizin and other constituents in licorice extract onlipopolysaccharide-induced nitric oxide production using knock-out extract. *Biochem Biophys Res Commun*, 417(1), 473-478.

[51] Moncada, S., Palmer, R. M., & Higgs, E. A. (1991). Nitric oxide: physiology, pathophysiology, and pharmacology. *Pharmacol Rev*, 43(2), 109-142.

[52] Blantz, R. C., & Munger, K. (2002). Role of nitric oxide in inflammatory conditions. *Nephron*, 90(4), 373-378.

[53] Kröncke, K. D., Fehsel, K., & Kolb-Bachofen, V. (1998). Inducible nitric oxide synthase in human diseases. *Clin Exp Immunol*, 113(2), 147-156.

Chapter 4

Standard Operating Procedures (SOP) for the Spectrophotometric Determination of Phenolic Compounds Contained in Plant Samples

Elba Lúcia Cavalcanti de Amorim,
Valérium Thijan Nobre de Almeida de Castro,
Joabe Gomes de Melo,
Allan Jonathan Chernichiarro Corrêa and
Tadeu José da Silva Peixoto Sobrinho

Additional information is available at the end of the chapter

1. Introduction

The quality control of raw materials and products from plants is one of the topics most discussed by universities and health surveillance agencies. One of the primary tools used to ensure the reliability of production processes is the use of Standard Operating Procedures (SOPs). SOPs sequentially describe the steps of a particular methodology so that it can be reproduced by different analysts, which minimises variations in their implementation and improves the standardisation of the final product.

Several techniques, such as high performance liquid chromatography, gas chromatography and mass spectrometry, can be used in SOPs to control the quality of plant phenolic compounds [1,2]. However, these compounds have a characteristic spectrum produced by the double bonds in the aromatic rings and substituent positions that facilitates their identification and the development of spectrometric analytical techniques is easily accomplished. In this sense, spectrophotometric methods are more practical, reproducible and inexpensive than other techniques and are therefore favoured for the development of analytical methodologies for such determinations.

In addition to producing compounds such as carbohydrates, lipids, proteins and nucleic acids directly involved in their essential growth functions, plants have an arsenal of enzymes capable of producing, processing and accumulating several other substances not necessarily related to the maintenance of their life [3]. All of these reactions can be defined as secondary metabolism, the products of which provide advantages for both survival and species perpetuation in the plant's ecosystem [4]. However, this protection has a cost for the plant because metabolic resources that could increase its biomass are used to produce these compounds. In addition to protection, secondary metabolites perform important ecological functions such as inhibiting the germination and growth of other plants, attracting both pollinators and seed-dispersing animals and providing chemical defences against microorganisms [5].

Phenolic compounds, which have one or more hydroxyl groups linked to an aromatic ring, stand out from other classes of plant secondary metabolites because they are widely distributed and have various ecological functions that are scientifically proven to have numerous pharmacological activities and are well represented by tannins, flavonoids and coumarins.

1.1. Tannins

Tannins are water soluble phenolic compounds with a molecular weight between 500 and 3000 Daltons and may be chemically classified into two groups: hydrolysable tannins and condensed tannins [6,7]. Hydrolysable tannins are connected by ester-carboxyl linkages, which undergo hydrolysis under acidic and basic conditions [8]. Figure 1 presents an example of hydrolysable tannin (gallotannin), connected through a polyol (usually β-D-glucose) with the hydroxyl group esterified by gallic acid. Polyphenols connected with ellagic acid are called ellagitannins [9].

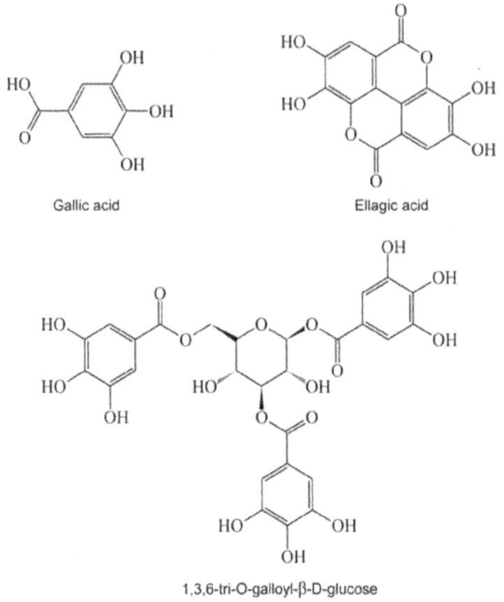

Gallic acid   Ellagic acid

1,3,6-tri-O-galloyl-β-D-glucose

Figure 1. Structure of gallic acid, ellagic acid and 1,3,6-tri-O-galloyl-β-D-glucose, a hydrolysable tannin.

Condensed tannins, also known as proanthocyanidins (Figure 2), can contain dozens of units of flavan-3-ols (catechin) or flavan-3,4-diols (leucoanthocyanidins). These units have a complex structure and are resistant to hydrolysis; however, they can be soluble in aqueous organic solvents because of their structure [7].

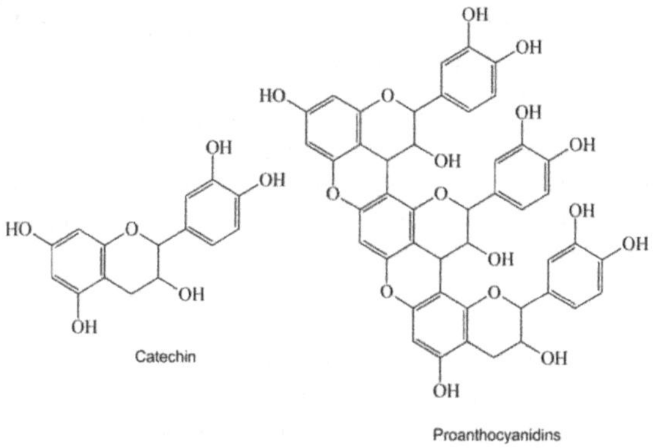

Figure 2. Basic structures of catechin and proanthocyanidins (condensed tannin).

Hydrolysable and condensed tannins may occur in the same plant simultaneously. However, the hydrolysable tannins are characteristic of Magnoliopsida herbaceous and woody plants and are restricted to certain taxonomic families. Ellagitannins have been used as taxonomic markers, particularly for Hemamelidaceae, Dilenidaceaa and Rosaceae. Condensed tannins have been identified in all plant groups, including Gymnosperms and Pteridophytes [10].

These secondary metabolites were initially identified by their astringent taste and capacity to bind proteins, which allows for the precipitation and formation of complexes with collagen skin fibres to increase their resistance to water and heat. Chemically speaking, hydrophobic interactions and hydrogen bonds between the phenolic groups in tannins and some macromolecules explain these features. However, the stability of the formed complexes only results after the formation of covalent bonds via the oxidation of tannins by quinones [11].

Since antiquity, plants containing tannins have been used medicinally as anti-inflammatory, antimicrobial, antitumor and antiviral agents and to treat both wound sand burns [7]. Tannins are also used to manufacture beverages and process animal skin into leather. Some researchers have shown that tannins protect plants against attack by herbivores and pathogens [12].

Although the use of tannin in the tanning industry has become restricted, interest in studying the ingestion of foods containing tannins to prevent diseases such as atherosclerosis or certain types of cancer has increased because of various epidemiological studies. Some studies report that the complexation of tannins with proteins gives them an important role in controlling bacteria, fungi and insects [13-15]. Other studies examined the inhibitory action of the enzyme reverse transcriptase [16] and the anticarcinogenic activity associated with green tea and diets rich in fruits containing tannins [17]. It is generally believed that the pharmacological activity of tannins occurs via their complexation with metal ions, antioxidant activity or the ability to complex with macromolecules.

Maytenus ilicifolia (Schrad.) Planch. (Celastraceae), popularly known as "espinheira-santa", is a species native to Brazil traditionally used to treat digestive disorders and the literature cites tannins as compounds that act to protect the stomach by helping to treat ulcers and gastritis [18-20]. In addition to these activities, *M. ilicifolia* has other pharmacological applications, such as anticancer, antimicrobial and antioxidant activity and treatment of the central nervous system [21]. For these reasons, *M. ilicifolia* was chosen as a reference species in this study.

1.2. Flavonoids

Flavonoids comprise a group of natural substances with great structural diversity and there are currently more than nine thousand known flavonoids that do not occur in humans but can be found in various plant parts such as the leaves, fruits, bark, roots, stems and flowers [22,23]. Flavonoids (Figure 3) are composed of a simple skeleton containing two phenol rings connected by a propionic chain; where ring A is the acetate derivative and both ring B and the three-carbon bridge are derived via a shikimate pathway, which may be associated with carbohydrates (heterosides), un associated (aglycones) or polymerised further (anthocyanins) [24].

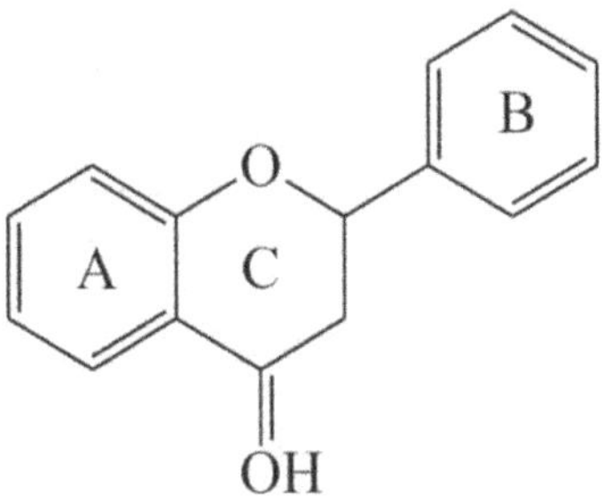

Figure 3. Basic structure of flavonoids.

This class of metabolites has several biological functions, such as defence against both herbivores and pathogens, the perpetuation of the species by attracting seed dispersing animals, protection from ultraviolet rays and allelopathy [24,25]. Flavonoids also possess important pharmacological properties, such as antioxidant, antiinflammatory, anti-thrombogenic, antimicrobial, anticancer, antidiabetic and hypocholesterolemic activities [23,26].

Studies show that flavonoids are chemical markers responsible for various pharmacological activities performed by the genus *Bauhinia* [27-29]. *Bauhinia forficata* Link (Fabaceae), popularly known as "pata-de-vaca", is a tree native to Brazil that prevails in the phytogeographical area of Mata Atlântica [30] and can also be found in Cerrado. Pata-de-vaca is used in folk medicine as a hypoglycemic, diuretic and antihypertensive agent [31,32]. Several plant-based products are sold in open markets, pharmacies and natural product stores [33]. Though not officially recommended, herbal products from the leaves of pata-de-vaca (*Bauhinia* L.) are popularly used for therapeutic purposes. This plant was used in our study as a reference species for flavonoids.

1.3. Coumarins

Coumarins are lactones of *O*-hydroxy-cinnamic acid derived from trans-cinnamic acid via oxidation-reduction and isomerisation to produce 1,2-benzopyrone. Coumarins are divided into simple coumarins, furanocoumarins, pyranocoumarins, dimeric coumarins and chromones (Figure 4) [34]. The difference between these classes is the position of the radical in the coumarin lactone ring, which varies between C-6, C-7 and C-8. Chromones represent a group of natural isomers to coumarin that may be linearly and angularly prenylated at C-6 and C-8, respectively, in furanochromones and pyranochromones, respectively [34].

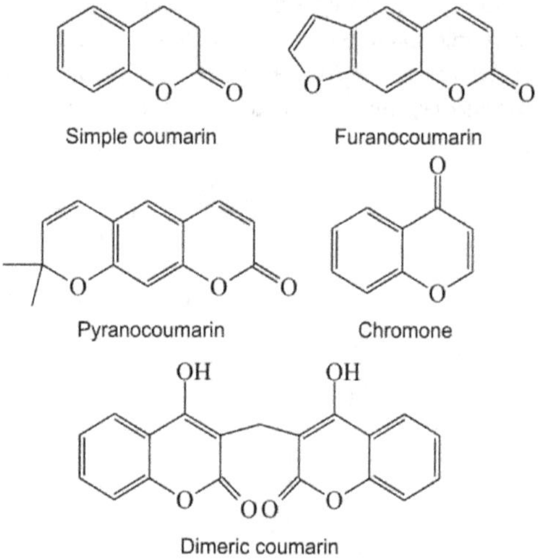

Simple coumarin   Furanocoumarin

Pyranocoumarin   Chromone

Dimeric coumarin

Figure 4. Basic structure of coumarins and chromones.

Coumarins are used as antioxidants, anti-HIV drugs, antispasmodics, spasmolytics, hypolipidemics, hypotensives and vasodilating agents [34]; however, they are also used in food flavouring, perfumes, tobacco and cosmetic products [35]. It is estimated that the daily human exposure to coumarins from cosmetics and perfumes is 0.04 mg/kg/day [36].

Coumarins are a class of secondary metabolites widely distributed throughout the Plantae kingdom and found in Fungi and Bacteria as well [37]. In plants, coumarins are found frequently in the families of Apiaceae, Rutaceae and Asteraceae, and less frequently in the families of Fabaceae, Oleaceae, Moraceae and Thymeleaceae [38].

Mikania glomerata Spreng. (Asteraceae), popularly known in Brazil as "guaco", has existed in the Brazilian Pharmacopoeia since 1929 and is used as an expectorant to treat respiratory problems. Most herbal products are marketed as some form of syrup; however, they are produced from fluid extracts and tinctures [39,40]. Chemical studies of this species show coumarins to be a major component that can be used as a chemical marker for the quality control of products based on guaco [41-43].

Coumarins have a characteristic UV spectrum due to the nature and position of their substituents, which facilitates both their identification and the development of analytical spectrophotometric techniques [11]. For these reasons, *M. glomerata* was chosen as the reference species to quantify the coumarin level.

2. Problem statement

Despite extensive literature presenting various analytical methods, the development of an SOP is often difficult for three reasons: 1) the work does not detail the difficulties and adjustments required to implement the methodology, 2) the steps are not clearly presented for reproduction and 3) the limits of interpretation are not discussed. One criterion recommended by the National Sanitary Surveillance Agency (Agência Nacional de Vigilância Sanitária - ANVISA) in Brazil for the standardisation of herbal drugs is the active compound content or chemical class, which is the total concentration of tannins for products based on *M. ilicifolia* (espinheira-santa) [44], flavonoids for *B. forficata* (pata-de-vaca) [45,46] and coumarins for *M. glomerata* (guaco) [44].

Thus, this paper presents research protocols adopted by our research group to study the levels of tannins, flavonoids and coumarins from plant extracts and the experimental application of these SOPs to analyse products sold in markets (pharmacies and natural product stores) as phytomedicines[1] or plant drugs[2] with high commercial value.

3. Standard operating procedures (POP)

The following SOPs describe the chemical classes to be analysed and the chemical basis of the methods. They provide a detailed list of all the reagents required for the preparation and describe the experimental procedure to be followed. Finally, there is a list of references used in the development of the SOP.

---

1 "All medicine is obtained using solely active raw vegetables. It is characterised by knowledge of the effectiveness and risks of their use, as well as the reproducibility and consistency of its quality. Its efficacy and safety are validated through ethnopharmacological surveys of use, documentation, technical and scientific publications or clinical trial phase 3"[44].

2 "Medicinal plant or their parts, after collection processes, stabilisation and drying and can be full, erasures, crushed or powdered" [44].

3.1. Standard operating procedure for the quantification of tannins

Description: Tannins are phenolic compounds with the ability to bind macromolecules, especially proteins. This class of compounds has traditionally been divided into two groups: hydrolysable and condensed tannins. Hydrolysable tannins are characterised by a central polyol, usually β-D-glucose, containing hydroxy groups esterified with gallic acid and ellagic acid. Condensed tannins are oligomers or polymers formed by the condensation of two or more molecules of flavan-3-ol or flavan-3,4-diol [3] [7].

Principle of the method: The phenolic compounds in the sample are oxidised using the Folin-Ciocalteu reagent. This reagent is a mixture of phosphotungstic and phosphomolybdic acids that are reduced by the oxidation of phenolic compounds in a mixture of tungsten and molybdenum oxides. The blue colour produced by the oxides has a maximum absorption at 760 nm and is proportional to the total phenolic concentration [47]. The tannin content is calculated as the difference between the total and waste phenol content.

Reagents:

(1) Tannic acid (0.1 mg/mL, w/v): Dissolve 10 mg of tannic acid in 100 ml of distilled water.

(2) Folin-Ciocalteu reagent (10%, v/v): Dilute 5 ml of Folin-Ciocalteu reagent with 45 mL of distilled water.

(3) Sodium carbonate Na_2CO_3 (7.5%, w/v): Dissolve 7.5 g of Na_2CO_3 in 100 ml of distilled water. If necessary, solubilising the solution on a heating plate and magnetic stirrer.

(4) Methanol (80%, v/v): Dilute 800 ml of methanol with 200 ml of distilled water.

The reagent volume is sufficient to examine a maximum of 100 analyses.

Preparation of samples: The powdered sample (500 mg) should be extracted with 50 mL of 80% methanol for 30 minutes on a hot plate. The extract should be filtered through filter paper into a 50 mL volumetric flask and the volume should be completed using the same solvent. The final extract concentration will be 10 mg/mL. If the products are liquid, they must be evaporated. The dried extract should be dissolved in 80% methanol for a final concentration of 1 mg/mL.

Calibration curve: The calibration curve must be prepared using 100-500 μL aliquots of the tannic acid solution, 500 μL of the Folin-Ciocalteu solution and 1 mL of the sodium carbonate solution. The final volume should be adjusted to 10 mL with distilled water. The final tannic acid concentration will be 1-5 μg/mL.

Measurement procedure: To quantify the total phenol concentration (that is, all of the phenols present in the sample), 500 μL of the extract must be transferred to a test tube. Next, 500 μL of the Folin-Ciocalteu solution, 1 mL of the sodium carbonate solution and 8 ml of distilled water are added. The samples remain at room temperature for 30 minutes. The spectrophotometer should be adjusted to a wavelength of 760 nm and the equipment must be rinsed with distilled water. To quantify the phenol waste, (i.e., the phenols present in the sample except for the proteins precipitated with the tannin) 500 mg of casein is weighed and transferred into a 25 ml Erlenmeyer flask before adding 5 ml of the extract and 5 ml of water distilled. After two hours (time required for the complexing of the tannins to the total protein), the extracts are filtered into a 10 mL volumetric flasks and its volume is adjusted with distilled water. The phenols are considered to be equal to the residue from the total phenol. These assays are performed at least in triplicate and the total phenolic content is expressed as milligrams of tannic acid equivalents per gram of sample or extract (mg TAE/g).

References:

Amorim E. L. C, Nascimento J. E., Monteiro J. M., Peixoto Sobrinho T. J. S, Araújo T. A. S., Albuquerque U. P. A simple and accurate procedure for the determination of tannin and flavonoid levels and some applications in ethnobotany and ethnopharmacology. Functional Ecosystems and Communities 2008; 2(1) 88-94 [47].

Santos S. C., Mello J. C. P. Taninos. In: Simões C. M. O., Schenkel E. P., Gosmanm, G., Mello J. C. P., Mentz L. A., Petrovick P. R. (ed.) Farmacognosia: da planta ao medicamento. Porto Alegre: Universidade Federal do Rio Grande do Sul; 2004. p.615-656 [3].

3.2. Standard operating procedure for the quantification of flavonoids

Description: Flavonoids are the most important and diverse phenolic compounds. Most flavonoids have 15 carbon atoms and consist of two phenol rings connected by a chain of three carbons to form a tricyclic compound [24].

Principle of the method: The aluminium ion (Al^{3+}) is reacted with the flavonoids in the sample to form the stable flavonoid-Al^{3+}complex, which has a yellow colour and intensity proportional to the flavonoid concentration. This reaction causes a bathochromic shift and intensification in the absorption, which can be measured without influence from other phenolic compounds present in the sample [48].

Reagents:

(1) Rutin (0.1 mg/mL, w/v): Dissolve 10 mg of rutin in 100 ml of methanol.

(2) Acetic acid solution (60%, v/v): Dilute 30 ml of acetic acid with 20 ml of methanol.

(3) Pyridine Solution (20%, v/v): Dilute 40 ml of pyridine with 160 ml of methanol.

(4) Aluminium chloride solution $AlCl_3$ (5%, w/v): Dissolve 5 g $AlCl_3$ in 100 mL of methanol. If necessary, complete dissolution via magnetic stirring.

(5) Methanol (80%, v/v). Dilute 80 ml of methanol with 20 ml of distilled water.

The reagent volume is sufficient to examine a maximum of 100 analyses.

Preparation of samples: The powdered sample (500 mg) should be extracted with 50 mL of 80% methanol on a hot plate for 30 minutes. The extract should be filtered through filter paper into a 50 mL volumetric flask and the volume should be adjusted with the same solvent. The final extract concentration will be 10 mg/mL. Liquid products must be evaporated. The dried extract should be dissolved in 80% methanol to obtain a final concentration of 1 mg/mL.

Calibration curve: The calibration curve must be prepared using 100-1000 μL aliquots of the rutin solution, 500 μL of the acetic acid solution, 2 mL of the pyridine solution and 1 ml of the reagent aluminium chloride solution. The final volume should be adjusted to 10 mL with 80% methanol. The final rutin concentration will be 1-10 μg/mL.

Measurement procedure: To quantify the flavonoids, 500 μL of the extract should be transferred to a test tube. Next, 500 μL of the acetic acid solution, 2 mL of the pyridine solution, 1 ml of the reagent aluminium chloride solution and 6 ml of 80% methanol will be added. The samples remain at room temperature for 30 minutes. The spectrophotometer should be adjusted to a wavelength of 420 nm and the equipment must be rinsed with distilled water. The test shall be performed at least in triplicate and the flavonoid content is expressed as milligrams of rutin equivalents per gram of sample or extract (mg RE/g).

References:

Peixoto Sobrinho T. J. S, Silva C. H. T. P., Nascimento J. E., Monteiro J. M., Albuquerque U. P., Amorim E. L. C. Validação de metodologia espectrofotométrica para quantificação dos flavonóides de *Bauhinia cheilantha* (Bongard) Steudel. Brazilian Journal of Pharmaceutical Sciences 2008; 44 (4) 683-689 [48].

Zuanazzi, J. A. S.; Montanha, J. A. Flavonóides. In: Simões C. M. O., Schenkel E. P., Gosmanm, G, Mello J. C. P., Mentz L. A., Petrovick P. R. (ed.) Farmacognosia: da planta ao medicamento. Porto Alegre: Universidade Federal do Rio Grande do Sul; 2004, p.577-614 [24].

3.3. Standard operating procedure for the quantification of coumarins

Description: Coumarins are lactones of O-hydroxy-cinnamic acid and are metabolites of phenylalanine. 1,2-benzopyrone is the simplest coumarin representative, others being furocoumarins, pyranocoumarins, dimeric coumarins and chromones [34].

Principle of the method: The Borntrager reaction is based on the solubility of free coumarin derivatives in polar organic solvents and the solubility of their soluble alkali phenolates. Coumarin absorbs at 280 nm; however, ionisation of phenolic hydroxyls in the molecule by alkaline hydroxide causes a bathochromic deviation to 320 nm, which is proportional to the coumarin concentration [40].

Reagents:

(1) 1,2-benzopyrone (1 mg/mL, w/v): Dissolve 10 mg of coumarin in 10 ml of distilled water.

(2) Lead acetate (5%, w/v): Dissolve 2,5 g of lead acetate in 50 ml of distilled water.

(3) Hydrochloric acid solution, HCl (0.1 M, v/v): Dilute 10 ml of concentrated hydrochloric acid with 1000 ml of distilled water.

(4) Methanol (80%, v/v): Dilute 80 ml of methanol with 20 ml of distilled water.

The reagent volume is sufficient to examine a maximum of 100 analyses.

Preparation of samples: The powdered sample (500 mg) should be extracted with 50 mL of 80% methanol for 30 minutes on a hot plate. The extract should be filtered through filter paper into a 50 mL volumetric flask and the final volume should be adjusted with the same solvent. The final extract concentration will be 10 mg/mL. Liquid products must be evaporated. The dried extract should be dissolved in 80% methanol for a final concentration of 1 mg/mL.

Calibration curve: The calibration curve must be prepared using 50-500 µL aliquots of the coumarin solution, 2 ml of distilled water and 500 µL of the lead acetate solution. The sample should be shaken and the final volume should be adjusted to 10 mL with distilled water before transferring 2 mL of this solution to a new test tube and adding 8 mL of hydrochloric acid solution. The final concentration of rutin will be 1-10 µg/mL.

Measurement procedure: To quantify the coumarins, 500 µL of the extract should be transferred to a test tube. Next, 2 ml of distilled water and 500 µL of lead acetate solution will be added. The sample is shaken and then 7 ml of distilled water are added before transferring 2 mL of this solution to a new test tube and adding 8 mL of hydrochloric acid solution. The samples remain at room temperature for 30 minutes. The spectrophotometer should be adjusted to a 320 nm wavelength and the equipment must be rinsed with distilled water. The test should be performed in at least triplicate and the total coumarin content is expressed as milligrams of coumarin equivalents per gram of the sample extract (mg CE/g).

References:

Kuster R. A. M., Rocha L. A. M. A. Cumarinas, coronas e cantinas. In: Simões CMO, Schenkel EP, Gosmanm, G, Mello JCP, Mentz LA, Petrovick PR. (ed.) Farmacognosia: da planta ao medicamento. Porto Alegre: Universidade Federal do Rio Grande do Sul; 2004, p. 537-556 [34].

Osório O. K., Martins J. L. S. Determinação de cumarina em extrato fluido e tintura de guaco por espectrofotometria derivada de primeira ordem. Brazilian Journal of Pharmaceutical Sciences 2004; 40 (4) 481-486 [40].

4. Results

Analysis of the active component levels in raw plant materials and phytomedicines is essential for the safety and efficacy of pharmaceutical products [49]. The quantification of active compounds in herbals is still only incidentally performed due to the presence of active phytocomplexes plants and their extracts [50], which complicates their analysis. Through this framework, the use of standardised extracts focusing on specific groups of active components ensures the chemical homogeneity of the product, which improves product quality [51]. The compounds selected for this quality adjustment process should be the same as the assets in the product [52].

In this way, five products containing *M. ilicifolia* (all plant drugs), four containing *B. forficata* (all plant drugs) and five containing *M. glomerata* (three plant drugs and two fluid extract) sold in pharmacies and health food stores in Recife/PE, Northeast Brazil were obtained.

Analysis of the active component concentrations were conducted as listed in the described standard operating protocols (SOPs) and the results are presented below.

4.1. Calibration curves

To quantify the active components, calibration curves with increasing concentrations pro-portional to their absorbance were constructed. A correlation equation was obtained from these curves (generally linear) of the type $y = ax + b$, where y corresponds to the absorbance of the sample and x the concentration. To convert the absorbance values   (nm) to sample concentration (µg/mL), it is necessary to place the sample absorbance into the equation as y. The correlation coefficient (R^2) shows the ability of the method to provide directly propor-tional results between the analyte concentration and the device response. The interval be-tween the lowest and highest scalar values, which is also called the linearity range, should be determined with both precision and accuracy. The correlation coefficient must be equal to or greater than 0.98.

The calibration curve constructed for tannic acid and tannins and used to quantify *M. ilicifo-lia* demonstrated a correlation equation of y = 0.067x + 0.01 and a correlation coefficient of R^2 = 0.996 (Figure 5).

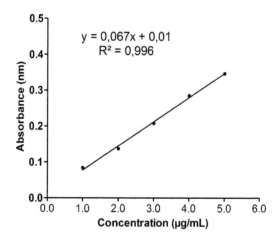

Figure 5. Calibration curve constructed using tannic acid concentrations of 1-5 µg/mL at 760 nm used to quantify the tannin content of *Maytenus ilicifolia* (Schrad.) Planch.

A calibration curve was constructed from rutin to quantify flavonoids in products from *B. forficata* and yielded the correlation equation y = 0.022 + 0.0039 x and correlation coefficient R^2 = 0.991 (Figure 6).

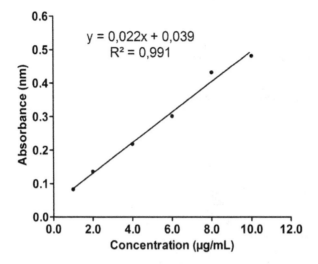

Figure 6. Calibration curve constructed from rutin for concentrations of 1-10 µg/mL at 420 nm used to quantify the flavonoids content in *Bauhinia forficata* Link.

The correlation equation and coefficient obtained from the calibration curve used to analyse coumarins in products containing *M. glomerata* were y = 0.049 x + 0.031 and R^2= 0.994 (Figure 7), respectively.

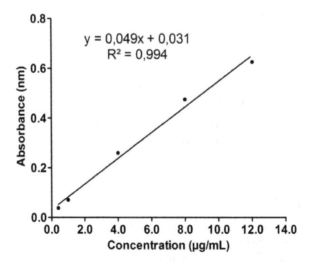

Figure 7. The calibration curve constructed using 1,2-benzopyrone in concentrations of 1-12 µg/mL using 320 nm excitation to quantify the coumarin content in *Mikania glomerata* Spreng.

4.2. Content of active principles

The results of quality control of tannins of *M. Ilicifolia*, flavonoids of *B. forficata* and coumarins of *M. glomerata* are shown in Table 1.

Specie / Marker	Sample	Concentration ± SD (mg/g)	CV (%)
Maytenus ilicifolia Tannins	MI1	12.57 ± 2.15a	17.12%
	MI2	4.04 ± 0.23b	5.75%
	MI3	5.61 ± 0.55bc	9.76%
	MI4	7.72 ± 0.84c	10.84%
	MI5	11.81 ± 1.00a	8.44%
Bauhinia forficata Flavonoids	BF1	4.89 ± 0.11a	2.33%
	BF2	7.27 ± 0.39a	5.41%
	BF3	50.38 ± 5.36b	10.64%
	BF4	65.98 ± 3.62c	5.49%
Mikania glomerata Coumarins	MG1	3.06 ± 0.20a	6.67%
	MG2	5.17 ± 0.59b	11.40%
	MG3	6.80 ± 0.24c	3.46%
	MG4	1.63 ± 0.20d	12.50%
	MG5	4.49 ± 0.20b	4.55%

Table 1. Results of quality control of tannins, flavonoids and coumarins contained in products based on *Maytenus ilicifolia* (Schrad.) Planch., *Bauhinia forficata* Link and *Mikania glomerata* Spreng. respectively, sold in pharmacies in Recife/PE, Northeast of Brazil.

Values are mean ± standard deviation. Values followed by the same letter in column are not statistically different (n = 6, p<0.05).

Analysis of variance (ANOVA) is one way to indicate significant differences (p<0.01) for the drugs of *M. ilicifolia*, which is made from five plants. Samples Mi1 (12.57 ± 2.15 mg TAE/g) and Mi5 (11.81 ± 1.0 mg TAE/g) both had higher concentrations of tannins and were not significantly different, whereas at least three of the other samples showed tannins (Figure 8). Comparing the average tannin concentration from different samples showed a low coefficient of variation (CV = 37.61%).

Analysis of four products containing *B. forficata* showed a significant difference (p<0.01). The sample Bf4 presented the highest flavonoid concentration (65.98 ± 3.62 mg RE/g), whereas samples Bf1 and Bf2 had the lowest concentrations (4.89 ± 0.11 and 7.27 ± 0.39 mg RE/g, respectively) with a content approximately 13 times lower. These results indicate that there is no standardisation regarding the flavonoid concentrations in products (Figure 9).

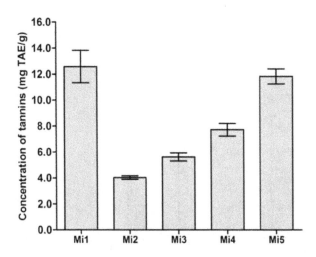

Figure 8. Concentration of tannin (mg TAE/g) contained in products from *Maytenus ilicifolia* (Schrad.) Planch. Sold in Recife/PE, Brazil.

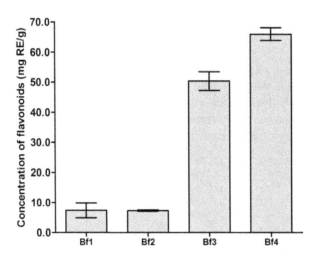

Figure 9. Concentration of flavonoids (mg RE/g) contained within *Bauhinia forficata* link. sold in Recife/PE, Brazil.

Of the five products from *M. glomerata*, three were plant drugs and two were fluid extracts. The plant drugs were extracted with ethanol as recommended by the Brazilian Pharmacopoeia 4th Edition to remove discrepancies from the results [53]. Both the extracts and liquids were evaporated to dryness. The one way ANOVA showed significant differences between the products ($p<0.01$) and sample Mg3 had the highest level (6.80 ± 0.24 mg CE/g), whereas sample Mg4 had the lowest level (1.63 ± 0.20 mg CE/g), with an approximately four times lower coumarin concentration.

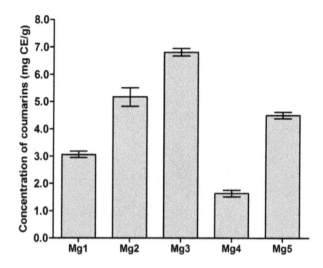

Figure 10. Concentration of coumarins (mg CE/g) contained in products from *Mikania glomerata* Spreng. sold in Recife/PE, Brazil.

The quantitative analysis of raw vegetables and phytomedicines is a fundamental quality control process that leads to security, stability, consistency and effectiveness in the produced phytomedicines [49]. It is important to emphasise the need for standardisation in analysing herbal medicines to determine the concentration of their active components in raw vegetable materials as well as for species identification.

5. Conclusion

This chapter provides easily reproducible standard operating procedures (SOPs) for the quality control of raw materials and herbal plants to ensure a minimal standard of quality in products sold. The implementation of these SOPs allows for the analysis of samples sold in establishments in Recife/PE and reveals an inconsistency in the concentration of tannins, flavonoids and coumarins within these products.

The low level of these metabolites may alter their effectiveness and more rigorous quality control and standardisation of these products is required to prevent compromising their therapeutic activity.

Author details

Elba Lúcia Cavalcanti de Amorim[1*], Valérium Thijan Nobre de Almeida de Castro[1],
Joabe Gomes de Melo[2], Allan Jonathan Chernichiarro Corrêa[1] and
Tadeu José da Silva Peixoto Sobrinho[3]

*Address all correspondence to: elba@ufpe.br

1 Department of Pharmacy, Federal University Pernambuco, Recife/PE, Brazil

2 Department of Biology, Federal Rural University of Pernambuco, Brazil

3 School of Medicine, Federal University of Tocantins, Palmas/TO, Brazil

References

[1] Aguilar-Sánchez, R., Ahuatl-García, F., Dávila-Jiménez, M. M., Elizalde-González, M.
P., & Guevara-Villa, M. R. (2005). Chromatographic and electrochemical determination of quercetin and kaempferol in phytopharmaceuticals. *Journal of Pharmaceutical
and Biomedical Analysis*, 38(2), 239-249.

[2] Matysik, G., & Wójciak-Kosior, M. (2005). Optimized Method for the determination
of Flavonoid Glycosides and Aglycones. *Chromatographia*, 61(1-2), 89-92.

[3] Santos, R.I. (2004). Metabolismo básico e origem dos metabólitos secundários. In: Simões CMO, Schenkel E.P., Gosmanm, G., Mello J.C.P, Mentz L.A., Petrovick P.R.
(ed.) Farmacognosia: da planta ao medicamento. Porto Alegre: Universidade Federal
do Rio Grande do Sul;, 403-434.

[4] Edwards, P. J., & Wratten, S. D. (1981). Ecologia das interações entre insetos e plantas. 1ª ed. São Paulo: Ed Pedagógica e Universitária; 78p.

[5] Harborne, J. B. (1993). Introduction to Ecological Biochemistry. 4ª ed. London Har-
court Brace and Company , 318p.

[6] Queiroz, C. R. A. A., Morais, S. A. L., & Nascimento, E. A. (2002). Caracterização dos
taninos da aroeira-preta (Myracrodruon urundeuva). *Revista Árvore*, 26(4), 485.

[7] Santos, S. C., & Mello, J. C. P. (2004). Taninos. In: Simões C.M.O, Schenkel E.P., Gosmanm, G, Mello J.C.P., Mentz LA, Petrovick P.R. (ed.) Farmacognosia: da planta ao
medicamento. Porto Alegre: Universidade Federal do Rio Grande do Sul, 615-656.

[8] Hagerman, A. E., & Butler, L. G. (1981). The specificity of proanthocyanidin-protein
interaction. *Journal of Biological Chemistry*, 256(9), 4494-4497.

[9]   Lewis, N. G., & Yamamoto, E. (1989). Tannins: their place in plant metabolism. In: Hemingway RW, Karchesy JJ. (Ed) Chemistry and significance of condensed tannins. New York: Plenum Press, 23-46.

[10] Heil, M., Baumann, B., Andary, C., Linsenmair, K. E., & Mckey, D. (2002). Extraction and quantification of "condensed tannins" as a measure of plant anti-herbivore defence? *Revisiting an old problem. Naturwissenschaften*, 89(11), 519-524.

[11] Bruneton, J. (1991). Elementos de Fitoquimica y Farmacognosia. 1ª ed. Zaragoza: Ed. Acribia Espanha , 594p.

[12] Harborne, J. B., Palo, R. T., & Robbins, C. T. (1991). Plant defenses against mammalian herbivore. C R C Press LLC , 192.

[13] Gobbo-Neto, L., & Lopes, N. P. (1991). Plantas medicinais: fatores de influência no conteúdo de metabólitos secundários., *Química Nova x*, 30(2), 374-381.

[14] Verpoorte, R. (1998). Exploration of nature's chemodiversity: the role of secondary metabolites as leads in drug development. *Drug Development Trends*, 3(5), 232-238.

[15] Wills, R. B. H., Bone, K., & Morgan, M. (2000). Herbal products: active constituents modes of action and quality control. *Nutrition Research Reviews*, 13-47.

[16] Kilkuskie, R. E., Kashiwada, Y., Nonaka, G., Nishioka, I., Bodner, A., Cheng, Y., & Lee, K. (1992). HIV and reverse transcriptase inhibition by tannins. *Bioorganic & Medicinal Chemistry Letters*, 2(12), 1529-1534.

[17] Chung, K., Wei, C., & Johnson, M. G. (1998). Are tannins a double-edged sword in biology and health. *Trends in Food Science and Technology*, 9(4), 168-175.

[18] Ferreira, P. M., Oliveira, C. N., Oliveira, A. B., Lopes, M. J., Alzamora, F., & Vieira, M. A. R. (2004). A lyophilized aqueous extract of Maytenus ilicifolia leaves inhibits histamine-mediated acid secretion in isolated frog gastric mucosa. *Planta*, 219(2), 319-324.

[19] Ming, L. C., Castro, D. M., & Delachiave, M. E. (1998). Plantas medicinais aromáticas e condimentares. Botucatu: Universidade Estadual Paulista.

[20] Pereira, A. M. S., Rodrigues, D. C., Cerdeira, R. M., & França, S. C. (1993). Isolamento de metabólitos de maytenus associadas à ação anti-úlceragástrica. 12º. Simpósio de Plantas Medicinais do Brasil, Curitiba.

[21] Santos-Oliveira, R., Coulaud-Cunha, S., & Colaço, W. (2009). Revisão da Maytenus ilicifolia Mart. ex Reissek, Celastraceae. Contribuição ao estudo das propriedades farmacológicas. *Brazilian Journal of Pharmacognosy*, 19(2B), 650-659.

[22] Martens, S., & Mithöfer, A. (2005). Flavones and flavone synthases. *Phytochemistry*, 66(20), 2399-2407.

[23] Nijveldt, R. J., Nood, E., Hoorn, D. E. C., Boelens, P. G., Norren, K., & Leeuwen, P. A. M. (2001). Flavonoids: a review of probable mechanisms of action and potential applications. *The American Journal of Clinical Nutrition*, 74(4), 418-25.

[24] Zuanazzi, J. A. S., & Montanha, J. A. (2004). Flavonóides In: Simões CMO, Schenkel EP, Gosmanm, G, Mello JCP, Mentz LA, Petrovick PR. (ed.) Farmacognosia: da planta ao medicamento. Porto Alegre: Universidade Federal do Rio Grande do Sul;, 577-614.

[25] Treutter, D. (2006). Significance of flavonoids in plant resistance: a review. *Environmental Chemistry Letters*, 4(3), 147-157.

[26] Harborne, J. B., & Williams, C. A. (2000). Advances in flavonoids in research since 1992. *Phytochemistry*, 55(6), 481-204.

[27] Argolo, A. C. C., Sant', Ana. A. E. G., Pletsch, M., & Coelho, C. B. B. (2004). Antioxidant activity of leaf extracts from Bauhinia monandra. *Bioresource Technology*, 95(2), 229-233.

[28] Silva, F. R. M. B., Szpoganicz, B., Pizzolatti, M. G., Willrich, M. A. V., & Sousa, E. (2002). Acute effect of Bauhinia forficata on serum glucose levels in normal and alloxan-induced diabetic rats. Journal of Ethnopharmacology., 83(1-2), 33-37.

[29] Sousa, E., Zanatta, L., Seifriz, I., Creczynski-Pasa, T. B., Pizzolatti, M. G., Szpoganicz, B., & Silva, F. R. M. B. (2004). Hypoglycemic effect and antioxidant potential of kaempferol-3,7-O-(α)-dirhammnoside from Bauhinia forficata leaves. *Journal of the Natural Products*, 67(5), 829-832.

[30] Vaz, A.M.S.F. (2012). Bauhinia in Lista de Espécies da Flora do Brasil. *Jardim Botânico do Rio de Janeiro.*, http://floradobrasil.jbrj.gov.br/2012/FB082666, accessed 27 June 2012).

[31] Damasceno, D. C., Volpato, G. T., Calderon, I. M. P., Aguilar, R., & Rudge, M. V. C. (2004). Effect of Bauhinia forficata extract in diabetic pregnant rats: maternal repercussions. *Phytomedicine*, 11(2-3), 196-201.

[32] Di Stasi, L. C., Oliveira, G. P., Carvalhaes, M. A., Queiroz-Junior, M., Tien, O. S., Kakinami, S. H., & Reis, M. S. (2002). Medicinal plants popularly used in the Brazilian Tropical Atlantic Forest. *Fitoterapia*, 73(1), 69-91.

[33] Melo, J. G., Nascimento, V. T., Amorim, E. L. C., Andrade-Lima, C. S., & Albuquerque, U. P. (2004). Avaliação da qualidade de amostras comerciais de boldo (Peumus boldus Molina), pata-de-vaca (Bauhinia spp.) e ginco (Ginkgo biloba L.). *Revista brasileira de farmacognosia*, 14(2), 111-120.

[34] Kuster, R. M., & Rocha, L. M. (2004). Cumarinas, cromonas e xantonas. In: Simões C M O, Schenkel E P, Gosmanm G, Mello JCP, Mentz LA, Petrovick PR. Farmacognosia: da planta ao medicamento. 5ª ed. Porto Alegre: Universidade Federal do Rio Grande do Sul;, 537-556.

[35] Mello, M.M. (2009). Desenvolvimento de uma metodologia por espectroscopia de fluorescência para quantificação de cumarina e 7hidroxicumarina em Drágeas e soro-sintético. Dissertação Universidade do Vale do Paraíba, São José dos Campos.

[36] Lake, B.G. (1999). Coumarin Metabolism, Toxicity and Carcinogenicity: relevance for human risk assessment. *Food Chemistry Toxicology*, 37(4), 423.

[37] Celeghini, R. M., Vilegas, J. H. Y., & Lanças, M. (2001). Extraction and quantitative HPLC analysis of coumarin in hydroalcoholic extracts of Mikania glomerata Spreng. ("guaco") leaves. *Journal Brazilian of Chemical Society*, 12(6), 706-709.

[38] Ribeiro, C. V. C., & Kaplan, M. A. C. (2002). Tendências evolutivas de famílias produtoras de Cumarinas em Angiospermae. *Química Nova*, 25(4), 533-538.

[39] Dias da Silva, J. L. S. (1926). Pharmacopéia dos Estados Unidos do Brasil. 1.ed., São Paulo:, Editora Nacional.

[40] Osório, A. C., & Martins, J. L. S. (2004). Determinação de cumarina em extrato fluido e tintura de guaco por espectrofotometria derivada de primeira ordem. *Brazilian Journal of Pharmaceutical Sciences*, 40(4), 481-486.

[41] Bolina, R. C., Garcia, E. F., & Duarte, M. G. R. (2009). Estudo comparativo da composição química das espécies vegetais Mikania glomerata Sprengel e Mikania laevigata Schultz Bip. ex Baker. *Revista Brasileira de Farmacognosia*, 19(1B), 294-298.

[42] Rocha, L., Lucio, E. M. A., França, H. S., & Sharapin, N. (2008). Mikania glomerata Spreng: Desenvolvimento de um produto fitoterápico. *Revista Brasileira de Farmacognosia*, (18), 744-747.

[43] Silva, C. R., Gomes, V. S., Kulkamp, I. C., & Kanis, L. A. (2008). Metodo espectroscópico para determinação de cumarina em xarope de Mikania glomerata Sprengel. *Revista Brasileira de Farmacognosia*, 18(4), 594-599.

[44] Brasil. Ministério da saúde. (2004). Agência Nacional de Vigilância Sanitária. Resolução da Diretoria Colegiada (RDC) N° 48, de 16 de março de, Dispõe sobre o registro de medicamentos fitoterápicos. Diário Oficial da União de 18.03.2004.

[45] Engel, I. C., Ferreira, R. A., Cechinel-Filho, V., & Meyre-Silva, C. (2008). Controle de qualidade de drogas vegetais a base de Bauhinia forficata Link (Fabaceae). *Brazilian Journal of Pharmacognosy*, 18(2), 258-264.

[46] Marques, G. S., Monteiro, R. P. M., Leão, W. F., Lyra, M. A. M., Peixoto, M. S., Rolim-Neto, P. J., Xavier, H. S., & Soares, L. A. L. (2012). Avaliação de procedimento para quantificação espectrofotométrica de flavonóides totais em folhas de Bauhinia forficata Link. *Química Nova*, 35(3), 517-522.

[47] Amorim, E. L. C., Nascimento, J. E., Monteiro, J. M., Peixoto, Sobrinho. T. J. S., Araújo, T. A. S., & Albuquerque, U. P. (2008). A simple and accurate procedure for the determination of tannin and flavonoid levels and some applications in ethnobotany and ethnopharmacology. *Functional Ecosystems and Communities*, 2(1), 88-94.

[48] Peixoto, Sobrinho. T. J. S., Silva, C. H. T. P., Nascimento, J. E., Monteiro, J. M., Albu-
      querque, U. P., & Amorim, E. L. C. (2008). Validação de metodologia espectrofoto-
      métrica para quantificação dos flavonóides de Bauhinia cheilantha (Bongard)
      Steudel. *Brazilian Journal of Pharmaceutical Sciences*, 44(4), 683-689.

[49] Bara, M. T. F., Cirilo, H. N., & Oliveira, V. (2004). Determinação de ginkgoflavo-
      nóides por cromatografia líquida de alta eficiência em matérias-primas e produtos
      acabados. *Revista Eletrônica de Farmácia*, 1(1), 1-7.

[50] Williamson, E.M. (2001). Synergy and other interactions in phytomedicines. *Phytome-
      dicine*, 8(5), 401-409.

[51] Capasso, R., Izzo, A. A., Pinto, L., Bifulco, T., Vitobello, C., & Mascolo, N. (2000).
      Phytotherapy and quality of herbal medicines. *Fitoterapia*, 71-58.

[52] Calixto, J. B. S. (2000). Efficacy, Safety, quality control, marketing and regulatory
      guidelines for herbal medicines (Phytotherapeutic agents). *Brazilian Journal of Medical
      and Biological Research*, 33(2), 179-189.

[53] (2005). Farmacopéia Brasileira. 4. ed. São Paulo: Editora Atheneu, parte II, sexto fascí-
      culo.

Chapter 5

Application of ISO 9001 Industrial Standard to Herbal Drug Regulation

Sunday Ameh, Florence Tarfa, Magaji Garba and
Karniyus Gamaniel

Additional information is available at the end of the chapter

1. Introduction

We noted earlier [1] that 1978 was the turning point in current public perception of traditional medicine (TM) following the famous WHO declaration at Alma-Ata. That declaration
ushered in a positive attitude that paved the way for the present global popularity of TM,
especially herbal medicine. We noted earlier also [2,3] that whereas herbal remedies are
called dietary supplements in the US, thereby shifting emphasis away from their medicinal
attributes, the Dietary Supplement Health Education Act of 1994 [4], which occasioned the
shift, actually helped to promote herbal medicine in the US, albeit indirectly, through the innovative provision it made for user information [5,6]. A similar situation obtained in Europe, where the net effect of the laws and rules passed in 2004 on herbal remedies had been
to promote their production and use [7, 8]. In terms of trade and economics of herbal drugs,
the following fact is notable: Although, Asia contributed only US$ 7.3 billion to herbal world
trade in 1999 [9], by 2005, a mere 6 years, China's contribution alone rose to US$ 14 billion
[10]. This stupendous growth was due to policies and programmes that favoured herbal
medicine – the cornerstone of Traditional Chinese Medicine (TCM). Similar situations as in
China held sway in Japan, South Korea and the Indian sub-continent, where government
policies also favoured herbal medicine. However, in many developing countries like Nigeria, a totally different picture obtained, not because policies were expressly against herbal
medicine, but in these countries there had been a lingering absence of proper policies and
laws supportive of traditional remedies. Another key fact on the political economy of herbal
drugs is that: Although, about 80% of people in developing countries depended on herbs,
these countries contributed only 7.2% to herbal drug trade in 1999. By contrast, the developed nations, where people relied less on herbs, contributed 55.2%. Asia, less Japan and

South Korea, contributed 37.6%. Equally interesting is the comparison of Brazil with Nigeria. Both are rich in medicinal plants and have high populations that depend substantially on herbs. But, while herbs contributed an unknown amount to the Nigerian economy in 2007, in Brazil it contributed US$ 160 million. By contrast, Nigeria's entire federal budget for health in 2007 was a mere US$ 800 million [2]. These findings earlier led us [11,12] to conclude that developing countries need strategies that will enhance the regulation of herbal drugs and promote their trade. The present article is an attempt to enunciate one of such strategies. It is particularly of note that the superior performance of Brazil in comparison with Nigeria indicates that with proper policies and strategies, herbs can indeed contribute substantially to any economy.

2. Methodology: Determinative Review of ISO 9001 and the Mandates of Nigeria's and Europe's DRAs

2.1. ISO 9001:2008 industrial standard – A synopsis

ISO 9001:2008 industrial standard or quality management system (QMS) is a document of about 30 pages with 8 clauses, published by and obtainable from the International Organization for Standardization (ISO), Basle, Switzerland, or from any of its national affiliates. The standard is designed to be met by any organization that i) needs to demonstrate its ability to consistently provide product or service that meets both customer and applicable statutory and regulatory requirements (collectively legal requirements); ii) aims to enhance customer satisfaction by effectively and continually improving its QMS; and iii) plans to provide continual assurance of conformity to customer and applicable legal requirements. These aims/ approaches (often called "QMS requirements" or "quality procedures") are generic and intended to be applicable to all organizations regardless of type, size and product provided. Wherever any requirement cannot be applied due to the nature of an organization and its product, such can be considered for exclusion. But wherever exclusions are made, claims of conformity to the standard are not acceptable unless such exclusions are limited to requirements within clause 7 of the standard, and such exclusions do not affect the organization's ability, or responsibility, to provide product that meets customer and applicable legal requirements. ISO 9001:2008 defines the minimum requirements for a well managed organization. In other words, noncompliance to an ISO 9001:2008 requirement puts at risk an organization's ability to consistently and efficiently satisfy the expectations of its customers/ stakeholders.

2.2. The six QMS requirements or "The Six Quality Procedures"

These procedures or requirements, as one may choose to call them, actually refer to sub-clause 4.1 (General requirements) under clause 4 (Quality Management System) of ISO 9001:2008. The sub-clause prescribes that organizations shall establish, document, implement, and maintain a QMS, and continually improve its effectiveness. To do so means that the organization shall operate its QMS with a view to carrying out (or meeting) the following six procedures (or requirements): determine the processes needed for the QMS, and their application throughout the organization; determine the sequence of the processes and their interactions; determine the criteria and methods for operating and controlling the processes; determine and ensure the availability needed resources and supporting information; check, measure and analyze the processes, where applicable; and implement actions to achieve planned results and continual improvement of the processes.

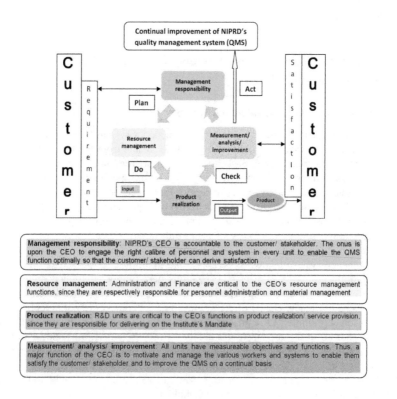

Figure 1. NIPRD's core business in the context of Plan-Do-Check-Act process-based QMS.[1]

The organization shall manage the processes above in accordance with ISO 9001:2008 requirements. It shall also define the type and extent of control to be applied to any outsourced process that can affect product conformity to requirements. ISO 9001:2008 specifically notes as follows:

---

1 Management responsibility corresponds to clause 5 of ISO 9001; while Resource management, Product realization and Measurement/ analysis/ improvement correspond to clauses 6, 7 and 8 respectively.

1. Processes needed for the QMS include the processes for management activities (clause 5), provision of resources (clause 6), product realization (clause 7), and measurement, analysis, and improvement (clause 8).

2. An outsourced process is a process the organization needs for its QMS, and which the organization chooses to have performed by an external party.

3. Ensuring control over outsourced processes does not absolve the organization of the responsibility to conform to customer and legal requirements.

The type and extent of control applied to an outsourced process can be influenced by factors such as: the potential impact of the outsourced process on the organization's capability to provide product that conforms to requirements; the degree to which the control over the process is shared; and the capability of the organization in achieving the necessary control via the application of sub-clause 7.4 (Purchasing). Philosophically, ISO 9001:2008 is formulated on the basis of management by objectives (MBO) and draws upon eight quality management principles. Ideally therefore, quality assurance covers activities in research, development, production and documentation. It embraces the rule: "do it right the first time". It involves regulating the quality of raw materials, the state of production line and works-in-progress, the product and related management processes. One of the most widely used paradigms for quality assurance management (QAM) is the "Shewhart cycle", also called "PDCA approach", meaning, "Plan-Do-Check-Act" [13,14]. The foregoing is illustrated in Figure 1 using NIPRD QMS processes as an example.

2.3. The eight quality management principles that underlie ISO 9001:2008

Like other ISO standards (Example: ISO 9004 - *Managing for Sustained Success*), ISO 9001:2008 is based on 8 quality management principles that are aligned with the philosophy and objectives of most quality award programmes in the world's most industrialized nations. The 8 principles are associated with the following themes:

1. Customer focus.

2. Leadership.

3. Involvement of people.

4. Process approach to management.

5. System approach to management.

6. Continual improvement.

7. Factual approach to decision making.

8. Mutually beneficial supplier relationships.

2.4. Key terminologies of ISO 9001:2008

2.4.1. Process approach to management

A process is an activity or operation that receives inputs and converts them to outputs. Practically all activities or operations involved in generating a product or providing a service are processes. For an organization to function, it must define and manage several inter-linked processes. Most often, the output of one process becomes the input into the next process. The systematic identification and control of the various processes employed within an organization, and the interactions between such processes, is termed "process approach" to management. Thus process approach to management is a way of obtaining a desired result, by controlling activities and related resources as a process. Process approach is a key element of all ISO 9000 standards, including ISO 9001:2008.

2.4.2. System approach to management

System approach to management is based on the premise that the efficiency and effectiveness with which an organization achieves its quality objectives are contributed and enhanced by identifying, understanding and managing all the interrelated processes within the organization as a system

2.4.3. Quality policy

Quality policy is a formal statement from the management of an organization that is linked to the nature of its business and its plans to meet the needs of its customers/ stakeholders. The policy is designed to be understood and followed at all levels and by all staff.

2.4.4. Quality objective

Quality objective is the factual or tangible basis upon which quality policy and plans for implementing the quality programmes of an organization are built. Quality objective should be SMART (ie: specific, measurable, achievable, realistic and time-bound). Each staff of the organization is expected to work towards measurable objectives.

2.4.5. Decision

Decision simply means the selection of one or more options from a multitude of options in tackling a given organizational task. As far as the QMS is concerned, an organization should make SMART decisions based on recorded data. An example of a SMART decision is: The QMS must be audited and evaluated regularly for conformance and effectiveness, so as to assure quality and continual improvement.

2.4.6. Traceability

Traceability is concerned with and refers to the fact that typically, recorded data are meant to show how and where raw materials and products were processed, in order to allow products and problems to be traced to their sources.

2.4.7. Product realization

Product realization refers to the scenario in which, when developing a new product, an organization plans the stages of development, with appropriate testing at each stage. The organization tests and documents whether the product meets design requirements, legal requirements, and user or customer needs.

2.4.8. Quality plan

Quality plan refers to a document specifying the QMS processes (including the product realization processes), and the resources to be applied to a specific product or project.

2.4.9. Monitoring and measurement

Monitoring and measurement refer to the scenario in which an organization must regularly review its performance through meetings and internal audits, and determine whether the QMS is working and what improvements can be made. The organization must have a documented procedure for internal audits and a procedure for dealing with past problems and potential problems. It must keep records of these activities and the resulting decisions, and monitor their effectiveness. It must have documented procedures for dealing with actual and potential non-conformances (problems involving suppliers, customers, or internal problems).

2.4.10. Continual improvement

Continual Improvement refers to the scenario in which an organization 1) makes sure no customer uses a bad product, 2) determines what to do with a bad product, 3) deals with the root cause of problems, and 4) keeps records to use as a tool to improve the QMS.

2.4.11. Customer requirements

Customer requirements refer to the attributes that the buyer of a product (or user of a service) wants. The core business of an organization is to determine customer requirements and to meet them, in accordance with sub-clause 5.2 (Customer focus).

2.4.12. Drug Regulatory Agencies (DRAs)

Drug regulatory agencies (DRAs) are organizations set up by the State on behalf of the general public with a Mandate to regulate drugs and related products and services. The Mandate of some DRAs may include production and distribution of certain goods like vaccines and orphan drugs. Either the State or the general public can be regarded as customer, stakeholder or shareholder. DRAs like all other organizations must have a system for communicating with customers or stakeholders about product information, inquiries, contracts, orders, feedback, and complaints. All DRAs are "service providers" but some produce and even distribute certain specific items, as mentioned above. Nigeria's National Agency for Food and Drug Administration and Control (NAFDAC) is a national DRA, while the European Medicines Evaluation Agency is a regional DRA.

2.4.13. Mandate

Mandate is a piece of legislation or instruction from a constituted authority to another constituted authority or body to carry out a named task. DRAs are mandated by the State to regulate drugs and health related products.

2.5. The new industrial revolution and the aim of this chapter

It is well established that the high state of development in the chemical/ pharmaceutical industrial sector in the US, Japan, South Korea, Britain, Germany and other European countries owes much to the powerful synergy between regulatory legislations, industrial standards and a focused political will. It is also manifest that the rapid, all-round industrial revolution in China in the past decade or so owes much to China's embrace of ISO standards, especially ISO 9001, as shown in Table 1 after a recent [15].

Country	Ranking	No. certificates	Pertinent remark
China	1	257,076	Relies mostly on ISO standard.
Italy	2	130,066	Relies mostly on ISO standard
Japan	3	68,484	Relies only partly on ISO standard
Spain	4	59,576	Relies substantially on ISO standard
Russia	5	53,152	Relies substantially on ISO standard
Germany	6	47,156	Relies only partly on ISO standard
UK	7	41,193	Relies only partly on ISO standard
India	8	37,493	Relies substantially on ISO standard
South Korea	9	28,935	Relies substantially on ISO standard
US	10	23,400	Relies only partly on ISO standard

*Source ISO Survey 2009 [15]. Most countries have their own national standards in addition to ISO standards. For example the UK is well known for its industrial standards pre-sufixed by BSI (British Standards Institution).

Table 1. The top 10 countries in ISO certification in 2009.

It must be stated that countries like Japan, Germany, Britain and US use their own national standards in addition to those of ISO. Based on the foregoing, we state that the specific aim of this article is: To examine the QMS requirements of ISO 9001:2008 and the requirements for regulating herbal drugs in Nigeria (a developing economy) and Europe (a developed economy), with a view to devising a framework that will better regulate herbal drugs and facilitate their trade worldwide. Such a framework will greatly benefit developing countries like Nigeria that are yet to benefit optimally from their comparative advantage in the abundance of spices, herbs and medicinal plants. In addition, marketers and users of herbs in consumer nations like the US, Canada, Germany, UK and France, where consumption now runs in to billions of US dollars, will also profit greatly from an improved and regularized world trade in herbs.

3. Results & discussion: A Framework for Efficient Herbal Drug Regulation (HDR)

3.1. Justification for establishing national or regional DRAs

Most or all countries have a national or regional agency that regulates the production, distribution and use of drug products. The process of regulation commences with the registration of the producer, the product, the distributor and in some cases the user. In some countries drugs, foods and dietary supplements are regulated by the same body (eg: Nigeria's NAF-DAC and US-FDA). The EU's EMEA however regulates only drug products. States or regions need to have DRAs in order to ensure order in the production, distribution and use of drugs. Without DRAs utter chaos and pandemonium will result in production (eg: manufacturers will do as they please without a uniform control), distribution (distributors and suppliers will do as they choose without a uniform order) and use (prescribers and users will do as they think without a uniform regime), which would allow incidences of counterfeit and expired drugs in drug distribution chain, drug abuse and emergence of drug resistant disorders, especially infective conditions like malaria and TB.

3.2. Comparative analysis of Nigeria's and EU's requirements for herbal drug regulation

A careful scrutiny of the requirements for registering and regulating herbal drugs in Europe and in Nigeria reveals their basic similarity, as shown in Table 2.

European Union (EU) – regulated by EMEA		Nigeria – regulated by NAFDAC	
Type of data	Details of data required	Regulatory aspect	Requirement
Product information: Summary of product characteristics	These include: name, strength, dosage form, list of excipients, shelf life, posology, indications, contraindications, and special precautions. These are used as basis for inserts or advertisement, which must undergo a process called "readability".	Legal status of applicant - manufacturer or marketer	Applicant must be certified by the Corporate Affairs Commission as a business. A marketer must show evidence of Power of Attorney.

European Union (EU) – regulated by EMEA		Nigeria – regulated by NAFDAC	
Type of data	Details of data required	Regulatory aspect	Requirement
Quality control data: Refer to GMP requirements for production.	These include: production must be in a GMP compliant, product must be produced with validated formula and method, there must be a product specification, stability studies must be carried out in the container proposed for marketing for purposes storage/ shelf-life, and dossiers must be provided for starting materials and finished product.	Analytical status of the product for registration.	The product must have: certificate of analysis, dossier containing data on ingredients, method of analysis, stability, dosage and safety precautions.
Safety data requirements	The data may be assembled from: animal or human studies, review of potential drug-drug interactions, side effects and contraindications. Others include: recognized monographs, data special groups - children, the elderly and mothers.	Pre-registration inspection of premises.	Manufacturing, storage and distribution premises must be GXP compliant. Marketers must provide convincing evidence of GXP
Traditional use evidence	Evidence that the product has been in use as medicine for 30 years or more (the last 15 must be in the EU. Notably, there is no requirement to prove efficacy (De Smet, 2005).	Post marketing surveillance plan/ report	Applicant may be required to provide a plan for reporting on the use of the product and of any adverse reactions.
-	-	Others, such as fees and waivers.	Fees are required at several stages of the registration but waivers are not expressly stated, thereby negating the concept and need for transparency (see Table 3 for extra requirements).

*The Table was drawn based on data gathered from references including Goldman [5]; De Smet [7, 8]; Ann Godsell Regulatory [16]; and various NAFDAC leaflets, including Akunyili [17]. Note that the requirements for registration in Nigeria are not necessarily less tasking, but their lack of explicitness can be a booby trap and a leeway for non-transparency. The necessity for explicitness and transparency is very important because some years ago the Director General of China's drug regulatory agency was sentenced to death for alleged corrupt practice [18]. In 2000 the entire Management of NAFDAC was sacked in similar grey circumstances.

Table 2. Requirements for herbal registration compared between EU and Nigeria.

But, while the EMEA approach is technically more explicit, though not necessarily more exerting than NAFDAC's, the latter is administratively much more cumbersome, and therefore more liable to inefficiency and abuse. Table 3 shows the extra bureaucratic demands of NAFDAC. We stated earlier that, although, 80% of people in developing countries like Nigeria depended on herbs, these countries contributed only 7.2% to herbal drug trade in 1999. By contrast, the developed nations, where people relied less on herbs, contributed 55.2%. This scenario is explained by the fact herbal drugs are better regulated in developed regions like the China, India, Japan and South East Asia, the EU and North America [2]

3.3. Justification for selecting ISO 9001:2008 for this study

Although most of the OECD countries and other highly industrialized economies, where herbal drugs are well regulated, have their own national standards, all do embrace ISO standards, especially ISO 9001:2008. For example, the British Standards Institution (BSI) is well known and widely adopted in many other countries worldwide, and although international in application, such national standards do not bear the tag "international". By contrast, the ISO family of standards bear the tag "international". ISO 9001:2008 is an international standard designed to address systemic change (ie: a change that affects an organization as a whole). The global popularity of ISO 9001:2000 - the predecessor of ISO 9001:2008, is attributable to the following factors: a) major purchasers require their suppliers to hold ISO 9001 certification [15, 19]; b) studies indicate significant financial benefits for organizations certified to ISO 9001 [19,20]; and c) similar superior operational performance of ISO certified firms has been severally confirmed [21-24]. As just noted, ISO 9001:2008 is an update of ISO 9001:2000, and we have selected it for this study by reason of its popularity and versatility, and because it is a process-based QMS that addresses systemic change affecting whole organizations like a national or regional drug DRA, like Nigeria's National Agency for Food and drug Administration and Control (NAFDAC), the US Food and Drug Administration (US-FDA) and the European Medicines Evaluation Agency (EMEA).

S/No	Extra requirement	Remark
1	Five (5) copies of the product dossier.	Probably unreasonable
2	Three (3) packs of the products samples.	Probably reasonable
3	Notarized original copy of the duly executed Power of Attorney from the product manufacturer.	Clearly unreasonable for all categories of applicants
4	Certificate of Manufacture issued by the competent health or regulatory authority in country of origin and authenticated by the Nigerian Mission in that country. Where there is no Nigerian mission, The British High Commission or an ECOWAS country Mission will authenticate.	Probably unreasonable for all categories of applicants
5	If contract-manufactured, Contract Manufacturing Agreement, properly executed and notarized by a Notary Public in the country of manufacture.	Clearly unreasonable for all categories of applicants
6	Current World Health Organization Good Manufacturing Practice Certificate for the manufacturer, authenticated by the Nigerian Mission.	Clearly unreasonable for all categories of applicants
7	Certificate of Pharmaceutical Products (COOP) duly issued and authenticated.	Clearly unreasonable for all categories of applicants
8	Current Superintendent Pharmacists license to practice issued by the Pharmacists Council of Nigeria (PCN).	Only probably reasonable

S/No	Extra requirement	Remark
9	Premises Registration License from PCN	Only probably reasonable
10	Certificate of Registration of brand name with trademark registry in the Ministry of Commerce here in Nigeria; Letter of invitation from manufacturer to inspect factory abroad, stating full name and location of plant.	Probably unreasonable for all categories of applicants
11	The applicable fee payable only if documents are confirmed to be satisfactory	Likely to be abused if the amount is high. The fee should be a token amount paid by all applicants
12	Nutraceuticals, medical devices and other regulated drug products have similar requirements, with minor variations. Specific details can be obtained from NAFDAC.	A sketch of the minor variations should be provided in print no matter how brief. Any information provided by NAFDAC should be printable for sake of transparency

*The information on NAFDAC were drawn from leaflets and NAFDAC's website (2010): www.nafdacnigeria.org/ The remarks are informed by current affairs and public perception of NAFDAC's role and activities including the wholesale reorganization of its Management in 2000.

Table 3. NAFDAC's extra requirements for registering herbal medicines.

3.4. A systematic review of the eight clauses of ISO 9001:2008 in relation to DRAs

3.4.1. A synopsis of the Mandate of DRAs and the eight clauses of ISO 9001:2008

ISO 9001:2008 is the most widely used QMS standard, with over a million certificates issued worldwide. Alas, it was revealed at the SON-NIPRD course in 2011, that only two public institutions in Nigeria have ISO 9001 certification! Yet, as stated earlier, ISO 9001:2008 defines the minimum requirements for a well managed organization. The standard is published by the International Organization for Standardization (ISO), Basle, Switzerland. National accreditation bodies like the Standards Organization of Nigeria (SON) provide accreditation to registrars who issue the ISO 9001 certificates to those they audit. ISO 9001:2008 is set out in eight clauses designated clauses 1 to 8. The structure and salient points/ directing principles of the clauses are tabulated below. A copy of ISO 9001:2008 is a prerequisite for this study. Similarly required, is a grasp of the requirements for registering and regulation herbal drugs in a developed economy like Europe; and in a developing country like Nigeria, as depicted in Table 2. It is well known that herbal drugs are better regulated in the developed than in developing countries. Table 3 suggests that undue bureaucracy or needlessly cumbersome requirements can hinder efficient regulation. Tables 4-13 show the structure and salient points/ directing principles of the 8 clauses.

Clause	Title and subtitles, with remarks	Salient points/ directing principles/ application to DRAs
1	**1. Scope** **1.1 General** **1.2 Application**	ISO 9001:2008 can be used to establish, and to update a DRA's QMS. A DRA, like other parastatals or private organizations must consider its unique operational environment and the dynamics and risks associated therewith.
2	**2. Normative references** (eg: ISO 9000:2005 is devoted to *QMS Fundamentals and Vocabulary*; and ISO 9004:2009 is devoted to *Managing for Sustained Success*)	A normative reference implies, unless otherwise stated, that the most recent versions of the separate documents should be referenced. DRAs would benefit immensely from such key references and compendia such as the *International Pharmacopoeia* and others like the *BP* and *USP*, and the WHO manual on *Quality Control Methods for Medicinal Plant Materials*.
3	**3. Terms and definitions** (see section 2.4 of this article on "Key terminologies of ISO 9001:2008)	The term "product" may also mean "service". "Legal requirements" means "statutory and regulatory requirements". Most DRAs are service providers only, while others may produce and distribute certain specialized health products.

*The Table is to be studied side by side with the contents of ISO 9001:2008 and Table 2, which is on regulatory requirements of DRAs.

Table 4. Clauses 1-3 of ISO 9001:2008 in relation to DRAs.

Clause	Title and subtitles, with remarks	Salient points/ directing principles/ application to DRA
4	**4. Quality Management System (QMS)** **4.1 General requirements** **4.2 Documentation requirements:** **4.2.1 General** – QMS documents must include: quality policy, quality objective, quality manual, documented procedures/ records specified by ISO 9001:2008, and documents/ records determined by the organization to be relevant for effective planning, operation and control of the QMS. **4.2.2 Quality manual** – this should include the scope of the QMS, SOPs and a description of the QMS processes. **4.2.3 Control of documents** - the documents required by the QMS must be established and controlled. This means that SOPs are to be established to define the controls needed. **4.2.4 Control of records** – records are a special type of documents and must be established and controlled. Here too, SOPs are to be established to define the controls needed. **Note:**1) A document is a piece of written, printed, or electronic matter that provides information or evidence. It may or may not exist	Clause 4.1 implies that the DRA must identify, manage and document the processes that make up its QMS – ie: the DRA must address the so called "Six Quality Procedures" and generate relevant documents, including: 1) quality manual, 2) quality policy, 3) quality objective, 4) process flowchart, and 5) work instructions. The DRA can achieve this by using a management strategy called "process approach", which means that it must manage: 1) the processes that make up its organization, 2) the interaction between these processes, and 3) the inputs and outputs that glue these processes together. The quality manual should: 1) describe how the QMS processes interact; 2) define the scope of the QMS (it should explain any reductions in the scope of the QMS and justify all exclusions/ reductions); and 3) document all procedures in the QMS or refer to them. It is most crucial that the DRA prepares, establishes and maintains a quality manual. The DRA must establish SOPs to define the controls needed: 1) to approve, review, update and re-approve documents prior to use; 2) to ensure that changes, current status, relevant versions of documents are identified; and 3) to prevent the unintended use of obsolete documents. The DRA must establish records to provide: 1) evidence that operations conform to QMS requirements; and 2) evidence that operations of the QMS are effective. Records must be ensured to be legible, readily identifiable and retrievable.

Clause	Title and subtitles, with remarks	Salient points/ directing principles/ application to DRA
	in a permanent form. 2) A record is a permanent	
	document of something that is	
	kept for evidence or information. It specifically bears the	
	history of events or arrangements, and is preserved in a	
	lasting form.	

*The Table is to be studied side by side with the contents of ISO 9001:2008 and Table 2, which is on regulatory requirements of DRAs.

Table 5. Clause 4 of ISO 9001:2008 in relation to DRAs.

Clause	Title and subtitles, with remarks	Salient points/ directing principles/ application to DRA
5	**5 Management Responsibility**	The DRA must be committed to developing and implementing a QMS, as well as, a commitment
	5.1 Management commitment	to continually improve the effectiveness of the QMS. The DRA can do this by 1) communicating
	5.2 Customer focus – the organization must ensure that	the importance of meeting "legal and customer requirements"; 2) establishing a quality policy
	its purpose/ focus (inclusive of customer/ stakeholder	and quality objectives; 3) conducting management reviews; and 4) by ensuring the availability of
	requirements) is understood and determined.	necessary resources. The "legal and customer requirements" of a DRA are implicit in its Mandate
	5.3 Quality policy – this should be:	– which may be an act, law or decree. In planning, the DRA must 1) ensure that quality objectives
	1) appropriate to the purpose of the organization; 2)	are established at the relevant functions and levels within the Agency; 2) ensure that quality
	focused on meeting requirements and continual	objectives are measurable and consistent with the quality policy; and 3) ensure that planning for
	improvement; 3) used as a framework for quality	the QMS meets the general requirements (clause 4.1) and quality objectives (clause 5.4.1), as
	objectives; 4) publicized and understood at appropriate	well as, maintains the integrity of the QMS.
	levels; and	In as much as operations must be carried out the DRA must ensure that the responsibilities and
	5) reviewed for continuing suitability .	authorities for such are defined and communicated appropriately. It is essential that a member
	5.4 Planning	of top management, irrespective of other duties, be appointed (as Quality Manager) and given
	5.4.1 Quality Objectives	the responsibility to: 1) ensure that the needed processes are established, implemented, and
	5.4.2 QMS Planning	maintained; 2) report to top management on the performance of the QMS; 3) report to top
	5.5 Responsibility, Authority, and	management on any need for improvement; and 4) ensure the promotion of awareness of
	Communication	Agency's Mandate. Most DRAs have a public relation office.
	5.5.1 Responsibility and Authority	For a DRA to be effective it must review its QMS at planned intervals to: 1) ensure an effective
	5.5.2 Management Representative	QMS; 2) assess possible opportunities for improvement; 3) evaluate the need for any changes;
	5.5.3 Internal Communication – it is crucial that the	and 4) consider the need for changes to the policy and objectives. The DRA must of course
	organization ensures that appropriate communication	maintain records of reviews as per clause 4.2.4. For a DRA, the inputs for review must include
	processes regarding the effectiveness	information on: 1) results of audits; 2) feedback from government and the public, eg - incidences
	of the QMS are established and implemented.	of counterfeit drugs; 3) status of preventive and corrective actions, eg – incidences of drug
	5.6 Management Review	abuse; 4) follow-up actions from earlier reviews; 5) changes that can affect the QMS; and 6)
	5.6.1 General	recommendations for improvement.
	5.6.2 Review Input – includes audit results, public	
	feedback, process performance, status of preventive/	
	corrective action, follow-up from previous management	
	review,	

Clause	Title and subtitles, with remarks	Salient points/ directing principles/ application to DRA
	changes that can affect the QMS, and recommendations for improvement. **5.6.3 Review Output** - includes decisions/ actions related to: 1) improvement of the QMS; 2) improvement in meeting Mandate; and 3) resource needs	

*The Table is to be studied side by side with contents of ISO 9001:2008 and Table 2, which is on regulatory requirements of DRAs.

Table 6. Clause 5 of ISO 9001:2008 in relation to DRAs.

3.4.2. The immediate historical antecedent of NAFDAC and the continuing relevance of ISO 9001

Nigeria's NAFDAC was created by decree in 1992/93 following the ethylene glycol disaster of 1991/92 in Langtang General Hospital, Plateau State, where ethylene glycol was used in the place of propylene glycol in preparing paracetamol elixir. The glycol had been purchased from a hitherto popular pharmacy shop located at Masalachin-Jumai Street, Jos. Prior to 1992/93, a department in the Federal Ministry of Health handled food and drug administration in Nigeria. Alas, in 2009 another ethylene glycol disaster occurred in Lagos. In this latter disaster a hitherto popular brand of paediatric mixture ("My Pikin") was found to contain ethylene glycol that had been purchased from an unregulated source. It is important to note that whereas the glycol implicated in the Lantang disaster was purchased from pharmaceutically regulated source, the glycol in the case of the Lagos disaster was purchased from a company that dealt in industrial chemicals associated with automobiles and cooling systems. The occurrence of this kind of disaster within less than two decades is matter of concern that calls for a more efficient programme for regulating drugs and industrial chemicals in developing countries. The US-FDA after whose image and likeness NAFDAC was created is known for efficiency mostly because it is supported by proper laws and strong institutions. Better laws and stronger institutions, including DRAs, are required to avoid or minimize this kind of disaster as seen in Nigeria. It seems instructive to mention the "Tylenol case" in the US, and how that case led to a new legislation. Between late September and early October 1982, seven persons in Chicago died after taking capsules of Tylenol (a brand of paracetamol), to which cyanide crystals had been added. The crystals had apparently been introduced into the capsules by someone who had removed bottles of Tylenol from several drugstores and then replaced them on the shelves. It took an intensive investigation by a team of over 100 agents, including FDA staff, to discover the mischief, which led to a 1982-legislation that required all over-the-counter drugs and medicines sold in the county (and later elsewhere in the US and beyond) carry manufacturers' seals which broken would be obvious. The rapid conclusion of the investigation led by the Illinois Attorney General himself (Tyrone C. Fahner) and the dispatch with which the new law was issued collectively testify to the inner workings of strong institutions – which developing nations lack.

Clause	Title and subtitles, with remark	Salient points/ directing principles/ application to DRAs
6	**6 Resource management**	The DRA must determine and provide the resources needed: 1) to implement, maintain and
	6.1 Provision of resources	continually improve the effectiveness of its QMS; and 2) to enhance the fulfilment of its
	6.2 Human resources	Mandate.
	6.2.1 General	By virtue of its role as a highly specialized agency, the DRA must ensure that all staff
	6.2.2 Competence, Training, and	irrespective of department whose work can impact DRA's Mandate are competent based on
	Awareness	appropriate education, skills, experience and abide by their professional ethics.
	6.3 Infrastructure	This implies that the DRA must: 1) determine the competency of staff; 2) provide training as
	Like any other public outfit the DRA must determine,	needed; 3) evaluate the effectiveness of the actions taken on training and skills acquisition ; 4)
	provide, and maintain infrastructure like buildings,	inform staff of their relevance within the QMS; 5) ensure staff know their contributions to
	workspace and associated utilities, and essential support	achieving quality objectives; and 6) maintain staff records of education, training, skill, and
	services.	experience in accordance with clause 4.2.4.
	6.4 Work Environment	The DRA must, of course, provide appropriate work environment for all staff whose work
	"Work environment" implies conditions under which work	impacts the DRA's Mandate.
	is performed, and includes physical aspects like weather	
	and noise pollution.	

*The Table is to be studied side by side with contents of ISO 9001:2008 and Table 2, which is on regulatory requirements of DRAs.

Table 7. Clause 6 of ISO 9001:2008 in relation to DRAs.

3.4.3. The making of stronger DRAs and the need for clearer demarcation of responsibilities

In most countries where DRAs are not a department of the Ministry of Health, they exist as a parastatal or as a special department within the Ministry (as in Japan), with conditions of service being slightly more favourable than in the rest of the Ministry. The idea is to give special incentives to the staff on account of hazards perceived to be peculiar to the job. In Nigeria, NAFDAC is well housed both at the federal and state levels and the staff earn about the same remuneration as the universities and research institutes. In most countries the DRAs have well equipped offices and laboratories, and those DRAs that produce and distribute goods are equipped with the necessary plant and storage facilities.

3.4.4. The inevitability of confusion in the absence of regulatory standardization

In Nigeria, NAFDAC previously handled certain aspects of manufacture/ distribution of vaccines until certain developments (or rather controversies over quality/ effectiveness of polio vaccines during the late 1990s/ early 2000s) led, first to the creation of a National Programme on Immunization (NPI); and latter to the transfer of the same functions from NPI back to the Federal Ministry of Health. It is obvious from the foregoing that institutions like NAFDAC and NPI would have performed better had they been certified. It seems also that one of the keys to ending the cycle of poverty and underdevelopment in some countries is to ensure that elite institutions like the DRAs are certified to appropriate ISO standards. Certifications of agencies like the Health Insurance Scheme and the Pension Commission will definitely reduce perceive current levels of corruption in such institution.

Clause	Title and subtitles, with remark	Salient points/ directing principles / application to DRAs
7	**7 Product realization** **7.1 Planning of product** realization Product realization typically implies that manufacturers 1) plan and develop the QMS processes needed for product realization; 2) keep the planning consistent with other requirements of the QMS; 3) document the plan in a suitable form; and 4) determine through the planning, the following: a) quality objectives and product requirements; b) need for processes, documents, and resources; c) verification (establishment of truth/ confirmatory evidence), validation (formal registration/ obtainment of official sanction), monitoring, measurement, inspection, and test activities; d) criteria for product acceptance; and e) records providing evidence that the processes and resulting product meet requirements. Since DRAs regulate manufacturers they too must be acquainted with clause 7. NOTE 1: Recall that "quality plan" (2.4.8 of this article) is a document specifying the processes, and the resources to be applied to a specific product, project, or contract. NOTE 2: An organization can apply the requirements of sub-clause 7.3 (vide infra) to the development of product realization processes7.2 Customer-Related Processes **7.2.1 Determination of** **Requirements Related to the** **Product** **7.2.2 Review of Requirements** **Related to the Product** **7.2.3 Customer Communication** The intensity and scope of communication depends on the product and the associated mandate. Thus the DRA must determine and implement the necessary arrangements for communicating with stakeholders on aspects like 1) product information; 2) inquiries and contracts; 3) customer/ stakeholder feedbacks -positive or negative	Some DRAs produce/ store/ distribute specialized and non-profit products like vaccines and orphan drugs. For such, all aspects of clause 7 apply. The DRAs of developed economies concentrate on regulating manufacturers, distributors and use of products. Different processes are involved in drug regulation but these often have some aspects in common. For example, the process of registering a manufacturer and that of registering a product are essentially the same, but they differ in their aims, point of action, who by, and so on. Some of the processes involved in "planning of service realization", which is the core business of a typical DRA, require a wide range of differing concepts, technicalities, approaches, specializations, and so on. For example, although the technical aspects of producing tablets of aspirin, diazepam, B-complex, erythromycin, and orphan drugs may be similar, the modes of their regulation and distribution are different. Given the involved Mandate of DRAs, different strategies must be developed to grapple with the differing nuances and intricacies associated with the regulation of the five products. Typically, questions that have answer buried in culture/ society rather than the lab do arise in drug regulation. Why, for example, despite the similarities between NAFDAC and EMEA, it is impossible to buy erythromycin or diazepam over-the-counter in Europe but not in Nigeria? To what extent do political, social and economic factors affect "planning of service realization" in different social environments? It well known that regulatory strategies that work in Europe often fail to work outside despite obvious legislative similarities between nations. The customers/ stakeholders of a typical DRA are the general public, manufacturers, suppliers and the government. DRAs that engage in production and distribution must determine customer requirements, which invariably include specified and unspecified but desirable attributes. Such DRAs must also determine the legal requirements applicable to the product. Other desirable requirements, including post-delivery activities like maintenance services, may be considered. DRAs that produce or distribute would normally review the product requirements before committing to supply in order to: 1) ensure that product requirements are defined; 2) resolve any requirements differing from those previously expressed; and 3) ensure its ability to meet the requirements. In the same vein when a DRA plans a regulatory strategy or legislation the plan should be graduated and made reasonable to its purpose and scope and with reference to the operating socioeconomic environment. The DRA must maintain the results of reviews, and any subsequent follow-up actions in accordance with 4.2.4. When the requirements are not documented, they must be confirmed before acceptance. But if product requirements are changed, the DRA must ensure relevant documents are amended and relevant personnel are made aware of the changed requirements. NOTE: In some situations a formal review is impractical for each order. In such cases reviews can cover relevant product information such as catalogues or adverts.

*The Table is to be studied side by side with contents of ISO 9001:2008 and Table 2, which is on the regulatory requirements of DRAs.

Table 8. Clause 7 of ISO 9001 in relation to DRAs (Product planning and Customer-Related processes).

Clause	Title and subtitles, with remarks	Salient points/ directing principles/ application to DRAs
7	**7.3 Design and Development**	The same principle followed in planning a physical product is followed in planning a
	7.3.1 Design/ Development Planning	service. The interfaces between the different groups involved must be managed to
	DRAs that produce or distribute must plan and control product	ensure effective communication/ clear assignment of responsibility. Design and
	design/ development. They must determine 1) the stages of	development review, verification and validation have distinct purposes. They can be
	design/development; 2) appropriate testing, review and validation	conducted and recorded separately or in any combination, as the DRA deems suitable
	for each stage; and 3) responsibility/authority for design/	for the product or the type of service.
	development.	A DRA would review the selected inputs for adequacy and resolve any incomplete,
	7.3.2 Design /Development Inputs	ambiguous, or conflicting requirements. Examples of application inputs include: (1
	In designing/ developing a physical good or a service, the DRA	applicable information derived from similar designs; and (2 requirements essential for
	must determine the needed inputs and keep records as per 4.2.4.	design and development. If a DRA is designing a policy to curb drug abuse in a
	The inputs must include: 1) functional and performance	particular locality, useful inputs for the design would include statistics like 1) the age,
	requirements; 2) applicable legal requirements; 3) applicable	gender and occupation of abusers; 2) the type of drugs abused; and 3) the success
	information derived from similar designs; and 4) requirements	rate of similar policies elsewhere. NOTE: Information for production and service can
	essential for design and development.	include details for product preservation.
	7.3.3 Design/ Development Outputs	A DRA must perform systematic reviews of design and development at suitable stages
	Where applicable, DRAs must	in accordance with planned arrangements (7.3.1) so as to: 1) evaluate the ability of
	document the outputs of the design/ development process in a	the results to meet requirements; and 2) identify problems and propose necessary
	form suitable for verification against the inputs to the process. The	actions. Reviews must include representatives of the functions concerned. Results of
	outputs must 1) meet or match design and development input	reviews and subsequent follow-up actions must be maintained as per 4.2.4. A DRA
	requirements; 2) provide information	would perform design and development verification in accordance with 7.3.1 to
	for purchasing, production and service; 3) contain or reference	ensure that output meets the design and development input requirements; and
	product acceptance criteria; 4) define essential characteristics for	maintain the results of such verification and subsequent follow-up actions. When
	safe and proper use; 5) be approved before their release	practical and desirable, validation must be completed before delivery or
	7.3.4 Design/ Development Review	implementation of the product. Results of the validation and of subsequent follow-up
	7.3.5 Design/ Dev. Verification	actions must be maintained as per 4.2.4. Just as some DRAs produce or distribute
	7.3.6 Design/ Dev. Validation	physical products, some DRA have their own testing facilities while others contract
	Validation activities are performed in accordance with 7.3.1 to	out such tests. Thus the purchase needs of DRAs differ with their Mandate. However,
	confirm that the resulting product is capable of meeting the	whenever purchasing is indicated the DRA must 1) ensure that purchased items
	requirements for its specified application or intended use.	conform to specified purchase requirements (Note: The type and extent of control
	7.3.7 Control of Des./ Dev Changes	applied to the supplier and purchased product depends upon the effect of the
	For either physical goods or policy,	product on the subsequent realization processes or the final product); 2) evaluate and
	DRAs must 1) identify design and development changes and	select suppliers based on their ability to supply goods in accordance with
	maintain records as per 4.2.4; 2) review, verify, validate and	requirements; 3) establish the criteria for selection, evaluation, and re-evaluation; and
	approve changes before implementation; 3) evaluate the changes	4) maintain the results of such evaluations and subsequent follow-up actions in
	in terms of their effect on constituent parts (raw material) and	accordance with sub-clauses 4.2.3 and 4.2.4.
	products (or policies) already delivered (or implemented).	

*The Table is to be studied side by side with contents of ISO 9001:2008 and Table 2, which is on the regulatory requirements of DRAs.

Table 9. Clause 7 of ISO 9001:2008 in relation to DRAs (Design and Development).

3.4.5. Some causes and signs of a malfunctioning DRA

Once the staff recruitment system can be skewed to favour persons, a serious non-compliance exists. Once the purchase processes can be demonstrated to have vested interest, a serious flaw exists in the QMS. Once there is a convincing evidence of maladministration, arbitrary treatment of personnel or executive high handed, a serious condition against performance exists.

Clause	Title and subtitles, with remarks	Salient points/ directing principles/ application to DRAs
7	**7.4 Purchasing**	Whether a DRA produces/ distributes it will have cause to purchase various items of commerce
	7.4.1 Purchasing Process	hence QMS requirements for purchases are required. Like other organizations a DRA would
	7.4.2 Purchasing Information	require and ensure the adequacy of the specifications of items to be purchased before
	All organizations irrespective of type of business will have	communicating the purchasing information to the supplier. Typically a DRA would establish
	cause to purchase a multitude of goods for the business. If	and implement inspection or other necessary activities for ensuring that purchased goods
	such goods are to meet their purposes criteria and	meet the specified purchase requirements. If a DRA or its customers/ stakeholders propose to
	processes must be developed their purchase. Thus	verify a good or service at the supplier's location, the intended verification arrangements/
	purchasing information should contain: 1) explicit	method must be stated in the purchasing information.
	description of goods: 2) approval criteria for the goods,	It is typically pertinent that a DRA 1) validates any production or service provision that
	procedures, processes, and associated equipment or	subsequent monitoring cannot verify. Such validations include processes where deficiencies
	accessories; and 3) profession/ qualification of staff	may become apparent only after product use or service delivery; 2) demonstrates through the
	associated with the goods.	validation the ability of processes to achieve the planned results; and 3) establishes validation
	7.4.3 Verification of Purchased Product	arrangements including, as applicable: a) criteria for process review and approval, b) approval
	7.5 Production and Service Provision	of equipment, c) qualification of staff, d) use of defined methods and procedures, e)
	7.5.1 Control of Production and	requirements for records, and f) re-validation. DRAs that produce/ distribute or have their own
	Service Provision	test facilities must 1) identify, where appropriate, the product by suitable means during
	A producing/ distributing DRA must plan and carry out	product realization; and 2) identify the product status with respect to monitoring and
	production and service provision under controlled	measurement requirements throughout product realization. DRAs may require that
	conditions, which include: 1) availa-	manufacturers of herbal products have the following where necessary and feasible: a)
	bility of data on needed inputs; 2) availability of necessary	chemically defined reference active crude extract (RACE), b) chemically defined marker
	work instructions; 3) availability/ usability of essential	substance (DMS) and TLC, HPLC or GC-MS fingerprints of RACE and DMS. Since traceability is a
	equipment; 4) availability/ usability of monitoring and	key requirement, DRAs need to enforce manufacturers to have the means of controlling the
	measuring equipment; 4) ability to implement monitoring	unique identification of the product at various stages of development, and of course maintain
	and measurement	records.
	activities; and 5) ability to implement product release,	Obviously, DRAs that produce/ distribute products or run test laboratories/ facilities must
	delivery, and post-delivery activities. DRAs that	exercise care with any customer property under their control. They must record and promptly
	do not produce/ distribute must nevertheless have	report any loss or damage to the customer. NOTE: Customer property may be physical or
	possess the ability to ensure that manufacturer/	otherwise.
	distributors have all it takes to adequately meet	As a standard practice, a DRA would: 1) assess and record the validity of prior results if the
	QMS requirements.	equipment/ method are found not to conform to requirements; 2) maintain records of the
	7.5.2 Validation of Processes for	results of calibration and verification; and 3) confirm or re-confirm the ability of any software
	Production and Service Provision	or programme used for monitoring or measurement before its initial use. To ensure the validity
	7.5.3 Identification and Traceability	of results, a DRA would normally:
	7.5.4 Customer Property	1. Calibrate and/or verify the measuring equipment at specified intervals or prior to use.

Clause	Title and subtitles, with remarks	Salient points/ directing principles/ application to DRAs
	7.5.5 Preservation of Product	2. Calibrate the equipment to national or international standards (or record other appropriate
	Preservation of product broadly includes: 1) identification,	basis).
	2) handling,	3. Adjust or re-adjust as necessary.
	3) packaging, 4) storage, and 5) protection	4. Identify the measuring equipment in order to determine its calibration status
	7.6 Control of Measuring and	5. Safeguard equipment from improper adjustments.
	Monitoring Equipment	6. Protect equipment from damage and deterioration
	As may be applicable, a DRA would:	
	1) Determine the type of monitoring	
	and measurements to be made,	
	and the equipment/ method to be	
	used in providing evidence of conformity	
	2) Use and control the monitoring and measuring devices	
	in order to ensure that measurement capability is	
	consistent with monitoring and measurement	
	requirements.	

*The Table is to be studied side by side with contents of ISO 9001:2008 and Table 2, which is on the regulatory requirements of DRAs.

Table 10. Clause 7 of ISO 9001:2008 in relation to DRAs (Purchasing/ Production/ Control of Equipment).

Clause	Title and subtitles, with remarks	Salient points/ directing principles/ application to DRAs
8	**8 Measurement, analysis and**	Given the overwhelming importance of measurement, analysis and improvement to the
	Improvement	Mandate of DRAs, a DRA would typically want to be sure, thorough and effective in the
	8.1 General	application of clause 8. To ensure effectiveness therefore, the DRA would routinely, or as may
	A producing/ distributing DRA would plan and implement	be necessary, determine through planning the need for, use of, and extent of use of applicable
	the monitoring, measurement, analysis, and improvement	methods, including statistical techniques. DRAs should view customer/ stakeholder perception
	processes it needs to: 1) demonstrate conformity to	as a key performance measurement of its QMS. For producing and/ or distributing DRAs
	product requirements; 2) ensure conformity of the QMS	especially, monitoring customer/ stakeholder perception can be obtained from: 1) customer/
	to planned arrangements;	stakeholder satisfaction surveys; 2) customer data on delivered product quality; 3) user opinion
	and 3) continually improve the effectiveness of the QMS.	surveys; 4) lost business analysis; 5) compliments; 6) warranty claims; and 7) dealer reports.
	Non-producing/ distributing DRAs	For thoroughness and effectiveness a producing/ distributing DRA must: 1) plan the audit
	must have the ability to ensure that manufacturers/	program; 2) consider the status and importance of the audited areas; 3) consider the results of
	distributors comply.	prior audits; 4) define the audit criteria, scope, frequency, and methods; and 5) select and use
	8.2 Monitoring and measurement	impartial and objective auditors. Non-producing/ distributing DRAs must have the ability to
	8.2.1 Customer Satisfaction	ensure that manufacturers/ distributors comply.
	DRAs must routinely: 1) monitor information on	To institute thoroughness and effectiveness, producing/ distributing DRAs must:
	customer/ stakeholder perception as to whether it is	1. Maintain records of the audits and their results.
	meeting	2. Ensure control of the audited areas.
	its Mandate; and 2) define the	3. Take actions without undue delay to eliminate detected nonconformities and their causes.
	methods for obtaining and using that information.	4. Verify through follow-up actions.
	8.2.2 Internal Audit	

Clause	Title and subtitles, with remarks	Salient points/ directing principles/ application to DRAs
	Internal audits must be conducted at planned intervals so that DRAs can determine if their QMS: 1) conforms to requirements of ISO 9001:2008; 2) conforms to planned arrangements as per sub-clause 7.1; and 3) is effectively implemented and maintained. In order to thoroughly address staff responsibilities and the requirements to be met by the audit exercise, DRAs must establish: 1) a documented procedure for planning audit; 2) a documented procedure for conducting audits; and 3) a documented procedure for recording and reporting audit results.	Again, non-producing/ distributing DRAs must have the ability to ensure that manufacturers/ distributors comply. NOTE: ISO 19011 (Audit guidance) should be consulted for further enlightenment quality auditing.

*The Table is to be studied side by side with contents of ISO 9001:2008 and Table 2, which is on the regulatory requirements of DRAs.

Table 11. Clause 8 of ISO 9001:2008 in relation to DRAs (Monitoring and measurement).

3.4.6. Remediation of a malfunctioning DRA

A national or regional DRA is a critical factor in socioeconomic development and wellbeing in at least two ways: i) by "guaranteeing the health of the nation" (as trumpeted in NAF-DAC's adverts); and by supporting the emergence of responsible manufacturers of regulated products. It is well known that the US-FDA more than any US organization has made the US the world leader in manufacture of health products. The prominence of India and China in world drug trade owes much to the vibrancy and relative efficiency of their DRAs. There is therefore a critical need for DRAs to be vibrant and responsible. The gravity with which China views the role of her DRA can be gauged by the death sentence passed on the Director General in 2007 for accepting a bribe [15].

Clause	Title and subtitles, with remarks	Salient points/ directing principles/ application to DRAs
8	**8.2.3 Monitoring and** **Measurement of Processes** 1) Apply suitable methods to monitor and, where applicable, measure the QMS processes. 2) Confirm through these methods the continuing ability of each process to satisfy its intended purpose. 3) When the planned results are not achieved, take correction and corrective action, as appropriate. **8.2.4 Monitoring and** **Measurement of Product**	Producing/ distributing DRAs need to 1) apply suitable methods for monitoring and measuring QMS processes; and 2) confirm through these methods the continuing ability of each process to satisfy its intended purpose. Non-producing/ distributing DRAs must have the ability to ensure that manufacturers/ distributors comply. NOTE: When determining "suitable" methods, consideration is given to the type and extent of monitoring or measurement for each process in relation to its impact on product conformity and on the effectiveness of the QMS. To better fulfil their Mandate producing/ distributing DRAs must 1) monitor and measure product characteristics so as to verify if product requirements are being met; 2) carry out the monitoring and measurements at the appropriate stages of product realization in accordance with planned arrangements; and 3) maintain evidence of conformity with the acceptance criteria.

Clause	Title and subtitles, with remarks	Salient points/ directing principles/ application to DRAs
	1) Monitor and measure product characteristics to verify if product requirements are being met.	It is again stressed that non-producing/ distributing DRAs must have the ability to ensure that manufacturers/ distributors comply.
	2) Carry out the monitoring and measuring at the appropriate stages of product realization in accordance with planned arrangements (see 7.1).	DRAs must ensure that product release and service delivery cannot proceed until all planned arrangements (see 7.1) have been satisfactorily completed, unless otherwise approved by a relevant authority, and where applicable, the customer.
	3) Maintain evidence of conformity with the acceptance criteria.	Where applicable, DRAs must deal with the nonconforming product by one or more of the following ways:
	4) Record the person responsible for authorizing release of product for delivery to the customer.	1. Take action to eliminate the detected nonconformity.
		2. Authorize its use, release, or acceptance by concession.
	8.3 Control of nonconforming product	3. Take action to preclude its original intended use or application.
		4. Take action appropriate to the effects, or potential effects, of the nonconformity when nonconforming product is detected after delivery or use has started
	DRAs must: 1) Ensure any nonconforming product is identified and controlled to prevent its unintended use or delivery.	To better fulfil their Mandate, DRAs must: 1) Ensure that any nonconforming product is identified and controlled to prevent its unintended use or delivery. 2) Establish a documented procedure to define the controls and related responsibilities and authorities for dealing with nonconforming product.
	2) Establish a documented procedure to define the controls and the related responsibilities/authorities for dealing with nonconforming product.	
	DRAs must maintain records of the nature of the nonconformity, and any subsequent actions, (including any concessions). When the nonconformity is corrected, DRAs must re-verify it to prove or show evidence of conformity.	

*The Table is to be studied side by side with contents of ISO 9001:2008 and Table 2, which is on the regulatory requirements of DRAs. Although a DRA may not possess certain facilities for measurements and monitoring, it should possess the ability or the means necessary to ensure that manufacturers/ distributors possess and use them in accordance with approved QMS guidelines.

Table 12. Clause 8 of ISO 9001 in relation to DRAs (Product characteristics/ Control of nonconformities).

In Nigeria, the entire NAFDAC Management was sacked on alleged acts of corruption in 2000. It seems to us that the following are essential for a DRA to perform optimally:

1. The laws creating/ amending a DRA should be well articulated as is the case with the US-FDA.

2. DRAs should be so well funded as not to rely on a plethora of frivolous fees as with NAFDAC.

3. Staffing of DRAs must be transparent - competence and integrity must be the decisive criteria.

4. DRAs should be audited frequently, at least yearly or twice yearly.

5. DRAs should have a Board of Governors to whom the Management reports

6. Parliamentary health committees should view DRAs as critical to socioeconomic well-being of the nation.

Clause	Title and subtitles, with remarks	Salient points/ directing principles/ application to DRAs
8	**8.4 Analysis of data**	DRAs should as a matter of practice:
	Whether producing/ distributing or not, as a rule,	1. Include the primary data generated by monitoring and measuring activities, and from other
	DRAs must determine, collect, and analyze appropriate	relevant sources in their analyses.
	data to demonstrate the suitability and effectiveness of	2. Analyze such primary data to provide secondary data on:
	their QMS, as well as, evaluate where continual	a. Customer satisfaction as per 8.2.1.
	improvement of the QMS can be made.	b. Conformity to product requirements as per 8.2.4.
	DRAs cannot enforce compliance among	c. Characteristics and trends of processes and products, including opportunities for preventive
	manufacturers/ distributors in an aspect of quality	action as per 8.2.3, 8.2.4, and 8.5.3.
	management in which they are themselves deficient.	d. Suppliers as per 7.4
	8.5 Improvement	DRAs are to continually improve the effectiveness of their QMS through:
	8.5.1 Continual Improvement	1. Quality policy
	8.5.2 Corrective Action	2. Quality objectives
	The standard practice for organizations is that:	3. Audit results
	1. Wherever a nonconformity or breach is detected,	4. Analysis of data
	corrective action must be taken to eliminate the cause	5. Corrective and preventive action
	of the nonconformity and to prevent its recurrence.	6. Management review
	2. Wherever corrective action is taken by an	For thoroughness and effectiveness, DRAs must establish a documented procedure (SOP) for
	organization, such action must be such as is	corrective action. Such a procedure must define requirements to:
	appropriate to the	1. Review nonconformities (including customer complaints).
	effects of the problem caused by the nonconformity or	2. Determine the causes of nonconformities.
	breach.	3. Evaluate the need for actions to prevent recurrence.
	8.5.3 Preventive Action	4. Determine and implementing the needed action.
	Organizations must:	5. Maintain records of the results of the action taken.
	1. Determine in advance the action	6. Review the effectiveness of corrective action taken
	that needs to be taken to eliminate	For thoroughness and effectiveness, DRAs must establish a documented procedure for
	the causes of potential non-	preventive action. Such a procedure must define requirements to:
	conformity, in order to prevent its occurrence.	1. Determine potential nonconformities and their causes.
	2. Ensure that preventive actions are appropriate to	2. Evaluate the need for actions to prevent occurrence.
	the anticipated effects of the potential problem.	3. Determine and implementing the needed action.
		4. Maintain records of the results of the action taken.
		Review the effectiveness of preventive action taken

*The Table is to be studied side by side with contents of ISO 9001:2008 and Table 2, which is on the regulatory requirements of DRAs. It must be stressed once again that if DRAs are to persuade manufacturers/ distributors to comply with the provisions of this and other clauses of ISO 9001:2008 industrial standard, they too must be conversant with and adept in them.

Table 13. Clause 8 of ISO 9001:2008 in relation to DRAs (Analysis of data/ Improvement).

3.4.7. Further remarks on clauses 7 and 8 of ISO 9001:2008

Although the principles of clauses 7 and 8 apply to all organizations, they are strictly speaking, the deeds and stuff intended for high profile institutions with elaborate concern and facilities for design and R&D, and with tall entrepreneurial ambition. Such organizations include the most successful pharmaceutical and biotechnology companies of the US, Europe, Japan and India; NASA, aircraft manufacturers, international airlines and 5-star hospitality concerns. However, in as much as DRAs must regulate the work and product of advanced pharmaceutical manufacturers, the onus is upon the DRAs themselves to be conversant with the entire provisions of these clauses and be as intellectually equipped as the manufacturer. This explains why it is often desirable that regulators have a stint in both academia and industry. In many countries, especially the US and India, top rate biomedical facilities/ institutions and personnel are to be found in the following four circles: i) the DRAs (eg: US-FDA); ii) health research institutions (eg: NIH); iii) the universities/ R&D institutions patronized by the DRAs; and iv) big transnational drug manufacturers (eg: Pfizer). We once again refer to the Nigeria polio vaccine controversy of the late 1990s/ early 2000s mentioned earlier, and ask the following question: When a DRA produces or distributes product as is the case in many developing economies, who regulates the DRA? Can subsequent revisions of ISO 9001or some other ISO standard provide an answer?

4. Conclusions

It is evident from the foregoing that all the eight clauses of ISO 9001:2008 apply to the Mandate of DRAs. However, most of what appears in clauses 7 and 8, the lengthiest of the clauses, relates more pertinently to high stake pharmaceutical manufacturers that have elaborate R&D than they do to the average DRA, which nevertheless should be thoroughly acquainted with the clauses. Some DRAs like the US-FDA and EMEA that have advance laboratories or access to such or that heavily fund R&D must be guided by the rigorous provisions of clauses 7 and 8. Needless to say, those DRAs that produce/ distribute products must be similarly guided to the extent of their relevance to the scope and size of their operations. The US-FDA, Japan's Ministry of Health and Social Services and EMEA are certified to appropriate performance standards and are known for their efficiency. By contrast NAFDAC and other developing national DRAs are not similarly certified and are less well known for efficiency, considering the rampancy of counterfeit drugs and other ills in their drug delivery systems. The DRAs of China, India and Southeast Asian countries compare quite well in many aspects with those of Europe, Canada and the US, and are by far more efficient than those of many African and South American countries. From the foregoing, and in view of the historical and international dimensions of phytotherapy, especially its galloping global patronage in recent times [1,2,11,12], it is necessary that there to be a minimum global standard to which DRAs should be certified. We propose ISO 9001 because of its global popularity, applicability and suitability. The standard provides the general climate for DRAs to efficiently discharge their Mandate. We project that a carefully planned application of ISO 9001 to herbal drug regulation will improve the production, distribution and usage of herbal drugs.

It will also boost the economy of developing economies that rely to a large extent on herbal drugs. But since the DRAs of many developing economies produce/ distribute certain products, there is a need for subsequent revisions of ISO 9001 to take cognisance of the question of who regulates the regulator that produces/ distributes? In the meantime we recommend that the Minister/ Secretary of Health and/ or the Parliamentary Committees of Health take note of this significant lacuna.

Acknowledgements

We gratefully acknowledge a copy of ISO 9001:2008 kindly furnished by the SON and the enlightenment offered by Engineer Timothy N. Abner, Dr. Justin B. Nickaf and Engineer. Shehu I. Maik during the NIPRD-SON workshop on ISO 9001:2008 held at Bolton White Apartments, Abuja, in November-December 2011.

Author details

Sunday Ameh[1*], Florence Tarfa[1], Magaji Garba[2] and Karniyus Gamaniel[3]

*Address all correspondence to: sjitodo@yahoo.com

1 Department of Medicinal Chemistry & Quality Control, National Institute for Pharmaceutical Research and Development (NIPRD), Idu Indusrial Area, Nigeria

2 Department of Pharmaceutical & Medicinal Chemistry, Ahmadu Bello University, Nigeria

3 Office of the Director General, NIPRD, Idu Indusrial Area, Nigeria

References

[1] Ameh, S. J., Obodozie, O., Inyang, U., Abubakar, M., & Garba, M. (2010). Current phytotherapy- a perspective on the science and regulation of herbal medicine. *Journal of Medicinal Plants Research*, 4(2), 072-081.

[2] Ameh, S. J., Obodozie, O., Inyang, U., Abubakar, M., & Garba, M. (2010). Current phytotherapy- an inter-regional perspective on policy, research and development of herbal medicine. *Journal of Medicinal Plants Research*, 4(15), 1508-1516.

[3] Ameh, S. J., Obodozie, O., Gamaniel, K., Abubakar, M., & Garba, M. (2011). Herbal Drug Regulation Illustrated with Niprifan® Antifungal Phytomedicine.

In: Eldin AB, editor. Modern Approaches to Quality Control, Rijeka, InTech, 367-382.

[4] DSHEA (1994). Dietary Supplements Health Education Act of 1994. Available: http://fda/Food/DietarySupplements/ucm109764.htm Accessed 2012 April 25.

[5] Goldman, P. (2001). Herbal medicines today and the roots of modern pharmacology. *Ann. Int. Med.,* 135(8), Pt 1, 594-600.

[6] Chineseherbsdirect.com (2010). What are Chinese Herbs? Available: http://www.chineseherbsdirect.com Accessed 2012 April 25.

[7] EDTHMP (2004). European Directive on Traditional Herbal Medicinal Products. Available: http://eur-lex.europa.eu/LexUriserv/LexUriserv.do?uri=CELEX: 32004L0024:EN:NOT Accessed 2012 April 25.

[8] De Smet, P. (2005). Herbal medicine in Europe- relaxing regulatory standards. *N. Eng. J. Med.,* 352(12), 1176-78.

[9] Mapdb.com (2003). Current status of medicinal plants. Available: http://www.mapbd.com/cstatus.htm Accessed 2012 April 25.

[10] WHO. (2008). Traditional Medicine. *WHO Fact sheet* [134], Revised: December World Health Organization, Geneva.

[11] Ameh, S. J., Obodozie, O. O., Chindo, B. A., Babalola, P. C., & Gamaniel, K. S. (2012). Herbal clinical trials - historical development and application in the 21st Century. Pharmacologia . DOI: 10.5567/pharmacologia.2012.121.131 Accessed 2012 April 25., 3, 121-131.

[12] Ameh, S. J., Obodozie, O. O., Babalola, P. C., & Gamaniel, K. S. (2011). Medical Herbalism and Herbal Clinical Research - A Global Perspective. *British Journal of Pharmaceutical Research,* 1(4), 99-123.

[13] Juran, J. M., & Godfrey, A. B. (1999). *Juran's Quality Handbook: The Complete Guide to Performance Excellence* (5th Edition), McGraw-Hill Professional, New York, USA, 1-1872.

[14] Pyzdek, T. (2003). Quality Engineering Handbook. 2nd Edition (Ed. Keller, P.), CRC Press, New York, USA, 1-744.

[15] ISO Survey (2009). Available: http://www.iso.org/iso/survey2009.pdf Accessed 2012 April 25.

[16] Ann Godsell Regulatory (2008). Pharmaceutical Good Manufacturing Practice for Herbal Drug Substances 2008 [cited 2010 April 8]. Available: http://www.pharmaceutical-int.com/article/category/treatment-herbal-medicines Accessed 2012 April 25.

[17] Akunyili, D. (2002). Herbal Preparations. *NAFDAC Consumer Safety Bulletin*, 1(2), 5-6.

[18] Gross, A., & Minot, J. (2007). Chinese Manufacturing: Scandals and Opportunities. Published in MX, November/ December, Pacific Bridge Medicals. Available: http://www.pacificbridgemedicals.com/ Accessed 2012 April 25.

[19] Corbett, C. J., Montes-sancho, M. J., & Kirsch, D. A. (2005). The financial impact of ISO 9000 certification in the United States: An empirical analysis. Management Science Available: http://personal.anderson.ucla.edu/charles.corbett/ paper/does_iso_pay.pdf Accessed 2012 April 25., 51(7), 1046-1059.

[20] Heras, I., Dick, G. P., & Casadesus, M. (2002). ISO 9000 registration's impact on sales and profitability - A longitudinal analysis of performance before and after accreditation. International Journal of Quality and Reliability Management Available: http://eps.udg.es/oe/webmarti/p774.pdf Accessed 2012 April 25., 19(6), 774-791.

[21] Naveh, E., & Marcus, A. (2007). Financial performance, ISO 9000 standard and safe driving practices effects on accident rate in the U.S. motor carrier industry. Accident Analysis & Prevention PMID 17166474Accessed 2012 April 25., 39(4), 731-742.

[22] Sharma, D. S. (2005). The association between ISO 9000 certification and financial performance. The international Journal of Accounting Available: http://masp.bus.ku.ac.th/files/ISO%209000%20and%20performamce.pdf Accessed 2012 April 25., 40, 151-172.

[23] Chow-chua, C., Goh, M., & Wan, T. B. (2002). Does ISO 9000 certification improve business performance? The International Journal of Quality & Reliability Management Available: http://www.emeraldinsight.com/journals.htm? articleid=840633&show=abstract Accessed 2012 April 25., 20(8), 936-953.

[24] Rajan, M., & Tamimi, N. (2003). Payoff to ISO 9000 registration. Available: http://www.iijournals.com/doi/abs/10.3905/joi.2003.319536Accessed 2012 April 25.

Quality Control in Food Science

Chapter 6

QA: Fraud Control for Foods and Other Biomaterials by Product Fingerprinting

Edoardo Capuano and Saskia M. van Ruth

Additional information is available at the end of the chapter

1. Introduction

Fraud can be generally defined as "the intentional deception made for personal gain or to damage another individual". In particular, *food fraud consists in the deliberate misdescription in order to deceive the consumers about the real nature of the product or of any of its ingredients*. It results in the mismatch between what a food product is and what it is claimed to be. Food fraud is a broad term that also involve criminal acts such as tax-avoidance and smuggling. In the following we will mainly discuss about economically motivated adulteration and mis-labelling i.e. food fraud issues falling in one of the following categories: 1) the substitution of an ingredient with a cheaper alternative (e.g., substitution of ethanol with methanol in wine or proteins with melamine in milk powders), 2) misdescription of the real nature of the product or one of its ingredients (e.g. counterfeiting, conventional products that are sold as added value products such as organic, fair trade, biodynamic), 3) incorrect quantitative in-gredient declaration and 4) implementation of non-acceptable process practices such as irra-diation, heating or freezing (e.g. thawed fish sold as fresh).

Food fraud can be implemented in any step of the food chain but it is mainly a food indus-try issue. In criminology, there are 3 elements of fraud opportunity (the crime triangle): vic-tim, fraudster and guardian [1]. The typical set-up is that where final consumers play the role of victims, food industry (but in general food producers, processors, traders or retailers) plays the role of the fraudsters and governmental control authorities, non-governmental and certification organizations play the role of the guardian. However, food producers can also be victim or guardian. They are victims when, for example, their products are counterfeited or simulated and guardian when they implements QA systems for the assessment of the au-thenticity of the raw materials. Nowadays food fraud represents a major problem that costs the EU food industry and governments hundreds of millions of euros every year. But the problem that food fraud poses is not merely an economic one: It is also a problem of public health because the adulteration can pose toxicological and hygienic risks to purchasers and consumers. In 2008, for example, Chinese milk was adulterated with melamine, an hazardous chemical, to increase milk nitrogen content causing 900 infants to be hospitalized with six deaths. Several other such examples can be given.

Since no one likes to be swindled, neither producers, traders, importers, retailers, and consumers, fraud prevention and detection is an important issue. Nowadays, authenticity of ingredients or products is mainly warranted by paper trailing. Analytical tests which can help to confirm the authenticity of ingredients/products compose a very useful complementary approach to paper trailing.

2. Fingerprinting approach: generalities and tools

Traditional strategies for the food fraud control have relied on the determination of the amount of a marker compound or compounds and the comparison of the obtained values for the test material with those established for the genuine material. The presence of an undesired adulterant can be uncovered by checking for its presence in the food material whereas the compliance of the food composition with the established legislative standards or with the amount of an ingredient as declared on the label can be simply proved by measuring the target compound or compounds. However, some aspects of food authenticity such as the geographical origin, the farming management systems (organic, free range..), or the application of some specific processes cannot be dealt with those traditional approaches. No single marker exists for the unequivocal authentication of an organic egg or a Dutch specialty cheese. Furthermore, based on conventional target analyses, an adulteration can be detected only if the adulterant is known beforehand and explicitly searched for by the analyst. Traditional quality control strategies are not designed to look for a near infinite number of potential contaminants so that new adulterants will not be unveiled until their presence in food is first acknowledged. For those reasons a more holistic approach is needed that is based on the measurement and the evaluation of several compounds at once, i.e. a fingerprinting approach. Moreover, in industrial and laboratory settings, there is always the need of implement screening methods that are able to reliably identify, in large numbers of samples, those that are potentially non-compliant before more detailed and accurate analysis with confirmatory methods are performed. A fingerprinting approach may, in many cases, provide rapid and high-throughput analyses well suited for screening purposes.

Fingerprint refers to the characteristic spectrum or image of a test material which can be related to its properties and thus to its authenticity in the same way as a human fingerprint is specific of a certain person and unequivocally identify him/her. The term thus recalls a comprehensive description of a test material that is carried out in a non-selective (or untargeted) way. Fingerprints can be generated through many analytical techniques. They can be obtained from chromatograms, spectroscopic measurements, spectral measurements or any other specific signal of complete spectra (Figure 1).

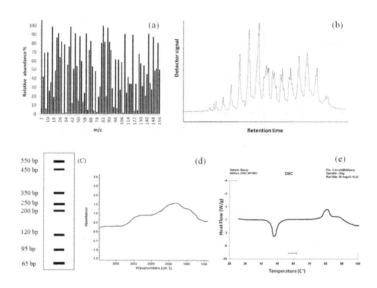

Figure 1. Analytical fingerprints: A mass spectrum (a), a chromatogram (b), a schematic representation of a DNA fingerprint on gel electrophoresis (c), an infrared spectrum (d) and a thermogram (e).

In a mass spectrum (Figure 1a), a collection of m/z and relative signal intensities is a chemical fingerprint of the material. Similarly, a chromatographic profile (Figure 1b) is a fingerprint of a more or less broad class of constituents of the material. The specific distribution of the restriction fragments of a selected DNA sequence on the electrophoretic gel (Figure 1c) is a genetic fingerprint of the test material. A NIR spectrum (Figure 1d) is a representation of the interaction of a test material with the infrared radiation whereas a thermogram (Figure 1e) is a representation of its interaction with thermal energy. (a) and (b) can be referred to as *chemical fingerprints*. They may be composed of as many groups of compounds as possible or alternatively of a specific group of compounds which requires higher level of purification and a selective extraction from the sample. (d) and (e) can be referred to as *physical fingerprints* even though chemical information can be obtained as well.

A fingerprinting approach implies that the whole information contained in the fingerprint (or a selected part of it) is used to infer about the properties of the system under study. To do that, a special statistical tool is necessary, i.e. chemometrics. Chemometrics can be defined as the science of extracting chemically relevant information from multivariate data by using statistical techniques to reduce the dimensionality of the dataset. It offers a tool to graphically summarise the analytical data to reveal relationships between samples and to detect characteristic patterns that can be used to identify a certain material. As a first step, an exploratory analysis is carried out in order to investigate the natural relations between the samples. This is carried out by so called unsupervised pattern recognition techniques because they do not require any prior knowledge of the properties of the samples. Examples of such techniques are: Hierarchical cluster analysis (HCA), cluster analysis (CA) and principal component analysis (PCA). PCA is the most widespread of those explorative tools. In a PCA model the original variables are transformed in new uncorrelated variables that arise from the linear combination of the original variables: the principal components (PCs). A number of PCs are extracted in sequence with each principal component accounting for the maximum of the residual variance in the data. The PCs extraction stops when most of the variance in the original data (typically around 90%) is explained. The new set of PCs define therefore a new space where the contribution of each original variables to each PC can be easily represented and the relationships between the original samples highlighted (Figure 2).

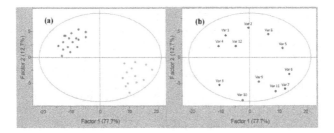

Figure 2. Plot of the first two dimensions in a typical PCA model. In a scores plot (panel a), samples are plotted in the space defined by the PCs. Similarities and differences between samples can be highlighted (in this case, two well separated groups of samples, red and green are apparent). In a loading plot (panel b) each variable (analytical response) is plotted on the new space defined by PCs. When score plot and loading plots are superimposed, information on the effect of the variable on samples properties can be obtained. When a variable is plotted close to a sample, this indicates that this variable shows relatively high concentration in this particular sample compared to the other samples. In the figure, variables 1,4,12 are higher in the samples of the red group and variables 6,7 and 11 are higher in the green group.

As a further step, multivariate methods are applied to either classify a certain product or quantify a certain property of the product. In the *classification models*, information about the class membership of the samples to a certain group (class or category) is used to classify new unknown samples in one of the known classes on the basis of its pattern of measurements. Classification models are useful, for instance, for the authentication of organic products or of geographical origin. Supervised pattern recognition techniques are used such: k nearest neighbours (kNN), soft independent modelling of class analogy (SIMCA), partial least square regression discriminant analysis (PLS-DA), linear discriminant analysis (LDA), support vector machine (SVM) and artificial neural network (ANN). Classification models may either build a delimiter between the classes so that they always assign a new object to the class to which it most probably belongs (suitable for limited and defined number of possible classes) or build a model for each class studied and then evaluate the fitting of new objects to each model (suitable for unlimited number of classes). In the *regression models*, a functional relationship is established between some quantitative sample property, the dependent variable, and a multivariate independent variables such as a raw chromatogram or a IR spectrum and the model is used to predict the property of interest in the unknown sample. Regression model are used, for instance, to quantify the level of adulteration in a food sample. For the building of regression models, multivariate regression methods such as principal component regression (PCR) and partial-least square regression (PLSR) are used.

The building of a classification (or regression) model comprises four essential steps: 1) Selection of a training set, which consist of objects of known class membership (or known quantitative values of a sample property) for which variables are measured. (2) Variable selection. Variables that contain information for the aimed classification are retained, whereas those encoding noise and/or with no discriminating power are eliminated. (3) Building of a model using the training set. A mathematical model is derived between the selected variables measured on the training set and their known categories (or quantitative values of the sample property). (4) Validation of the model. The model is validated in order to evaluate the reliability of the classification achieved either using an independent test set of samples (external validation) or the training set (cross validation).

The fingerprinting techniques are gaining more and more popularity over the past years thanks to advancements in the analytical instruments that are able to generate enormous amount of data at once and the application of chemometrics techniques. Herewith, fingerprinting techniques are classified in five broad categories according to the kind of fingerprint that can be obtained: *Mass spectrometry (MS) fingerprinting, chromatographic fingerprinting, electrophoretic fingerprinting, spectroscopic fingerprinting, and other fingerprinting*. This classification is shown in Table 1.

MS fingerprinting	Chromatographic fingerprinting	Electrophoretic fingerprinting	Spectroscopic fingerprinting	Other fingerprinting
PTR-MS	LC (HPLC, LC-MS..)	CE (CZE, CIF…)	NMR	DSC
ICP-MS	GC (GC-FID, GC-MS..)	Gel electrophoresis (isoelectric focusing, DNA electrophoresis…)	Fluorescence spectroscopy	Electronic nose
IR-MS			IR (NIR, MIR, FTIR)	Microarray technologies, reverse PCR
Direct infusion and ambient MS (ESI, MALDI-TOF, DART…)				

Table 1. Classification of fingerprinting techniques. For abbreviations, see text.

3. MS fingerprinting

MS is a powerful analytical technique that measures the mass-to-charge ratio of ions. The samples are first ionised, the ions are separated and their relative abundance assessed based on the intensity of the ions flux. MS produces therefore a mass spectrum representing the fingerprint of the sample components (Figure 1a). A number of different MS set-ups are possible based on the ionisation technique and the mass analyser used. MS can be used alone or they can be coupled with separation techniques. In this section, the stand-alone MS techniques will be dealt with in details whereas the application of MS as coupled with separation techniques will be dealt with in the next sections.

Stand-alone MS fingerprinting techniques that proved to be very useful for the fraud control and prevention are: proton transfer reaction MS (PTR-MS), inductively coupled MS (ICP-MS), isotope ratio mass spectrometry (IRMS), and direct infusion MS techniques.

Proton Transfer Reaction Mass Spectrometry (PTR-MS)

PTR-MS is a relatively new technique that is rapidly gaining popularity in the food analysis. PTR-MS allows quantitative on-line monitoring of volatile organic compounds. The volatile compounds are softly ionized by means of hydroxonium ions that are generated in an external ion source operating in pure water vapour. Only the volatile compounds that have a higher affinity for the ions are protonated and then accelerated by an electric field to the reaction chamber where they are separated and quantified. Because of this soft chemical ionisation the fragmentation of the parent compounds is limited and the interpretation of the spectra are much easier. Other major advantages of this technique are the great sensitivity with detection limits as low as few part per trillion, volume (pptv) and the possibility to monitor the food samples in real time, without any work up procedure. As a result, a fingerprint of all the volatile compounds comprised in a well definite mass range is obtained. The main disadvantage of this technique is that compounds are characterized only via their masses which is insufficient for their unequivocal identification.

PTR-MS has been extensively used in several aspects of food fraud control. It proved, for example, very successful for the geographical authentication of foods. The EU has long recognized the importance of differentiating food products on a regional basis. The normative framework introduced by the EU comprises the EU Regulations 509/2006 and 510/2006 and the EU Regulation 1898/2006. The EU Regulation introduced three geographical indications to a food product: protected designation of origin (PDO), protected geographical indication (PGI) and traditional specialities (TSG). In a study of 2008, the geographical origin (country) of butter samples was successfully predicted in 88% of the cases based on PTR-MS fingerprint and PLS-DA [2]. Recently, volatile fingerprint generated by PTR-MS has been used to discriminate between the Boeren Leidse specialty cumin cheeses with EU PDO from other 29 cumin cheese manufactured in the Netherlands [3]. The volatile fingerprint coupled with a PLS-DA model allowed the correct classification of 96% of the traditional boeren leidse cheese samples and 100% of the other commercial cheese samples. Another typical added value that is protected by the EU regulations is represented by the monovarietal extra virgin olive oil (EVOO), i.e. oil that is produced out of just one variety of olive trees. Frauds can be committed by mixing the more valuable monovarietal virgin olive oil with cheaper oils or by mixing different monovarietal olive oils. Volatile fingerprint of virgin olive oil obtained by PTR-MS and subjected to PLS-DA proved successful in discriminating among 5 different monovarietal EVOO from Spain with 100% sensitivity (% of objects of the modelled class correctly accepted by the model) and specificity (% of object, extraneous from the modelled class, correctly refused by the model) close to 100% [4].

In conclusion, PTR-MS is a rapid and low cost analytical technique that can be also fully automated and implemented on-line. Recently, the coupling of the time of flight (TOF, see below in this section) mass analyser to PTR-MS instruments has generated PTR-TOF-MS which is characterized by a high sensitivity with limits of detection down to few pptv and a high time resolution. The technique has been recently applied to discriminate among PDO labelled hams from Spain and Italy [5].

Inductively coupled plasma mass spectrometry (ICP-MS)

ICP-MS provides quantitative measurements of a wide range of metals and non-metals (inorganic elements) at trace and ultratrace concentration level (ppt). In this technique, the sample (even solid or liquid) is decomposed to neutral elements in a high-temperature argon plasma and the single elements are separated based on their mass/charge ratio and analysed. The great advantage of this technique compared to others (e.g. atomic spectroscopy) is that more than one element can be analysed at once so that a multi-elemental fingerprint is obtained in a very fast and sensitive way. The multi-elemental composition of animal and vegetal tissues can provide valuable information on the characteristics of the soil where a crop has been cultivated and on plants composition of the animal diet. The multi-element fingerprint is thus a valuable marker of the geographical origin of food. For instance, the authenticity of Tropea red onion, an onion Italian variety that achieved the PGI certification by the European Union as "Cipolla Rossa di Tropea Calabria" can be proved by means of multi-elemental analysis by ICP-MS and multivariate statistics [6]. All the statistical models applied (LDA, stepwise LDA, SIMCA, ANN), allowed a success rate of prediction >90% for the genuine samples. Moreover, the availability of nutrients from the soil strictly depends on the fertilization strategies and the pest and weed control management systems. In organic farming synthetic fertilizers are not permitted and the pest and weed control is based exclusively on natural products. It has been thus proposed that the multi-elemental fingerprint might be a marker for organically cultivated crops as compared to conventionally cultivated ones. Laursen *et al.* managed to discriminate between organic and conventional wheat, barley and faba beans (but not potatoes) based on the profile of 25 elements measured by ICP-MS [7].

Isotope ratio mass spectrometry (IRMS)

IRMS is a technique that can measure the ratio of the stable isotopes of the constituents of a biological material. Light elements like carbon, nitrogen, hydrogen, oxygen and sulphur stable isotopes ratios are most frequently assessed with this technique. Those ratios vary according to specific food production factors and geo-climatic conditions. Carbon stable isotope ratio depends, for example, from the plant composition of ruminant diets and can then be used to authenticate feeding regime or the farming management system (organic, free-range). Nitrogen stable isotope ratio is on the other hand depending on the type of fertilizers used in agriculture and is thus much useful for the authentication of farming practices for vegetal products and crops. Oxygen isotope ratio is instead highly dependent on the distance from the ocean and the altitude above sea level and could then be used for the authentication of the geographical origin of a food product.

The stable isotope fingerprint has been successfully used for the authentication of geographical origin and the farming practice. Normally the data are measured for many different elements and analysed with multivariate statistics. As an example, Fontina PDO cheese can be discriminated with good success from other cheeses based on stable isotopes $^2H/^1H$, $^{13}C/^{12}C$, $^{15}N/^{14}N$ and $^{34}S/^{32}S$ and PCA analysis [8]. However, frequently the isotope ratios (or a selection of them) are combined with other markers (elements) to improve the accuracy of the classification models. IRMS is often combined with ICP-MS for simultaneous elemental analysis. Stable isotope analysis combined with multi-elemental analysis has proven ideally suited to determine geographical origin of foods. The most accurate measurements of the isotope ratios is obtained by dual inlet (DI) IRMS. However, the purchasing and operating costs of a DI-IRMS instrument coupled with the time-consuming sample preparation are major disadvantages for the diffusion of this technique. The introduction of continuous flow (CF) IRMS instruments offers on-line, rapid and automated sample preparation, greater cost-effectiveness and easier interfacing with other preparation techniques.

Direct infusion mass spectrometry

Direct infusion MS techniques are based on the direct injection of the sample in the ion source without or with small sample pre-treatment. This allows for rapid analysis suited for high-throughput screenings. Electrospray ionisation (ESI), matrix assisted laser desorption ionization (MALDI) and direct analysis in real time (DART) are typical ionization techniques used for direct infusion MS. They are coupled with a variety of mass analysers, e.g. time of flight (TOF), Fourier Transform Ion Cyclotron Resonance (FT-ICR), single quadrupole (Q) and ion trap (IT) in many different set-ups.

ESI is a typical soft ionisation technique that is particularly suited for the determination of the molecular mass of large molecules (proteins, peptides, polysaccharides, triglycerides), because the ionisation does not bring about the fragmentation of the molecule. The liquid in which the analyte is contained is dispersed by electrospray to a fine aerosol. The droplets shrink as the solvent evaporates till solvated ions desorb from their surface. ESI-MS has proven to be very helpful in the authentication of vegetable oils. Lipid composition of vegetable oils depends on their botanical origin and the way they are processed. Fatty acids (FAs) and/or triglycerides (TGs) profile can thus help authenticate the type of oil, its origin, its quality grade and potential adulteration. Direct infusion ESI-MS has been for example used to predict the olive oil quality according to European Union marketing standards based on fatty acids and LDA analysis [9]. In the same research, the percentage of either EVOO and VOO in binary mixture with other lower grade oils was predicted with 5–11% average prediction errors by using PLS and multilinear regression (MLR). Samples were 1:50 diluted in an alkaline 85:15 (v/v) propanol/methanol mixture and directly infused into the MS system. Triglycerides analysis has some advantage over the analysis of the fatty acids profile for authentication or fraud control. Indeed, different oils can have specific TG fingerprint despite showing the same fatty acids composition. The triglyceride profiles, obtained using Q-TOF-ESI-MS was used to predict adulteration of olive oils with other vegetable oils.

The adulteration with hazelnut oil was predicted at a level of 10% v/v [10]. This adulteration is difficult to detect at levels below 20% by conventional methods due to the compositional similarity between the two oils. Similarly, PCA and HCA methodologies, applied to the ESI(+)-MS data were able to readily detect adulteration of EVOO with ordinary olive oils, at levels as low as 1% w/w [11]. Mono-, di- and triglycerides together with vitamins and antioxidants were detected and quantified with this method. Direct infusion ESI-MS has been used to authenticate other food commodities. The chemical fingerprint generated by direct infusion ESI-Q-TOF-MS in the negative mode can be used to discriminate between genuine whisky from Scotland and US, from counterfeited whisky produced in Brazil [12] and between alembic (the most valuable) and industrial cachaças (Brazilian sugarcane spirit) as well as the fraudulent addition of sucrose to the spirit [13]. Finally, direct-infusion ESI-QqQ-TOF-MS and atmospheric pressure photoionization (APPI)-QqQ-TOF-MS have been used for Iberian ham typification. APPI is a soft ionization technique based on a photoionisation mechanism. Five types of Iberian hams were successfully classified. Applying a PLS-DA model [14].

MALDI is another soft ionisation technique that proved very useful in the analysis of macromolecules, especially proteins. In MALDI the molecules are desorbed from the support matrix and ionised by means of a UV laser beam in a complex process mediated by the support matrix itself. MALDI is mainly coupled with a time-of-flight (TOF) mass analyser which separate the ions based on their flying time to the detector, which on turns depends on their m/z ratio. An example of application of MALDI-TOF-MS for authentication issues is represented by the fast method developed by Wang *et al.* for the fingerprinting of honey proteins [15]. The mass spectra were used to build up a database library to be used for authentication purpose. The protein fingerprint was thus successfully used to authenticate the geographical origin of commercial honeys produced in the US and other countries. In a similar fashion, peptide fingerprinting obtained by MALDI-TOF has been converted in a biological bar code for the authentication of high quality Campania white wines [16].

An innovative technique for food fingerprinting is represented by the direct analysis in real time (DART)-MS. DART is an ambient ionisation technique i.e. in which ions are formed outside the mass spectrometer without sample preparation or separation. The samples, either gaseous, liquid or solid are ionised in open air under ambient conditions. This means that organic compounds can be directly, and in real time, determined without time-consuming analytical protocols and thus with high sample throughput. DART coupled with TOF-MS has been used to obtain the fingerprint of the triglycerides from olive oil [17]. This method, coupled with LDA allowed the discrimination between EVOO, olive oil and olive oil pomace and the detection of hazelnut oil in EVOO at 6% v/v. DART-TOF-MS with solid phase micro extraction (SPME) pre-concentration of the analytes has been also reported to allow discrimination between trappist and non-trappist beers based on volatiles and phenolic compounds [18]. A combination of DART-TOF-MS and chemometrics was used for animal fat (lard and beef tallow) authentication [19]. TGs and polar compounds were extracted and analyzed. Mass spectral records were processed by PCA and stepwise LDA. The LDA model developed using TAG data enabled the classification of lard and beef tallow samples but also detection of admixed lard and tallow at adulteration levels of 5 and 10% w/w.

Additional ambient ionisation techniques have been recently proposed for authentication and fraud control by product fingerprinting. For instance, easy sonic spray ionisation (EASI)-MS fingerprinting of fatty acids and phenolic compounds have been used for the authentication of olive oil geographical origin [20].

4. Chromatographic fingerprinting

Chromatographic techniques aim at resolving complex mixtures in well separated compound. Based on the detection system, each single compounds generates a signal that can be used for the qualitative and quantitative analysis of the mixture. The graphical representation of such signal as a function of time is referred to as a chromatogram and can be thought of as the fingerprint of one or more classes of compounds occurring in the sample. Different strategies are available to obtained multivariate data matrices from chromatographic analyses (Figure 3). The fingerprint can be composed by the set of concentrations of the separated compounds based on an identification/calibration/quantification procedure as depicted in the path (a) of Figure 3. Alternatively, the fingerprint can be represented by the set of peak areas/heights (b). In this case the identification of each single peak is not necessary. Finally, it can be represented by the whole chromatogram that is handled as a continuous signal (c). In this case, the multivariate dataset is composed by as many variables as the sampling points the chromatogram is made up of (each data point of the chromatogram represents an individual variable). However, the application of chemometrics on raw chromatographic data requires specific data pre-processing techniques. In fact, problems related to the peak alignment or baseline shifts are particularly critical when a raw chromatogram is used as a data set.

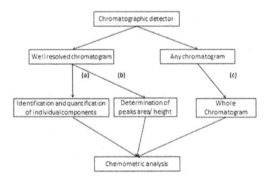

Figure 3. Schematic representation of the strategies to obtain multivariate dataset from a chromatogram for chemometric analysis.

Liquid chromatography

In liquid chromatography, the mixture components are separated as they pass through a column based on their selective partition behaviour between a stationary phase (column material) and a mobile liquid phase. Depending on the type of stationary phase, compounds can be separated based on their size, charge, molecular mass, hydrophobicity etc. The most popular LC technique is high performance liquid chromatography (HPLC) that is a straightforward, robust and reproducible technique. HPLC has been used for the analysis of a wide range of food compounds such as vitamins, proteins, carbohydrates, TGs, additives, secondary plant metabolites. A typical example of the application of HPLC based fingerprint for fraud control is the authentication of the organic eggs by means of the carotenoids profile [21]. Carotenoids are a group of fat-soluble pigments that occur in the egg yolk in concentrations of about 10 mg kg^{-1}. In animals carotenoids are entirely of dietary origin. Since the feeding regime of organic hens is clearly different from that of conventionally reared hens, the carotenoids fingerprint in eggs were used to discriminate between production systems. The carotenoids profile was determined by HPLC with UV detection, the single carotenoids quantified and the resulting concentrations used to build up a classification model by kNN. Almost all the conventional eggs and all the organic ones were correctly classified in external validation. The robustness of the method has been recently improved by testing eggs produced in several EU and non-EU countries. An example of HPLC fingerprint based on raw chromatographic data is in [22]. The authors applied PLS to the full TGs chromatogram profiles of vegetable oils to predict the % of olive oil in the mixtures with errors not exceeding 10%. Liquid chromatography can also be coupled with MS which allows higher resolution and higher sensitivity for metabolites occurring in relatively low amount. As an example, an untargeted method for proteins analysis based on LC-QTOF-MS has been developed which allowed to detect the fraudulent addition of cheaper vegetal proteins (from soy and pea) to skimmed milk powders based on the different peptides profile [23].

Gas Chromatography

In gas chromatography, the mixture is first vaporised in a heated chamber and then the mixture components are separated as they travel through the column transported by the flow of an inert gas (helium, nitrogen or hydrogen) based on their selective interaction with the column material. GC is a very popular separation technique mainly used for the analysis of volatile compounds. However a wide spectrum of compounds can be rendered volatile by proper derivatisation and thus analysed by GC. The analysis of fatty acids and triglycerides is usually carried out by GC with flame ionisation detector (FID) previous derivatisation in fatty acids methyl esters (FAME) and TG trimethylethers, respectively. FID is a general detector capable of high sensitivity and robustness. Fatty acids composition of animal tissues and animal products strongly depends on the feeding regime. FAs composition of fish muscle fat is affected by animal diet/feeding, the geographical area of catch and the marine conditions and is thus different between farmed and wild fishes. The discrimination between wild and farmed Atlantic salmon (*Salmo salar* L.) and Wild Turbot (*Psetta maxima*) has been reported based on FAs analysis and chemometrics [24-25]. The fatty acid fingerprint obtained by GC-FID followed by PLS-DA analysis has been also reported for the authentication of organic eggs and of organic feeds [26-27]. In the last case 90% of the analysed samples were correctly classified in their proper group in external validation. GC-FID can also be used for the TG profiling. TG fingerprinting by GC-FID has been for example reported for the authentication of three fat classes (animal fats, fish oils, recycled cooking oils) [28]. The TGs fingerprint was subjected to multivariate analysis (PLS-DA) and allowed the correct classification of 96% of the fat samples.

GC coupled with MS represents the method of choice for the analysis of volatile compounds because of its high reproducibility. On the other hand, GC-MS analysis requires careful sample cleaning and is quite expensive and time-consuming. The volatile fingerprint of coffee obtained by GC-TOF-MS after SPME has been reported for the geographical authentication of coffee [29]. SPME preconcentration of volatiles followed by GC-MS analysis coupled with PCA analysis allowed the detection of adulteration of ground roasted coffee with roasted barley [30]. The adulteration is detectable at level of 1% w/w in mixtures of dark roasted barley and coffees. Metabolomics studies can be also fruitfully performed by GC-MS. The fingerprint of a large range of metabolites obtained by GC-MS has been used to discriminate between mechanical separated meat (MSM) from hand-deboned meat [31]. MSM could be detected in raw meat mixtures down to a level of 10%.

5. Electrophoretic fingerprinting

Electrophoretic techniques are able to separate a complex mixture under a spatially uniform electric field, based on electrophoretic mobility of its components that depends, in turn, from their hydrodynamic properties and charge. Positively charged molecules move towards the anode and negatively charged molecules towards the cathode at a different rate based mainly on their mass to charge ratio. Smaller molecules move faster than larger ones.

Gel electrophoresis

In a gel electrophoresis, a gel is used as a medium for the movement of the charged particles under the applied electric field. Agar and polyacrylamide are typical medium used in gel electrophoresis. Proteins and nucleic acid fragments are usually separated by gel electrophoresis. Gel electrophoresis is of major importance for the genomic fingerprint of a sample material. Genomic fingerprints are obtained when properly amplified targeted or untargeted DNA or RNA fragments are separated by electrophoresis thus providing patterns that can be associated to sample properties (specie, variety and the like). Unlike the fingerprints discussed in the previous (and the next) sections, DNA fingerprint shows somehow different characteristics. The single features of the fingerprint are not quantitative variables (physical or chemical variables allowed to take on quantitative values, e.g. area of a peak in a chromatogram, signal intensity for a m/z or absorbance at a fixed wavelength in a IR spectra) but rather categorical variables, i.e. electrophoretic bands that can be either present or absent (see Figure 1 (c)). The sample identification is thus mainly carried out by checking for the presence (or absence) of one or more target bands. Multivariate analysis of the DNA fragments patterns is rarely performed.

Genomic fingerprinting mainly relies on polymerase chain reaction (PCR) based techniques. PCR is based on the amplification of a target DNA sequence by means of a thermostable DNA polymerase. The process consists of several cycles where the DNA molecule is denaturated, specific primers (small DNA sequences) anneal to the target DNA sequence and the DNA polymerase synthetizes a new DNA fragment delimited by the two primers. In each cycle the number of DNA molecules increases exponentially. A PCR-derived fingerprint can be obtained in different ways. In PCR-RFLP (restriction fragment length polymorphism) the amplified region is digested with an endonuclease and the resulting DNA fragments are separated by electrophoresis and properly visualised. The pattern of fragment represents a fingerprint of the DNA sequence that has been amplified. In multiplex PCR, two or more DNA fragments are simultaneously amplified by means of different target primer pairs, separated by electrophoresis and visualised. In RAPD (random amplification of polymorphic DNA) random DNA fragments are amplified by means of arbitrarily created primers. After separation, the DNA fragments will give rise specific patterns on the gel. Finally, in single-strand conformation polymorphism (SSCP), DNA sequences are amplified, denatured and the resulting single strand DNA molecules separated by electrophoresis based on their specific secondary structures.

PCR-based fingerprinting techniques have been widely used for species identification. For instance, the identification of ten species of salmon genus in a wide range of commercial products can be accomplished by PCR-RFLP based on the amplification of a specific region of the mitochondrial *cytochrome b* gene followed by polyacrylamide gel electrophoresis (PAGE) [32]. Similarly, PCR-RFLP has been used to identify 15 species of gadoid fishes based on the amplification of a small region of the *cytochrome b* gene and three restriction enzymes [33]. Gadidae family is one of the most commercially important fish family comprising species as Atlantic cod (*Gadus morhua*), the pollack (*Pollachius pollachius*) and the haddock (*Melanogrammus aeglenus*). Duplex PCR targeting the *cytochrome b* gene can be used to detect cow milk in buffalo mozzarella at a level of 1%. Buffalo mozzarella is labelled with PDO and can be produced only with pure water buffalo milk (*Bubalus bubalis*) [34]. In an original approach, the multiplex PCR fingerprint of the 16S and 23S rDNA genes of the lactic bacteria naturally occurring in milk has been used to discriminate the geographical origin of PDO mozzarella cheese [35]. The PCR fingerprint was subjected to cluster analysis (neighbour-joining algorithm) which allowed a fair discrimination of the samples.

Genomic fingerprinting shows a unique potential for the species or variety authentication in food products. The introduction of PCR has notably increased the potential of this approach. However, compared to other fingerprinting techniques, genomic fingerprinting is relatively time-consuming and labour-intensive. Its applicability to fraud issues other than genetic identification is limited. Furthermore, food processing may degrade the DNA molecule and lower its recovery thus negatively affecting the results of a analysis when applied to heavily processed foods.

Capillary electrophoresis

Capillary electrophoresis (CE) is the electrophoretic technique that shows a notable potential for food fraud detection based on product fingerprint. CE is a family of separation techniques that separate charged analytes based on their electrophoretic mobility: capillary zone electrophoresis (CZE), capillary isoelectric focusing (CIF), capillary gel electrophoresis, capillary electrochromatography. An electric field is applied to the ends of a capillary column. The ions migrate through the column in the same direction pulled by the electrosmotic flow and are separated based on their electrophoretic mobility. The signal that is generated when the mixture components are detected as they are eluted from the column is referred to as a capillary electropherogram. Multivariate dataset can be obtained from electropherogram in the same way as depicted in Figure 3. However, only strategy (a) has been used so far for authentication and fraud control purposes. CE are capable of rapid, low cost and high resolution analysis with little consumption of mobile phase. Main disadvantages of the technique are the low reproducibility (compared to other separation techniques) and low sensitivity that makes CE not suitable for the analysis of compounds occurring in trace amounts. CE represents a good alternative for the multiple detection of inorganic and organic acids. Many fruits and vegetables is rich in organic acids occurring in varying quantities in different fruits types, giving each fruit a unique organic acid profile. These profiles can be thus used to authenticate a vegetable product or identify the addition of another fruit type. For example the organic acids content measured by CE and LDA has been used to classify Spanish white wines [36].

6. Spectroscopic fingerprinting

Spectroscopy is the study of the interaction between a material and radiated energy. The graphical representation of such interaction is what is referred to as a spectrum i.e. a plot of the response of interest as a function of the wavelength or the frequency of the radiation used (see Figure 1d). Such a spectrum is by its very nature a fingerprint of the target material and contains information that are multivariate in nature. The extraction of the chemically relevant information from such a fingerprint requires the application of multivariate statistical techniques. The whole spectrum is used (or part of it) to obtain a multivariate dataset for further chemometric analysis in the same way as described for raw chromatograms (see Figure 3c). Spectral fingerprinting can be used either to classify and discriminate between samples or to quantify a certain compounds. According to the nature of the radiating energy (infrared, visible, ultraviolet, x-rays) and the nature of the interaction between energy and matter (absorbance, emission, scattering, resonance) different kind of spectra can be obtained. In the following we will mainly focus on nuclear magnetic resonance (NMR), fluorescence spectra and infrared (IR) spectra.

NMR

NMR spectra are generated by the absorption of radiofrequency radiation by atomic nuclei with non-zero spin in a strong magnetic field. Such absorption is affected by the surroundings of the atomic nucleus so that precise information about the molecular structure of a sample can be obtained. The atomic nuclei with non-zero spin that are most frequently used in NMR are ^1H, ^{13}C even though ^{15}N, ^{17}O, ^{19}F and ^{31}P can be also employed.

Generally, NMR is superior to other spectroscopic technique because of the much richer and more detailed information that can be gathered from the NMR spectra, at least with high resolution instruments that use frequencies above 100 MHz. Those information can be used for the simultaneous quantitative determination of a number of compounds without any prior separation. Furthermore the NMR spectrum can be considered a molecular fingerprint of the test material and subjected to multivariate analysis. The main disadvantage of this technique is the elevated costs of the instruments and the running costs. Nowadays, low resolution NMR instruments are available that use frequency ranging from 10 to 40 MHz. Those instruments are much cheaper and easy to use but do not provide the same detailed information as the high resolution instruments. NMR instruments are also capable of good accuracy but the sensitivity is lower compared to MS.

A recent study on the quality control of cola beverages using NMR is exemplar of the potential application of this technique for food authentication and fraud control [37]. ^{1}H NMR spectroscopy was used to discriminate with high success between premium and discount cola brands. This is important in the light of possible counterfeiting. The whole NMR spectra were used in combination with PCA. In addition, the information contained in specific regions of the NMR spectra combined with multivariate calibration (PLS) allowed the quantification of several cola ingredients (caffeine, aspartame, acesulfame-K, and benzoate) which concentration must comply with regulatory limits. NMR has been also used for the authentication of the geographical origin of olive oils. ^{1}H NMR spectra of the bulk olive oil, its corresponding unsaponifiable fraction, and a subfractions of the unsaponifiable fraction (alcohol, sterol, hydrocarbon, and tocopherol fractions) were used to classify olive oils according to their origin [38]. The unsaponifiable fraction had to be extracted to avoid the signal to be masked by that from the TGs in the bulk oil. The adulteration of virgin olive oil with a wide range of seed oils can be detected at level as low as 5% by means of combined ^{1}H and ^{31}P NMR spectra and discriminant analysis provided that the virgin olive oil are fresh (as reflected by their high 1,2-diglycerides to total diglycerides ratio) [39]. In this case the multivariate analysis was performed on 13 compositional parameters derived from the spectra rather than on the whole NMR spectral fingerprint. ^{13}C NMR spectra have been used for the authentication of fish and fish products. Discrimination between farmed and wild salmon is possible based on the NMR spectra of the muscle lipids and neural networks (PNN) and support vector machines (SVM) multivariate analysis [40]. Using the peak intensities of 12 selected chemical shifts an excellent discrimination is obtained by using PNN and SVM (98.5 and 100.0%, respectively). The authentication of different gadoid species was also achieved based on the NMR spectra of muscle lipids and Bayesian belief networks (BBN) with successful classification of 100% [41]. However, ^{1}H NMR spectroscopy can also provide useful information for the authentication of wild fish. In Figure 4, the PLS-DA scores plot for the ^{1}H NMR data measured in the authors' group on frozen, smoked and canned salmons both wild and farmed is presented. The score plot shows a clear separation of the two groups in distinct regions of the three dimensional plot. The results of the classification model (leave 5 out internal validation) were extremely positive with 100% of the wild samples (29 samples) and almost 100% of the farmed samples (60 out of 62 samples) correctly classified.

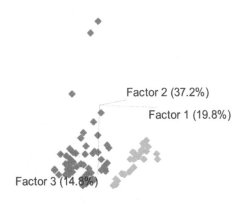

Figure 4. PLS-DA scores plot for the ¹H NMR data on wild and farmed salmon (frozen, canned and smoked). Red=farmed salmons; green=wild salmons

Fluorescence spectroscopy

Fluorescence spectra are normally obtained by exciting the test material. With radiations at a fixed wavelength and recording the intensity of the emitted radiation over a range of wavelengths. However, a 3D spectrum can be obtained by recording the emission spectra at different excitation wavelengths: the so called fluorescence excitation-emission matrix (EEM) which provides more information about the fluorescent compounds occurring in the sample. In synchronous fluorescence scan (SFS) the whole fluorescence landscape can also be achieved by scanning the excitation and the emission wavelengths simultaneously keeping a fixed wavelength interval (the so-called offset). Products that contains natural (or added) fluorophores are suitable for Fluorescence spectroscopy. Tryptophan, tyrosine and phenylalanine residues are fluorophores typically present in a variety of foods along with vitamin A, riboflavin (vit B2), NAD, NADH and compounds originating from Maillard reaction/lipid oxidation. Fluorescence spectra provide information about the amount of those compounds and on the way the fluorophore environment interacts with them. Traditionally, the fluorescence spectra have been treated by means of univariate approaches i.e. taking advantage of one specific wavelength or the derived fluorescence peak features. Nowadays the multivariate information contained in the fluorescence spectra is processed by chemometric techniques. When EEMs or SFS spectra are produced, decomposition methods such as two-way PCA, TUCKER and parallel factorial analysis (PARAFAC) are necessary to extract information from such a multi-way dataset (the data can be arranged in a cube instead of a matrix as in standard multivariate data sets). In the right-angle fluorescence spectroscopy the incidence angle between the excitation and the emission radiation is 90°. Only liquids and diluted solutions can be analysed and an attenuation of the signal intensity at high absorbance (> 0.1) is observed. To overcome this problem the front-face fluorescence (FFF) has been developed where only the surface of the material is analysed and the incidence angle is around 56° to minimise the artefacts from the excitation radiation reflected or scattered by the sample. Solid and powdered samples as well as bulk liquids can be analysed by FFF.

Fluorescence spectra are a promising tool to verify the egg freshness. Albumen samples stored for 1,2,3 and 4 weeks can be discriminated by means of the Maillard reaction products fluorescence and factorial discriminant analysis (FDA) with high success rate [42]. Vitamin A fluorescence together with FDA allows discrimination among egg yolk samples stored for different times [43]. Similarly, the freshness of fish can be predicted based on NADH and tryptophan fluorescence spectra. NADH fluorescence spectra can be also considered as a promising tool for the discrimination between frozen-thawed fish and fresh fish. The NADH emission spectra show a typical maximum at 455 nm in fresh fish and at 379 nm in frozen-thawed fish. The multivariate analysis (FDA) of the NADH spectrum allowed the correct classification of 100% of the analysed samples [44]. The authenticity of edible oils has also been extensively investigated by fluorescence spectroscopy. Chlorophyll and vitamin E are important fluorophores in olive oils and contribute greatly to oil colour and stability during storage. Refining processes decreases the content of chlorophyll and vitamin E with a corresponding change in the fluorescence spectrum. However, the discrimination between virgin and refined olive oil is mainly based on the fluorescence of lipid oxidation products (more abundant in the less resistant refined oils). A fast screening method has been also developed to detect adulteration of EVOO with olive-pomace oil [45]. It is based on the EEMs and it is able to detect adulteration at a level of 5%. Similarly, the discrimination between olive oils according to their overall acidity are also possible with fluorescence spectroscopy [46]. In this case, the maximum differentiation between the oils was obtained in the region 429-545 nm of the spectrum and allowed 100% correct classification of lampante olive oil (acidity >3.3%, not edible) from virgin olive oil with lower acidity (<3.3%). Finally, SFS with multiple regression analysis has been reported to for the detection of adulteration of EVOO with olive oil to a level as low as 8.4% when a 80 nm wavelength interval is used [47].

The great advantage of fluorescence spectroscopy is the rapidity, the limited costs and the non-destructive nature of the analysis. The sensitivity is also much greater than that of other techniques because the fluorescence signal has in principle no background.

Infrared spectroscopy

Infrared spectra are produced by measuring the intensity of the absorbance of infrared light by a sample as function of the wavelength. The absorption of infrared light is ascribed to transitions in the vibrational energies of the molecules contained in a sample. Each functional group of a molecule shows characteristic IR absorption at specific frequency ranges regardless of the interaction of the functional group with the rest of the molecule. However, interaction between atoms within a molecule may sometimes affect the position of characteristic bands in a IR spectra depending on the surroundings of the functional group. IR spectra can thus provide qualitative information about the nature of the functional group present in a food sample and quantitative information on their amount. When the effect of all the functional groups is taken together, the whole spectrum represents a molecular fingerprint that can be used to verify the nature of the sample. The IR region of the electromagnetic spectrum can be divided in 3 portion: The far IR (FIR, 400-10 cm^{-1}) has the lower energy and induces rotational transitions in the molecules. The mid IR (MIR, 4000-400 cm^{-1}) induces fundamental vibrational transitions in the molecules. The near IR region (NIR, 14000-4000 cm^{-1}) also induces transitions in the vibrational energies of the molecules. However, the transitions of the vibrational energy induced by the NIR portion of the spectrum are more complex than those induced by the MIR region. Overtones (transitions from the fundamental vibrational level over two or higher energy levels) and combination modes (arising from the interaction of two or more vibrations taking place simultaneously in different functional groups) give rise to very complex bands in the NIR spectrum that can give more complex structural information than MIR. On the other hand, NIR spectra are less selective than MIR spectra because of the superposition of different overtones and combination bands. A raw spectrum contains background information and noise beside valuable information. To remove those interferences as well as those coming from scattering, to normalise the effect of particle size and light distance, pre-processing methods such as smoothing, derivative, standard normal variate transformation (SNC), multiplicative scatter correction (MSC) or wavelet transforms (WT) are required. Recently, the introduction of the Fourier transform technique in IR (FTIR) has further increased the application range of the IR spectroscopy in the food field. In such a case the spectrum is obtained by mean of an interferogram in which multiple frequencies are measured simultaneously. The resulting interferogram is then deconvoluted using proper algorithms in order to have the original spectrum. The advantages of that technology is a faster analysis and a higher throughput and a better alignment of spectrum obtained by repetitive scans.

IR spectroscopy have been successfully applied to detect adulteration of juices, purees and syrups with cheaper juice concentrates. Adulteration of orange juice with orange pulpwash, grapefruit juice or synthetic sugars/acids mixture can be detected at a level as low as 50 g/kg by NIR [48]. Similarly, the adulteration of strawberry or raspberry juice with apple juice can be detected at level> 10% by transmittance NIR coupled with PLS [49]. MIR spectra have been used to detect adulteration of pure pomegranate juice with grape juice (2%-14% v/v) [50] and to predict the percent fruit content in strawberry jam [51]. Adulteration of honey and maple syrup can also be detected by NIR and MIR spectroscopy. NIR and FTIR have been successfully applied for the detection and quantification of cane and beet sugars in maple syrup [52]. Attenuated total reflectance (ATR)-FTIR coupled with LDA and PLS was used to discriminate the type of adulterant in three different honey varieties. A success rate of prediction of 100% was achieved for honey samples adulterated with 7-25% w/w of simple (glucose, fructose, sucrose) and complex (beet and cane invert) sugars [53]. NIR and MIR have also been employed for the authentication of lard and fats. Lard adulteration can be detected in cake [54] and in chocolate [55]. The adulteration of shortening with lard can be detected at levels ranging from 0 to 100% and a standard error of calibration (SEC) of 1.75 by using the regions 1.117-1.097 cm^{-1} and 990-950 cm^{-1} of the NIR spectrum. Adulteration of olive oils has also attracted much attention due to the economic value of the product. Adulteration of EVOO with palm oil can be detected by FTIR and PLS in concentration varying from 1.0 to 50.0% w/w [56]. The region 1500-1000 cm^{-1} of the MIR spectra was used for the regression model. The adulteration of EVOO with sunflower, corn, soyabean and hazelnut oil can be detected at level as low as 5% by using FTIR and LDA [57]. In this latter case, the normalized absorbance of peaks and shoulders areas were used in the model as predictors. The standard of identity for butter require that no vegetal oil nor margarine is added to the product. The presence of margarine can be detected by NIR coupled with PLS in the range 0-100% with a standard error of calibration after validation (SECV) <1.2% [58]. IR spectroscopy has been also widely used to predict and control meat quality. The discrimination between fresh and frozen-thawed beef can be accomplished by IR spectroscopy due to modification of the myofibrillar proteins and the corresponding change in their water holding capacity [59].

Infrared spectroscopy is a well-established technique for fast, high-throughput and non-destructive analysis of food and other biological samples. The analysis can be easily implemented on-line, can be automated and does not requires trained personnel to be carried out. It is little expensive and environmental friendly since does not require solvents, chemicals and does not produce waste. However, even though the analysis per se (collection of the spectrum) is fast, post-processing (pre-processing of the spectra and model building) of the input data can be laborious and time-consuming. The calibration models are usually built against reference analytical methods so that the measurement errors accumulated and the total predictive error increases. Finally, the classification or regression models are theoretically valid only on the instruments with which the training and the calibration has been carried out. The transfer of a multivariate model to other instruments affects its precision and accuracy compared to the original ones.

A case study on NIRS and adulteration.

As an example of the potential of the NIR Spectroscopy for the detection of adulteration, the results of an investigation that has been carried out in the authors' research group will be shown. NIR spectra were used to detect the presence of nitrogen replacers in milk powders. The compositional standards for milk powders require that the amount of milk proteins in milk solids-not-fat should be at least equal to 34% m/m, unless declared. The low prices of some nitrogen containing compounds make them attractive as potential adulterants to increase the level of apparent proteins in milk powders. The Kjeldahl method (official reference method for proteins content) measures the total amount of N irrespective of whether it comes from proteins or not. Expensive and time-consuming analytical methods such as enzyme-linked immunosorbent assay (ELISA), LC-MS/MS and GC-MS/MS are necessary for confirmatory analysis of melamine and its analogues in milk powders. To prove the potential of NIR spectroscopy for the detection of such adulteration, 33 skim milk powders were randomly adulterated with adulterants ammonium chloride, caprolactam, diammonium phosphate and polyvinylpyrrolidone (PVP) in order to produce an increment of 0.10, 0.50, 1.00 and 2.00% in the (apparent) proteins content of the milk powder. The samples were measured by NIR spectroscopy and the spectra subjected to PLS-DA analysis. A few milk powders were randomly selected and adulterated by melamine, ammelide and urea to test the robustness of the predictive models.

A PLS-DA model was first developed to predict the type of adulterant. The training set consisted of 80% genuine milk powders (26 samples) and 80% adulterated samples (19 samples from each adulterant) which were randomly selected. The remaining 20% of the samples, and those adulterated with the non-modelled adulterants melamine, ammelide and urea were used for external validation. The success rate of prediction was 100% in cross-validation and 78% for the external validation set (Table 2). Three out of 6 samples adulterated with melamine, ammelide and urea were correctly predicted as adulterated.

Class item	Genuine powder	+ NH$_4$Cl	+ caprolactam	+ (NH$_4$)$_2$HPO$_4$	+ PVP	No match
PLS-DA model based on training set						
Genuine powder	26	-	-	-	-	-
+ NH$_4$Cl	-	19	-	-	-	-
+caprolactam	-	-	19	-	-	-
+ (NH$_4$)$_2$HPO$_4$	-	-	-	19	-	-
+PVP	-	-	-	-	19	-
External validation						
Genuine powder	7	-	-	-	-	-
+ NH$_4$Cl	-	4	-	-	1	-
+caprolactam	-	-	3	-	1	1
+ (NH$_4$)$_2$HPO$_4$	-	-	-	4	-	1
+PVP	-	-	-	-	3	2
External validation based on melamine, ammelide and urea						
+melamine	-	-	-	-	-	2
+ammelide	2	-	-	-	-	-
+ urea	1	-	-	-	-	1

Table 2. Prediction results of PLS-DA model for the type of adulterant in milk powders

A PLS-DA model was then developed to discriminate generally between genuine and adulterated samples. The training set and the validation set were built in the same way as previously described. The PLS-DA scores plot is presented in Figure 4. The prediction results are reported in Table 3.

In external validation only one genuine sample was wrongly predicted as adulterated. One adulterated sample was incorrectly predicted as genuine (PVP added at its lowest concentration) and 3 adulterated samples could not be classified. Samples adulterated with melamine, ammelide and urea were all correctly predicted as adulterated.

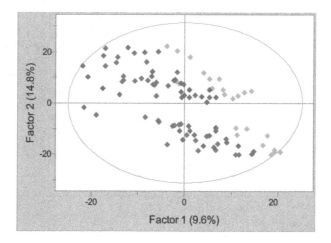

Figure 5. PLS-DA scores plot of IR spectra for genuine and adulterated milk powders. Red = adulterated powders; green=genuine powders.

Class Item	Genuine powder	Adulterated powder	No match
		Internal validation	
Genuine powder	24	2	-
Adulterated powder	0	68	8
		External validation	
Genuine powder	6	1	0
Adulterated powder	1	22	3

Table 3. Prediction results of PLS-DA model for genuine versus adulterated milk powders.

NIRS combined with chemometrics proved to be a promising tool for the cost-effective detection of adulteration of milk powders with a range of nitrogen replacers. The reliability of the classification models can be improved by the careful selection of those regions of the NIR-visible spectrum which showed the best discrimination power between genuine and adulterated samples.

7. Other fingerprintings

Differential scanning calorimetry (DSC)

Differential scanning calorimetry is a themoanalytical technique that measures the amount of heat required to increase the temperature of a sample relative to a reference material. When the amount of heat absorbed/released is plotted as a function of temperature a thermal spectrum of the sample is obtained from which kinetic and thermodynamic information such as the heat capacity and the enthalpy of any phase transition (fusion, evaporation, glass transition etc) the sample undergoes in the temperature span of the experiments can be determined. Those physical properties depends in turn on compositional and structural properties of the samples.

DSC has been mainly applied for the authentication of fats/oils. The level of adulteration of canola oil with lard, beef tallow and chicken fat as well as that of virgin coconut oil with palm kernel oil (PKO) and soybean oil can be predicted by the analysis of the DSC thermogram and stepwise multilinear regression (SMLR) [60]. The melting profiles of cow, goat, sheep, camel, horse and water buffalo milk fat samples were also determined by DSC. Differences in the DSC profiles for the fat fraction of milk of different species can be attributed to their fatty acid/TAG composition. In general, the melting point of the fats decreases with decreasing chain length and increasing degree of unsaturation of the fatty acids in the milk. The thermograms were subjected to PCA analysis which showed a clear distinction of the four milk samples analysed. The loadings plots of the heat flow data showed that the data are most influenced between the temperatures of 13° and 24° C [61].

Sensor technology

Sensor technology is often referred to as electronic nose technology. In this technology the volatile compounds present in the headspace of a sample are detected by an array of semi-selective sensors. Normally each sensor is sensitive to all the volatile but each in a peculiar way. There are many sensors for EN instruments such as metal oxide sensors, conducting polymer sensors, quartz crystal membrane sensors, or mass spectrometers (MS-EN) available on the market. The sensor's response is then transformed in a spectrum that represents a fingerprint of the volatile compounds of the tested sample. Electronic nose analysis are often cheaper and faster than GC analysis and the sample preparation is usually quite simple. The technique, however, does not have the same sensitivity of other techniques. Furthermore, single volatile compounds cannot be identified and the signal is sensitive to water vapour.

Electronic nose has been used mainly for the detection of adulteration in fats/oils. Rapid detection of pork and lard in food samples for halal authentication (compliance with Islamic dietary rules) are reported with electronic nose [62]. Under Jewish and Islamic dietary laws, foods containing porcine-based ingredients such as lard are strictly prohibited from consumption. Electronic nose and chemometric analysis was applied for the detection of adulteration of olive oil samples with sunflower and olive-pomace oil at levels as low as 5% [63]. Application are also reported for the authentication of the geographical origin of Italian wines [64], and emmenthal cheese [65].

Transcriptomics

Transcriptomics is a post-genomic technique that consists in the simultaneous measurements of all the transcripts (mRNA molecules) in a given organism, or of a specific subset of transcripts present in a particular cell type. Unlike genome, transcriptome varies according to the environmental conditions and represents the genes that are actively expressed in a certain cell at a certain time. Transcriptome is usually obtained by DNA microarray technologies and reverse PCR. The set of all the mRNA produced (and hence of the genes actively expressed) represents a fingerprint of that target cell/organism and can thus use for fraud detection and authentication purposes. At the present the potential of transcriptomics in this respect is still underexplored.

8. Fingerprinting options for other biomaterials

Biofuels are an important environmental-friendly alternative to fossil fuels. The term biodiesel refers primarily to FAME obtained after transesterification of triglycerides with methanol. The methyl esters can be produced from many different triglyceride sources, primarily rapeseed oil but also sunflower oil, soybean oil, palm oil, linseed oil, tallow, and used frying oil. Blends of biodiesel with conventional petrodiesel fuel represent a common utilization of biodiesel. The ability to predict retail biodiesel blend percent composition is important to detect adulterations. It has been reported that biodiesel from different sources can be discriminated by direct infusion ESI-MS and multivariate statistics [66]. In addition, the % of rapeseed or salmon biodiesel in petrodiesel in concentrations ranging from 0.5% to 10% can be predicted with good accuracy by applying a PLS model. Similarly, the feedstock source of blends of biodiesel and conventional diesel, as well as the % composition of the blend can be predicted applying a kNN and a PLS model respectively to the total ion current chromatograms from gas chromatography–quadrupole mass spectrometry (GC–qMS) using a polar column [67]. The precision of the prediction was between 4-5%. Furthermore, the addition of residual oil (non-transesterified residual vegetable oil) is one of the easiest ways of adulterating biofuels. Synchronous fluorescence combined to LDA can be used to discriminate between diesel oils, biodiesels and biodiesel adulterated with residual oil and the % of residual oil can be predicted with good accuracy when a PLS model is used [68].

Perfume counterfeiting is an illegal practice that causes huge economical loss to the perfume industry and pose potential health risk to consumers who might be exposed to harmful chemical from counterfeited products. Traditionally, the quality control analyses for perfume focuses on volatile and semi-volatile compounds and are performed by GC based techniques. Recently, more straightforward methods have been proposed for the fast authentication of premium perfumes and detection of adulteration/counterfeiting. A fingerprint of the polar compounds can be achieved by direct infusion EASI-MS (see section 3) [69]. The samples are sprayed onto a glass rod and directly exposed to the ionisation source of the MS system. An almost instantaneous, simple and reproducible fingerprint of the polar compounds in the product is obtained that allows a complete discrimination between authentic and counterfeited products. A fast discrimination between authentic and counterfeited products can be also obtained by fingerprinting of the polar compounds by ESI-MS in the positive ion mode and chemometric analysis previous extraction of few μL of the sample in a 1:1 methanol/water solution [70]. Even more recently, a fast, simple and low-cost method for the authentication of perfume based on a commercial electronic olfactory system (EOS) equipped with thin film metal oxide semiconductors has been proposed [71]. The PCA analysis of the R/R_0 values (resistance of the sensor in the presence of the volatile compounds relative to that of the sensor balanced in air) generated by 6 sensors based on different metal oxide semiconductors can unequivocally discriminate between authentic and counterfeited perfumes. The prior removal of ethanol from the samples is necessary for the correct discrimination of the samples.

Essential oils are also widely employed for their fragrance in perfumery but also in cosmetics and household products. One of the most common fraud is the blend of valuable essential oils with other less valuable alternatives. As an example, the valuable Rosewood essential oil, obtained from the trees of *Aniba rosaeodora* Ducke and employed in fine perfumery, can be blended with the far cheaper synthetic linaool, obtained by re-distillation of Rosewood leaf oil. The ESI-MS fingerprint in the positive ions mode of the polar compounds extracted by an acidified 1:1 water methanol solution can easily detect adulteration of Rosewood oil with synthetic linaool at concentration as low as 10% v/v [72]. A PCA model is necessary to extract the relevant information from the fingerprint.

Direct infusion MS can be used to authenticate wood as well. Venturi easy ambient sonic spray ionization (V-EASI)-MS fingerprint of a very simple methanolic extract of wood chips or directly acquired from the freshly scratched wood surface may help to control the illegal logging and trade of the noble Mahogany tropical wood and its falsification [73]. V-EASI-MS is a novel ambient ionization MS technique characterized by sonic spray ionization and a self-pumping system based on the Venturi effect. It allows the direct analysis of solid or liquid samples. Ionization is assisted by compressed nitrogen and the apparatus is thus free of electrical discharge, thermal interferences since no heating, voltage or radiation is used. The introduction of fast and high-throughput analytical techniques for wood authentication is especially valuable since the classical controls are based on time-consuming morphological evaluations. Recently an original and fast approach for the authentication of wood species has been proposed. It is based on the analysis of the volatile compounds measured by a low-cost conductive polymer-based portable electronic nose formed by an array of only three gas sensors and/or the elemental fingerprint measured by laser-induced breakdown spectrometry (LIBS) which performs a multielemental and direct analysis even in solid samples [74].

The assurance of quality of herbal supplements and medicines is a major concern for the phytopharmaceutical and the food industry. The identification of the herbal drug and the presence of adulterant is a mandatory test to ensure the quality, the efficacy and the safety of a medical preparation or an herbal supplement. Among a variety of quality control methods, chromatographic fingerprinting has gained more and more attention recently and have been used to authenticate a large number of herbal products. They are accepted by many international organization for the quality control of herbal medicine but are relatively time-consuming. More recently, spectroscopic techniques have been explored to rapidly authenticate herbal products. For instance, different species of *Echinacea, e.g., E. purpurea, E. angustifolia,* and *E. pallida* are used for commercial preparations to prevent or cure the common cold, flu, and several other diseases due to their nonspecific stimulating effect of the immune system. It is also well known that *Echinacea* preparation are commonly adulterated with roots of *Parthenium integrifolium* L. This adulteration can be detected by NIRS at a minimum of 10% of adulteration [75]. The method requires just the milling of the sample and can be carried out within 1 minute.

The list of potential applications of products fingerprinting is not limited to the cases discussed above and many other examples may be provided. In the authors' research group for instance, PTR-MS and ICP-MS are used for the authentication of the geographical origin of flower bulbs. Counterfeiting of pharmaceuticals is another area where the application of fingerprinting techniques has proved of great help. The topic is so huge that we would address the interested readers to specialized publications.

9. Conclusions

Product fingerprinting combined with chemometrics represents a valuable tool for fraud detection and control for food products and other biomaterials. A fingerprinting approach is particularly useful:

• For the authentication of products for which target analyses based on specific markers are not available

• For the detection of adulteration based of yet unknown adulterants

• For a fast and high-throughput screening of the samples before more elaborated confirmatory analysis are applied.

At the same time a fingerprinting approach may substantiate nutritional, sensory or other product qualities.

LC, GC, and IR spectroscopy are already common instrumental platforms available in most QA laboratories and they will continue to provide valuable support for food fraud prevention. IR and other spectroscopic techniques have the great advantage of providing fast, high-throughput and non-destructive analyses with limited costs. They can be easily automated and adapted for *in-line* or *in-situ* analysis which makes these techniques well suited for implementation in the industrial setting. MS and NMR are not as common in QA laboratories, principally because of their high costs but they may become more important in routine QA testing because of their superior performances. However, even though the costs of MS and NMR instruments is still very high, the cost per sample can be very low if a high samples turnover can be achieved.

From an analytical point of view, a further improvement is expected in the future from the broader application of multi-dimensional separation techniques such as GCxGC or LCxLC which provide enhanced resolution and an higher number of peaks. Ultra-performance liquid chromatography (UPLC) and CE may also provide rapid separation with limited costs. The application of novel (or still underexploited) ambient ionisation MS techniques that allow the rapid analysis of liquid and solid samples with little, if any, preparation will be particularly valuable in the future.

The applicability and the reliability of a fingerprint approach also depends from the correct and tailored usage of the relevant and appropriate chemometric tools. For the development of regression and/or classification models, special care should be devoted to ensure:

- The representativeness of the classes considered, in order to cover all the possible source of variability for the class at stake.

- A robust validation of the model (external validation to be preferred over internal validation).

- The use of the appropriate chemometric tools depending on the problem at stake. Whereas a few pattern recognition techniques are frequently used (PLS-DA, SIMCA, LDA..), some other such as classification and regression trees (CART), quadratic discriminant analysis (QDA) are still underexploited despite the good results that they can provide.

Another key aspect is represented by the validation of methods based on fingerprinting and chemometrics that is essential for their application in a commercial context. Whereas standards exist for the validation of regular analytical methods (see for instance, Commission Decision 2002/657/EC and ISO 17025), internationally accepted protocols for the validation of methods based on fingerprinting techniques and chemometric classification models are lacking at the present. Such protocols should indicate the performance characteristics that have to be checked and the criteria to be met in order to verify the compliance of the method with the performance characteristics.

Acknowledgements

We acknowledge Martin Alewijn, Grishja van der Veer and Pan Weijing for the work on NIR spectroscopy and milk powder and Angela Dura de Miguel, Arjen Lommen and Maikel Rozijn for the work on ^{1}H NMR and fish. We also acknowledge the Dutch ministry of agriculture, economic affair and innovation for the funding of this book chapter.

Author details

Edoardo Capuano[1*] and Saskia M. van Ruth[1]

*Address all correspondence to: edoardo.capuano@wur.nl

1 RIKILT – Institute of Food Safety, Wageningen University and Research Centre,, The Netherlands

References

[1] Felson, M. (1998). Crime and everyday life. 2nd ed. Thousand Oaks, Calif. Pine Forge Press.

[2] Macatelli, M., Akkermans, W., Koot, A., Buchgraber, M., Paterson, A., & van Ruth, S. (2009). Verification of the geographical origin of European butters using PTR-MS. DOI: 10.1016/j.jfca.2008.10.009.

[3] Galle, S. A., Koot, A., Soukoulis, C., Cappellin, L., Biasioli, F., Alewijn, M., & van Ruth, S. (2011). Typicality and Geographical Origin Markers of Protected Origin Cheese from The Netherlands Revealed by PTR-MS. *Journal of Agricultural and Food Chemistry*, 59(6), 2554-2563.

[4] Ruiz-Samblas, C., Tres, A., Koot, A., van Ruth, S., Gonzales-Casado, A., & Quadros-Rodriguez, L. (2012). Proton transfer reaction-mass spectrometry volatile organic compound fingerprinting for monovarietal extra virgin olive oil identification. *Food Chemistry*, 134(1), 589-596.

[5] Del Pulgar, J. S., Soukoulis, C., Biasioli, F., Cappellin, L., Garcia, C., Gasperi, F., Granitto, P., Mark, T. D., Piasentir, E., & Schuhfried, E. (2011). Rapid characterization of dry cured ham produced following different PDOs by proton transfer reaction time of flight mass spectrometry (PTR-ToF-MS). *Talanta*, 85(1), 386-393.

[6] Furia, E., Naccarato, A., Sindona, G., Stabile, G., & Tagarelli, A. (2011). Multielement Fingerprinting as a Tool in Origin Authentication of PGI Food Products: Tropea Red Onion. DOI: 10.1021/jf201556e.

[7] Laursen, K. H., Schjoerring, J. K., Olesen, J. E., Askegaard, M., Halekoh, U., & Husted, S. (2011). Multielemental Fingerprinting as a Tool for Authentication of Organic Wheat, Barley, Faba Bean, and Potato. *Journal of Agricultural and Food Chemistry*, 59(9), 4385-4396.

[8] Pillonel, L., Bütikofer, U., Rossmann, A., Tabacchi, R., & Bosset, J. O. (2004). Analytical methods for the detection of adulteration and mislabeling of Raclette Suisse and Fontina PDO cheese. *Mitteilungen aus Lebensmittel Untersuchung und Hygiene;*, 95-489.

[9] Lerma-Garcia, M. J., Herrero-Martinez, J. M., Ramis-Ramos, G., & Simo-Alfonso, E. F. (2008). Evaluation of the quality of olive oil using fatty acid profiles by direct infusion electrospray ionization mass spectrometry. *Food Chemistry*, 107(3), 1307-1313.

[10] Gomez-Ariza, J. L., Arias-Borrego, A., Garcia-Barrera, T., & Beltran, R. (2006). Comparative study of electrospray and photospray ionization sources coupled to quadrupole time-of-flight mass spectrometer for olive oil authentication. *Talanta*, 70(4), 859-869.

[11] Alves , J. de O., Neto, W. B., Mitsutake, H., Alves, P. S., & Augusti, R. (2010). Extra virgin (EV) and ordinary (ON) olive oils: distinction and detection of adulteration

(EV with ON) as determined by direct infusion electrospray ionization mass spectrometry and chemometric approaches. DOI: 10.1002/rcm.4590.

[12] Moller, J. K. S., Catharino, R. R., & Eberlin, M. N. (2005). Electrospray ionization mass spectrometry fingerprinting of whisky: immediate proof of origin and authenticity. *Analyst*, 130-890.

[13] De Souza, P. P., de Oliveira, L. C. A., Catharino, R. R., Eberlin, M. N., Augusti, D. V., Siebald, H. G. L., & Augusti, R. (2009). Brazilian cachaça:"Single shot typification of fresh alembic and industrial samples via electrospray ionization mass spectrometry fingerprinting. *Food Chemistry*, 115(3), 1064-1068.

[14] Gonzalez-Dominguez, R., Garcia-Barrera, T., & Gomez-Ariza, J. L. (2012). Iberian ham typification by direct infusion electrospray and photospray ionization mass spectrometry fingerprinting. *Rapid Communications in Mass Spectrometry*, 26(7), 835-844.

[15] Wang, J., Kliks, M. M., Quw, Jun. S., Shi, G., & Li, Q. X. (2009). Rapid determination of the geographical origin of honey based on protein fingerprinting and barcoding using MALDI TOF MS. *Journal of Agricultural and Food Chemistry*, 57-10081.

[16] Chambery, A., del Monaco, G., di Maro, A., & Parente, A. (2008). Peptide fingerprint of high quality Campania white wines by MALDI-TOF mass spectrometry. DOI: 10.1016/j.foodchem.2008.08.031.

[17] Vaclavik, L., Cajka, T., Hrbek, V., & Hajslova, J. (2009). Ambient mass spectrometry employing direct analysis in real time (DART) ion source for olive oil quality and authenticity assessment. *Analytica Chimica Acta*, 645(1-2), 56-63.

[18] Cajka, T., Riddellova, K., Tomaniova, M., & Hajslova, J. (2011). Ambient mass spectrometry employing a DART ion source for metabolomic fingerprinting/profiling: a powerful tool for beer origin recognition. *Metabolomics*, 7-500.

[19] Vaclavik, L., Hrbek, V., Cajka, T., Rohlik, B. A., Pipek, P., & Hajslova, J. (2011). Authentication of Animal Fats Using Direct Analysis in Real Time (DART) Ionization −Mass Spectrometry and Chemometric Tools. *Journal of Agricultural and Food Chemistry*, 59(11), 5919-5926.

[20] Riccio, M. F., Sawaya, A. C. H. F., Abdelnur, P. V., Saraiva, S. A., Hadda, R., Eberlin, M. N., & Catharino, R. (2011). Easy Ambient Sonic-Spray Ionization Mass Spectrometric of Olive Oils: Quality Control and Certification of Geographical Origin. *Analytical Letters*, 44(8), 1489-1497.

[21] van Ruth, S. M., Alewijn, M., Rogers, K., Newton-Smith, E., Tena, N., Bollen, M., & Koot, A. (2011). Authentication of organic and conventional eggs by carotenoid profiling. *Food Chemistry*, 129-1299.

[22] de la Mata-Espinoza, P., Bosque-Sendra, J. M., Bro, R., & Cuadros-Rodriguez, L. (2011). Olive oil quantification of edible vegetable oil blends using triacylglycerols chromatographic fingerprints and chemometric tools. *Talanta*, 85-177.

[23] Cordawener, J. H. G., Luykx, D. M. A. M., Frankhuizen, R., Bremer, M. G. E. G., Hooijerink, H., & America, A. H. P. (2009). Untargeted LC-Q-TOF mass spectrometry method for the detection of adulterations in skimmed-milk powders. *Journal of Separation Science*, 32-1216.

[24] Axelson, D. E., Standal, I. B., Martinez, I., & Aursand, M. (2009). Classification of Wild and Farmed Salmon Using Bayesian Belief Networks and Gas Chromatography-Derived Fatty Acid Distributions. *Journal of Agricultural and Food Chemistry.*, 57-7634.

[25] Busetto, M. L., Moretti, V. M., Moreno-Rojas, J. M., Caprino, F., Giani, I., Malandra, R., Bellagamba, F., & Guillou, C. (2011). Authentication of Farmed and Wild Turbot (Psetta maxima) by Fatty Acid and Isotopic Analyses Combined with Chemometrics. DOI: 10.1021/jf0734267.

[26] Tres, A., O'Neil, R., & van Ruth, S. M. (2011). Fingerprinting of fatty acid composition for the verification of the identity of organic eggs. *Lipid technology*, 23-40.

[27] Tres, A., & van Ruth, S. M. (2011). Verification of Organic Feed Identity by Fatty Acid Fingerprinting. *Journal of Agricultural and Food Chemistry*, 59(16), 8816-8821.

[28] van Ruth, S. M., Rozijn, M., Koot, A., Perez-Garcia, R., van der Kamp, H., & Codony, R. (2010). Authentication of feeding fats: Classification of animal fats, fish oils and recycled cooking oils. *Animal Feed Science and Technology*, 155(1), 65-73.

[29] Risticevic, S., Carasek, E., & Pawliszyn, J. (2008). Headspace solid-phase microextraction-gas chromatography-time-of-flight mass spectrometric methodology for geographical origin verification of coffee. *Analytical Chimica Acta*, 617-72.

[30] Oliveira, R. C. S., Oliveira, L. S., Franca, A. S., & Augusti, R. (2009). Evaluation of the potential of SPME-GC-MS and chemometrics to detect adulteration of ground roasted coffee with roasted barley. *Journal of Food Composition and analysis*, 22(3), 257-261.

[31] Jiye, A., Surowiec, I., Fraser, P., Patel, R., Halket, J., & Bramley, P. (2010). Metabolomic approach to the identification of robust markers for the detection of mechanically separated meat (MSM) in meat products. http://www.foodbase.org.uk/results.php?f_report., *FSA final technical report*.

[32] Russell, V. J., Hold, G. L., Pryde, S. E., Rehbein, H., Quinteiro, J., Rey-Mendez, M., Sotelo, C. G., Perez-Martin, R. I., Santos, A. T., & Rosa, C. (2000). Use of Restriction Fragment Length Polymorphism To Distinguish between Salmon Species. *Journal of Agricultural and Food Chemistry*, 48-2184.

[33] Calo-Mata, P., Sotelo, C. G., Pérez-Martín, R. I., Rehbein, H., Hold, G. L., Russel, V. J., Pryde, S., Quinteiro, J., Rey-Méndez, M., Rosa, C., & Santos, A. T. (2003). Identification of gadoid fish species using DNA-based techniques. *European Food Research and Technology*, 217-259.

[34] Bottero, M. T., Civera, T., Anastasio, A., Turi, R., & Rosati, S. (2002). Identification of cow's milk in "buffalo"cheese by duplex polymerase chain reaction. *Journal of Food Proteins*, 65-362.

[35] Bonizzi, I., Feligini, M., Aleandri, R., & Enne, G. (2006). Genetic traceability of the geographical origin of typical Italian water buffalo Mozzarella cheese: A preliminary approach. *Journal of Applied Microbiology*, 102(3), 667-673.

[36] Garrido-Delgado, R., Lopez-Vidal, S., Arce, L., & Valcarcel, M. (2009). Differentiation and identification of white wine varieties by using electropherogram fingerprints obtained with CE. *Journal of Separation Science*, 32(21), 3809-3816.

[37] Maes, P., Monakhova, Y. B., Kuballa, T., Reusch, H., & Lachenmeyer, D. W. (2012). Qualitative and Quantitative Control of Carbonated Cola Beverages Using ^{1}H NMR Spectroscopy. DOI: 10.1021/jf204777m.

[38] Alonso-Salces, R. M., Heberger, K., Moreno-Rojas, G. M., Bellan, M. G., Reniero, F., & Guillou, C. (2010). Multivariate analysis of NMR fingerprint of the unsaponifiable fraction of virgin oliveoils for authentication purposes. *Food Chemistry*, 118(4), 956-965.

[39] Vigli, G., Philippidis, A., Spyros, C., & Dais, P. (2003). Classification of Edible Oils by Employing ^{31}P and ^{1}H NMR Spectroscopy in Combination with Multivariate Statistical Analysis. A Proposal for the Detection of Seed Oil Adulteration in Virgin Olive Oils. DOI: 10.1021/jf030100z.

[40] Aursand, M., Standal, I. B., Prael, A., Mc Evoy, L., Irvine, J., & Axelson, D. E. (2009). 13C NMR Pattern Recognition Techniques for the Classification of Atlantic Salmon (Salmo salar L.) According to Their Wild, Farmed, and Geographical Origin. DOI: 10.1021/jf8039268.

[41] Standal, G. B., Axelson, D. E., & Aursand, M. (2010). ^{13}C NMR as a tool for authentication of different gadoid fish species with emphasis on phospholipid profiles. *Food Chemistry*, 121(2), 608-615.

[42] Karoui, R., Kemps, B., Bamelis, F., De Ketelaere, B., Decuypere, E., & De Baerdemaeker, J. (2000). Development of a rapid method based on front face fluorescence spectroscopy for the monitoring of egg freshness: evolution of thick and thin egg albumens. DOI: 10.1007/s00217-005-0204-x.

[43] Karoui, R., Kemps, B., Bamelis, F., De Ketelaere, B., Merten, K., Schoonheydt, R., Decuypere, E., & De Baerdemaeker, J. (2006). Development of a rapid method based on front-face fluorescence spectroscopy for the monitoring of egg freshness: 2 -evolution of egg yolk. DOI: 10.1007/s00217-005-0179-7.

[44] Karoui, R., Thomas, E., & Dufour, E. (2006). Utilisation of a rapid technique based on front-face fluorescence spectroscopy for differentiating between fresh and frozen-thawed fish fillets. . Food Research International; ., 39-349.

[45] Guimet, F., Ferre, J., & Boque, R. (2005). Rapid detection of olive-pomace oil adulteration in extra virgin olive oils from the protected denomination of origin"Siurana using excitation-emission fluorescence spectroscopy and three-way methods of
analysis. *Analytica Chimica Acta*, 544-143.

[46] Poulli, K. I., Mousdis, G. A., & Georgiou, C. A. (2005). Classification of edible and
lampante virgin olive oil based on synchronous fluorescence and total luminescence
spectroscopy. DOI: 10.1016/j.aca.2005.03.061.

[47] Dankowska, A., & Malecka, M. (2009). Application of synchronous fluorescence spectroscopy for determination of extra virgin olive oil adulteration. DOI: 10.1002/ejlt.
200800295.

[48] Twomey, M., Downey, G., & Mc Nulty, P. B. (1995). The potential of NIR spectroscopy for the detection of the adulteration of orange juice. .Journal of the Science of
Food and Agriculture , 67-77.

[49] Contal, L., Leon, V., & Downey, G. (2002). Detection and quantification of apple
adulteration in strawberry and raspberry purees using visible and near infrared
spectroscopy. DOI: 10.1255/jnirs.345.

[50] Vardin, H., Tay, A., Ozen, B., & Mauer, L. (2008). Authentication of pomegranate
juice concentrate using FTIR spectroscopy and chemometrics. *Food Chemistry*,
108-742.

[51] Fugel, R., Carle, R., & Schieber, A. (2005). Quality and authenticity control of fruit
purees, fruit preparations and jams: a review. *Trends in Food Science and Technology*,
16-433.

[52] Paradkar, M. M., Sivakesava, S., & Irudayaraj, J. (2002). Discrimination and classification of adulterants in maple syrup with the use of infrared spectroscopic techniques.
DOI: 10.1002/jsfa.1332.

[53] Sivakesava, S., & Irudayaraj, J. (2002). Classification of simple and complex sugar
adulterants in honey by midinfrared spectroscopy. *International Journal of Food Science
and Technology*, 37-351.

[54] Syahariza, Z. A., Che Man, Y. B., Selamat, J., & Bakar, J. (2005). Detection of lard
adulteration in cake formulation by Fourier transform infared (FTIR) spectroscopy.
Food Chemistry, 92-365.

[55] Che Man, Y. B., Syahariza, Z. A., Mirghani, M. E. S., Jinap, S., & Bakar, J. (2005). Analysis of potential lard adulteration in chocolate and chocolate products using Fourier
transform infrared spectroscopy. *Food Chemistry*, 90-815.

[56] Rohman, A., & Che Man, Y. B. (2010). Fourier transform infrared (FTIR) spectroscopy
for analysis of extra virgin olive oil adulterated with palm oil. *Food Research International*, 43(3), 886-892.

[57] Lerma-Garcia, M. J., Ramis-Ramos, G., Herreo-Martinez, J. M., & Simo-Alfonso, J. M. (2010). Authentication of extravirginoliveoils by Fourier-transform infrared spectroscopy. *Food Chemistry*, 118(1), 78-83.

[58] Koca, N., Kocaoglu-Vurma, N. A., Harper, W. J., & Rodriguez-Saona, L. E. (2010). Application of temperature controlled attenuated total reflectance-mid-infared (ATR-MIR) spectroscopy for rapid estimation of butter adulteration. *Food Chemistry*, 121-778.

[59] Downey, G., & Beauchene, D. (1997). Discrimination between fresh and frozen-then-thawed beef m. Longissimus dorsi by combined visible-near infrared reflectance spectroscopy: A feasibility study. *Meat Science*, 45-353.

[60] Marina, A. M., Che Man, Y. B., Nazimah, S. A. H., & Amin, I. (2009). Monitoring the adulteration of virgin coconut oil by selected vegetable oils using differential scanning calorimetry. *Journal of Lipid Science*, 16(1), 50-61.

[61] Smiddy, M. A., Huppertz, T., & van Ruth, S. (2012). Triacylglycerol and melting profiles of milk fat from several species. *International Dairy journal*, 24(2), 64-69.

[62] Nurjuliana, N., Che Man, Y. B., & Mat Hashim, D. (2011). Analysis of Lard's Aroma by an Electronic Nose for Rapid Halal Authentication. *Journal of the American Oil Chemical Society*, 88-75.

[63] Oliveros, M. C. C., Pavon, J. L. P., Pinto, C. G., Laespada, M. E. F., Cordero, B. M., & Forina, M. (2002). Electronic nose based on metal oxide semiconductor sensors as a fast alternative for the detection of adulteration of virgin olive oils. *Analytica Chimica Acta*, 459-219.

[64] Penza, M., & Cassano, G. (2004). Chemometric characterization of Italian wines by thin-film multisensors array and artificial neural networks. *Food Chemistry*, 86-283.

[65] Pillonel, L., Ampuero, S., Tabacchi, R., & Bosset, J. O. (2003). Analytical methods for the determination of the geographic origin of Emmental cheese: Volatile compounds by GC/MS-FID and electronic nose. *European Food Research and Technology*, 216-179.

[66] Eide, I., & Zahlsen, K. (2007). Chemical Fingerprinting of Biodiesel Using Electrospray Mass Spectrometry and Chemometrics: Characterization, Discrimination, Identification, and Quantification in Petrodiesel. *Energy & Fuels*, 21-3702.

[67] Schale, S. P., Le , T. M., & Pierce, K. M. (2012). Predicting feedstock and percent composition for blends of biodiesel with conventional diesel using chemometrics and gas chromatography-mass spectrometry. *Talanta*, http://dx.doi.org/10.1016/j.talanta. 2012.03.050.

[68] Corgozinho, C. N. C., Pasa, V. N. D., & Barbeira, P. J. S. (2008). Determination of residual oil in diesel oil by spectrofluorimetric and chemometric analysis. *Talanta*, 76(2), 479-484.

[69] Haddad, R., Catharino, R. R., Marques, L. A., & Eberlin, M. N. (2008). Perfume fingerprinting by easy ambient sonic-spray ionization mass spectrometry: nearly instan-

taneous typification and counterfeit detection. *Rapid Communication in Mass Spectrometry*, 22-3662.

[70] Marques, L. A., Catharino, R. R., Bruns, R. E., & Eberlin, M. N. (2006). Electrospray ionization mass spectrometry fingerprinting of perfumes: rapid classification and counterfeit detection. *Rapid Communication in Mass Spectrometry*, 20(24), 3654-3658.

[71] Cano, M., Borrego, V., Roales, J., Idigoras, J., Lopes-Costa, T., Mendoza, P., & Pedrosa, J. M. (2011). Rapid discrimination and counterfeit detection of perfumes by an electronic olfactory system. *Sensors and Actuators B: Chemical*, 156(1), 319-324.

[72] Souza, R. C. Z., Eiras, M. M., Cabral, E. C., Barata, L. E. S., Eberlin, M. N., & Catharino, R. R. (2011). The Famous Amazonian Rosewood Essential Oil: Characterization and Adulteration Monitoring by Electrospray Ionization Mass Spectrometry Fingerprinting. *Analytical Letters*, 44-2417.

[73] Cabral, E.C., Simas, R.C., Santos, V.G., Queiroga, C.L., da Cunha, V.S., de Sa, G.F., Daroda, M.J., & Eberlin, M.N. (2012). Wood typification by Venturi easy ambient sonic spray ionization mass spectrometry: the case of the endangered Mahogany tree. *Journal of Mass Spectrometry*, DOI 10.1002/jms.2016.

[74] Cordeiro, J. R., Martinez, M. I. V., Li, R. W. C., Cardoso, A. P., Nunes, L. C., Krug, F. J., Taixao, T. R. L. C., Nomura, C. S., & Gruber, J. (2012). Identification of Four Wood Species by an Electronic Nose and by LIBS International. *Journal of Electrochemistry*, doi:10.1155/2012/563939.

[75] Laasonen, M., Harmia-Pulkkinen, T., Simard, C. L., Michiels, E., Rasanen, M., & Vuorela, H. (2002). Fast identification of Echinacea purpurea dried roots using near-infrared spectroscopy. *Analytical Chemistry*, 74-2493.

Chapter 7

Novel Analytical Tools
for Quality Control in Food Science

Christian W. Huck

Additional information is available at the end of the chapter

1. Introduction

Due to the fast technological and data treatment advancements new insights into food can be considered. The application of these novel analytical techniques belongs to the responsibility of food chemists and analysts. Thereby, an increase in efficiency is based on an improved lower limit of detection (LOD), selectivity to separate analytes of interest and speed of analysis.

High-performance liquid chromatography (HPLC) belongs to the traditional separation techniques applied to a broad range of hydrophilic and hydrophobic ingredients in both the reversed-phase (RP) [1] as well as normal-phase (NP) [2] mode. In a conventional HPLC system the inner diameter of the separation column, which is the core of the separation unit, is 4.6 mm. During the last decade miniaturization down to 20 μm allowed to increase on one side the sensitivity and on the other side speed of analysis could be enhanced dramatically. Therefore, novel stationary phases mainly based on polymers have been designed and brought to the market to enable both the separation of low and high-molecular weight analytes [3]. As an alternative separation technique capillary electrophoresis (CE), which separates analytes due to their different ion mobility based on charge and molecular weight in an electric field within a fused silica capillary having an inner diameter of approximately 200 μm can be applied [4]. Thereby, the appearance of the electroosmotic flow (EOF) can influence the separation efficiency by either speeding up the separation process or by improving the resolution. Capillary electrochromatography (CEC) is a hybrid technique of both HPLC and CE in which both pressure and an electrical field are applied and enables extreme high resolution. The drawback of this separation method is the fact, that real samples can hardly be analysed due to the disturbance by the matrix [5]. In many cases the analyte of interest is only available in very low concentrations. Therefore, selective enrichment and purification steps are the method of choice, which can be accomplished by solid-phase extraction (SPE). Therefore, a material designed for a special analytical question is filled into a cartridge or pipette tip and the sample of interest is put onto the material in liquid form [6]. In the following, analytes of interest can interact with the functional groups of the stationary phase and compounds being not of interest can simply be washed away. In the final elution step, only some micro liters of liquid are required to elute the analytes of interest from the stationary phase being available in relatively high concentrations for the following analytical steps. The following analytical procedure can be either a separation or spectroscopic method. Spectroscopic methods at this stage of the analytical procedure either include mass spectrometry (MS) and/or vibrational spectroscopy, respectively. In MS most of the samples are analysed applying electrospray ionization (ESI) as an interface with different types of mass detectors including e.g. time of flight (TOF), ion trap, ion cyclotron and quadrupoles. As an alternative, matrix assisted laser desorption ionization time of flight mass spectrometry (MALDI-TOF/MS) can be applied for the determination of high molecular weight compounds including proteins, peptides and lipids. For the analysis of low molecular ingredients < 1000 Da the so called matrix-free laser desorption ionization (mf-LDI) MS technique must be applied [7].Vibrational spectroscopy in the field of food analysis is mainly applied in the mid (400 – 4000 cm^{-1}) as well as in the near infrared (4000 – 12000 cm^{-1}) of the electromagnetic spectrum. In combination with chemo metrical algorithms these methods can be used for the authentication of the material on one hand, on the other hand quantitative analysis allows to control selected quality parameters [8].

In the following a systematic analytical approach is introduced, which allows combining the different analytical techniques in a synergistic manner to get deeper insights into the composition and origin of food samples.

2. Systematic analytical approach

The key technologies described in the above chapter can be combined according to the scheme depicted in Figure 1. In this approach extraction of the material for the further analytical steps and individual procedures can be linked to sample enrichment/purification, separation, vibrational spectroscopy and mass spectroscopy followed by database analysis. The different parts are described in the following sub-chapters.

2.1. Sample enrichment/purification

In many cases interesting analytes are only available in extremely low concentrations and/or in very complex matrices, respectively. Therefore, pre-concentration steps based on solid-phase extraction (SPE) can be very helpful. Nano-materials such as nanotubes, fullerenes, diamond offer excellent physiochemical properties due to a high ratio of surface to size, which results in a high capacity and allows analyte detection with high sensitivity down to the femtomole range in the case when mass spectrometry is applied for detection. Especially carbon nano materials can be easily further derivatised with a number of different functional groups including reversed-phase (RP), normal-phase (NP), ion exchange (IEX), immobilized affinity (IMAC) and so on depending on the specific demand. As an alternative they can be incorporated into a polymer matrix for highly selective extraction by certain compound characteristics. For the practical handling pipette tips have been tested to be most suitable and this special type of SPE is called "hollow monolithic incorporated tip" as it has an open flow channel in the middle enabling an easy pipetting procedure. For the highly efficient pre-concentration of phosphopeptides nano particular TiO_2, ZrO_2 and mixtures thereof are incorporated into a polymer matrix as depicted in Figure 2 [9]. By this technique hundreds of microliters can be flushed over the system and finally elution of the desired compounds to be analysed is carried out with only a few microliters causing a dramatic increase in concentration from which further analytical investigations can benefit due to the easier handling of the systematic investigation.

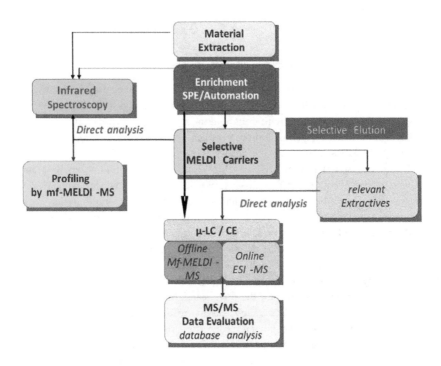

Figure 1. Multidimensional analytical approach

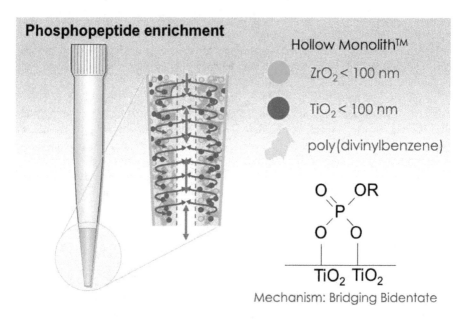

Figure 2. TiO$_2$, ZrO$_2$ incorporated into a polymer matrix for phosphopeptide enrichment

Immobilisation of such polymers into pipette tips with trypsin can be used for fast digestion of peptides and proteins within only a few minutes ensuring high capacity and sequence coverage (Figure 3) even in the high-throughput mode using robotic pipetting systems [10]. In comparison to this quite young approach the conventional digestion procedure lasts approximately 24 hours and doesn't show in any case better results by higher sequence coverages. For this reason this approach is of high interest for the routine analysis and/or diagnostics, respectively. As a carrier glycidylmethacrylate-co-divinylbenzene (GMA/DVB) polymerized in pipette tips was chosen. The major advantages of in-tip digestion are easy handling and small sample amount required for analysis. Microwave-assisted digestion was applied for highly efficient and time saving proteolysis. Adaption to an automated robotic system allowed fast and reproducible sample treatment. Investigations with matrix-assisted laser desorption/ionization time-of-flight mass spectrometry (MALDI-TOF/MS) and liquid chromatography coupled to electrospray-ionization mass spectrometry (LC-ESI/MS) attested high sequence coverages (SCs) for the three standard proteins, myoglobin (Myo, 89%), bovine serum albumin (BSA, 78%) and alpha-casein (α-Cas, 83%). Compared to commercially available trypsin tips clear predominance concerning the digestion performance was achieved. Storability was tested over a period of several weeks and results showed only less decrease (<5%) of protein sequence coverages. The application of microwave-assisted in-tip digestion (2 minutes) with full automation by a robotic system allows high-throughput analysis (96 samples within 80 minutes) and highly effective proteolysis.

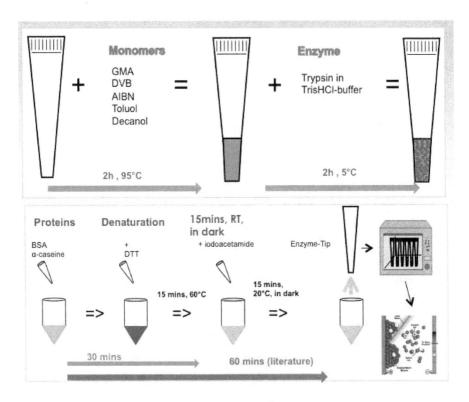

Figure 3. Trypsin immobilized pipette tips for high-throughput analysis of peptides

2.2. Selective MELDI-carriers

Material enhanced laser desorption ionisation (MELDI) is a method, which is based on the conventional matrix assisted laser desorption ionisation time of flight mass spectrometric (MALDI-TOF/MS) detection with the significant difference that before LDI MS step a selective enrichment procedure is carried out for the distinct analysis of a certain compound class. Compared to other similar techniques in this field, this approach benefits from the physical properties of the material itself (pore size, surface area, capacity, etc.) and its chemical derivatisation/functionalisation. In the past this technique was proven to be highly efficient for the analysis of biomarkers following an optimised strategy (Figure 4). In the first step a selected material including e.g., nanotubes, fullerenes, nano-crystalline diamond, polymers, cellulose, etc., which are derivatised with functional groups (C18, IMAC (immobilised metal affinity chromatography), IEX and others) is activated and the serum sample of interest is incubated. During this step, selective binding of molecules according to their functional group is achieved and finally undesired components can be washed away applying an optimised protocol. In the next step the incubated material is put onto a conventional steel target used in MALDI-TOF/MS, a matrix substance is added (e.g., sinapinic acid) and finally the mass spectrum is generated by the laser desorption ionisation process. The result is a mass spectrum being characteristic for a patient and/or the nutrition profile. Multivariate analysis (MVA) can be applied for further data analysis and interpretation, a clustering into certain stages of an illness can be achieved, respectively. From the mass spectrum potent biomarker molecules can be selected and identified by further analytical steps. The biomarker itself and/or the profile of the corresponding mass spectrum can be used for the screening of certain diseases, stages therefrom, allergies, nutrition effects and so on [7].

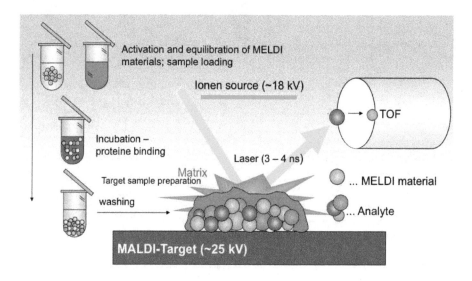

Figure 4. Principle of material enhanced laser desorption ionization (MELDI)

For the analysis of low-molecular weight compounds (MW < 1000 Da) the conventional MELDI approach is replaced by the matrix-free (mf) MELDI approach for which the addition of a matrix substance is not required so that no disturbing peaks appear. In this approach a conventional steel target with a 50 nm thick titanium oxide layer can be applied fulfilling all requirements for a successful laser desorption ionization process [11].

As an alternative the incubated analytes of interest can be selectively eluted from the functinalised carrier material and further analysed by liquid chromatography (LC) or capillary electrophoresis (CE).

2.3. Liquid chromatography, capillary electrophoresis and electrochromatography

Novel materials used in miniaturised liquid chromatography (μ-LC) are mainly polymer based, e.g. poly(1,2-bis(p-vinylphenyl)ethane). These polymers possess the huge advantage that chemical (composition of the polymer) and physical parameters including mainly porosity can be adjusted [12]. Extensive investigations on polymerisation time and temperature have been carried out enabling a tailored design of micro-, meso- and macro-pore distribution [13, 14]. This results in the applicability of such capillaries with an inner diameter between 20 and 200 μm for even the separation of high- and low-molecular weight compounds. These capillaries can be highly successfully applied analysing peptides, proteins, oligonucleotides, DNA fragments as well as "small molecules" such as phenols, flavonoids, catechins, acids etc. Figure 5 shows as an example the separation of olive oil ingredients. This separation is characterised by a very high ratio of flow to back pressure, which is of high interest to perform extremely rapid Coupling to mass spectrometry enables a highly efficient analysis even of crude samplesoffering all the possibilities of collision induced dissociation (CID) and database search [15].

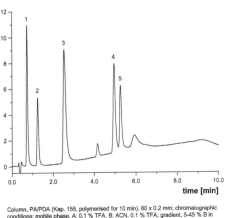

Column, PA/PDA (Kap. 155, polymerised for 10 min), 80 x 0.2 mm; chromatographic conditions: mobile phase, A: 0.1 % TFA, B: ACN, 0.1 % TFA; gradient, 5-45 % B in 10 min; flow rate, 8 μl/min; temperature, RT; detection, UV 210 nm; Peak identification: (1) Hydroxytyrosol, (2) Tyrosol, (3) Caffeic acid, (4) Vanillin and (5) Oleuropein.

Figure 5. Separation of olive oil ingredients using a monolithic capillary column. Conditions: capillary 80 x 0.2 mm; mobile phase, A: 0.1% TFA; B: CAN; gradient, 5-45%B in 10 min; Flow rate 8 μl/min; temperature, RT; detection, UV 210 nm. Peak assignment, (1) hydroxytyrosol, (2) tyrosol, (3) caffeic acid, (4) vanillin, (5) oleuropein.

As an alternative separation method capillary electrophoresis (CE) and /or electrochromatography (CEC) can be applied. In CE separation of analytes is achieved due to their different ion mobility based on charge and molecular weight in an electric field within a fused silica capillary having an inner diameter of approximately 200 μm [4]. As has already been remarked the electroosmotic flow (EOF) has a main influence on the separation and can be used for speeding up. In CEC both an electrical field and high pressure are applied resulting in high resolution. This technique can be applied to check the identification and purity of standards compounds with very high efficiency. For the reproducible separation and analysis of food ingredients such as phenols, acids, peptides, lipids, coating of the capillary´s inner wall was shown being advantageous as irreversible analyte adsorption by free hydroxyl-groups from the silanole of the fused silica capillary can be avoided. Latex-diol

and fullerene coated capillaries were successfully introduced and as a detection system on-
line hyphenation to MALDI-TOF/MS was shown to be highly efficient not only for the investigation of flavonoids but also for peptides, especially phosphorylated (Figure 6) [16, 17].
This system can be used for the investigation of the casein profile in milk offering the advantage over all other more classical analysis tools that in this case also higher phosphorylated species can be separated and detected. From the ratio of different phosphorylation
degrees several interpretations concerning the quality but also the origin of the milk can be
carried out.

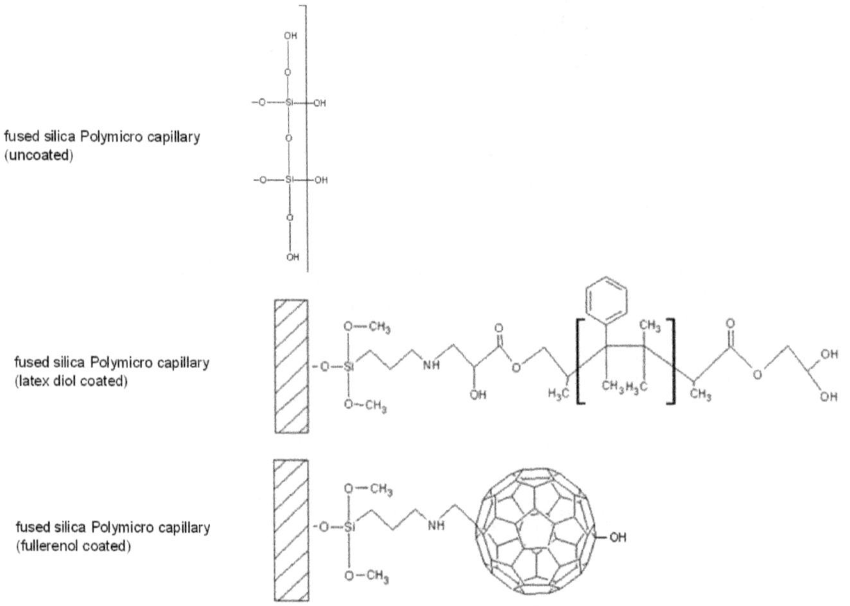

Figure 6. Inner capillary wall coatings applied in CE and CEC

2.4. Vibrational spectroscopy

For quality control both mid- (MIR, 400 – 4000 cm^{-1}) and near-infrared (NIR, 4000 – 12000
cm^{-1}) can be conducted. In MIR fundamental stretching and bending vibrations occur, in
NIR the corresponding overtones and combination vibrations are detected. This means that
NIR-spectra can contain a lot of more vibrational information, which is an advantage for the
analysis of highly complex samples. Therefore, during the last decade several applications
in the field of food analysis were developed in the NIR region. Samples can be analysed either in transmission, reflectance and interactance mode (Figure 7) so that liquid as well as
solid samples can be investigated. Due to the quite broad bands compared to MIR, chemo-
metrical spectra treatment is required for establishing adequate calibration models and to

analyse data. These are mainly multivariate (MVA) methods allowing to correct baseline, atmospheric noise etc. For qualitative analysis in most cased principal component analysis (PCA), for quantitative partial least square regression (PLSR) are applied [18].

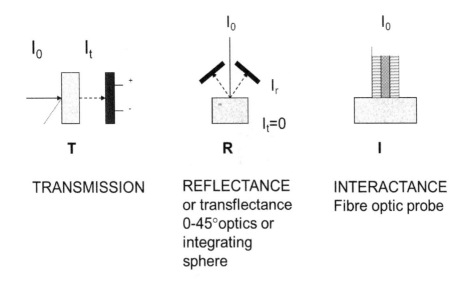

Figure 7. Sample measurement modes in NIR

An impressive example for the successful implementation in the food related production is the quality control of wine. It has been shown that NIR can be used to identify grapes, vines, age by qualitative (Figure 8) and its ingredients (acids, carbohydrates, pH etc.) simultaneously, non-invasively within a few seconds by quantitative analysis [19]. Another big advantage of this method can be found by the fact that the sample is not destroyed and can therefore be used for further purposes including following analytical steps.

Quantitative NIRS methods, which allow determining the carbohydrate, total acid, tartaric acid, malic acid, pH in grape variety and the polyphenol content in grapes were established [19]. The method can control the quality already at a very early stage during the wine production and allows improvement of its quality by this. Grapes of 12 different vines (*Weißburgunder, Chardonnay, Ruländer, Silvaner, Müller Thurgau, Gewürztraminer, Sauvignon, Lagrein, Grossvernatsch, Blauburgunder, Cabernet, Merlot*) were harvested in autumn 2000 and squeezed. The obtained grape variety was thermo stated at 23°C and analyzed quantitatively by NIRS in the transflection mode using an optical thin layer thickness of 1 mm. In order to establish a calibration model 252 spectra of samples with lower and upper concentration as a reference were recorded. 76 % of all spectra were randomly used for calibration, 24% for validation. Data preparation was carried out in order to minimize technical influences, which mainly cause a drift in baseline. Quantitative analysis was carried out by partial least square regression (PLSR).

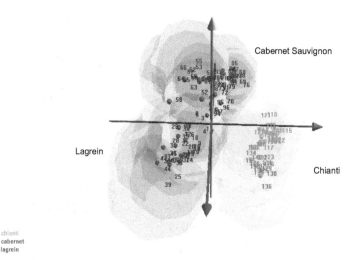

Figure 8. Factor plot of 141 specta of different wines (Lagrein, Chianti, Cabernet Sauvignon). Conditions: Normalisation, 1. derivative; wavenumber range, 4500 - 10000 cm⁻¹; thickness 3 mm; scans, 10; temperature, 23°C.

Carbohydrates. Data preparation comprised normalization between 0 and 1 and following calculation of the first derivative using a wavenumber range from 4500 - 7548 cm⁻¹. The PRESS function showed that 3 factors were needed for the calculation of the model. Calculation with 3 factors resulted in a good conformity between SEE and SEP. Linear regression between true and predicted values resulted in a value for the correlation coefficient of R^2=0.99 for calibration and R^2=0.99 for validation. Results for SEE and SEP: 0.13° KMW and 0.11 °KMW, the BIAS value is 2.30×10^{-15}.

Total acids. PLSR in a concentration range between 5 and 11 g/l included normalization between 0 and 1, full multiplicative scatter correction (MSC) and calculation of the 1st derivative (Taylor 3 points) between 4500 and 7548 cm⁻¹. 3 factors were necessary to obtain a minimum for PRESS and an agreement between SEE (0.60 g/l) and SEP (0.61 g/l) of nearly 100%.The highly linear model allows determining the total acid content with a prediction error of 0.61 g/l.

Tartaric acid. After normalization, performing of the 1st derivative over between 4500 and 7308 cm⁻¹, four factors were used for creation of the highly linear model depicted in Figure 6c with R^2=0.91 for calibration and R^2=0.87 for validation). Despite the small concentration range between 3.1 and 6.7 g/l used for calibration this system allows to determine the tartaric acid content in grape variety with an absolute error of estimation of 0.40 g/l and prediction of 0.54 g/l.

Malic acid. Malic acid often shows 2-5 times higher values compared to tartaric acid. Calibration between 2.9 and 7.0 g/l after normalization between 0 and 1 and calculation of a second smoothened derivative was carried out using three factors, SEE and SEP showing acceptable agreement.Absolute values for SEE, and BIAS were 0.43 g/l and $-4.25 \times 10^{-15.}$ Straight line for calibration showed a linearity of $R^2 = 0.89$ and allowed a prediction of the malic acid content with an absolute error of 0.55 g/l.

pH. Normalization and calculation of the smoothed 2nd derivative between 4500 and 7308 cm^{-1} showed an optimum for BIAS at five factors. Despite the narrow calibration range of pH 3.09 - 3.74 the calibration equation shows a R^2 of 0.82.

In order to enable the determination of these parameters with only one single measurement, simultaneous analysis of the carbohydrate, total acid, tartaric acid, malic acid content and pH was achieved by performing normalization (between 0 and 1) and calculating its 2nd derivative (Taylor 3 points). Four factors over a wavenumber range from 4500 to 7308 cm^{-1} showed 73-100% agreement between SEE and SEP. Linear regression showed high linearity for each investigated parameter with slightly lower values for R^2. Compared to the above-described single analysis this method allows a quantitative analysis of all parameters at once within a few seconds. Values for SEP are slightly increased (Table 1).

Polyphenols mainly influence taste, sensory properties and color of a wine. Therefore, a rapid method to analyze its quantity is important. The method according to Folin - Ciocalteu was used as a reference method (see Materials and Methods). Gallic acid-1-hydrate was used as reference standard in a concentration range from 0 to 4.93 µg/ml with equidistant steps. 24 gallic acid-1-hydrate solutions in a concentration range between 0.442 and 7.08 mg/ml were measured in the transmission mode threefold and in random order by NIRS. Evaluation using PLSR was achieved by dividing 72-recorded spectra randomly into a calibration (54 spectra) and validation (18 spectra) set. Data pretreatment comprised normalization between 0 and 1 and calculation of the 1st derivative (Savitzky-Golay) between 4008-7512 cm^{-1}. Using three factors, the PRESS function showed a minimum and a good agreement between SEE (0.45 mg/ml) and SEP (0.46 mg/ml). Linear regression between predicted and true values allowed to predict the gallic acid-1-hydrate concentration between 0 and 7 mg/ml with $R^2 = 0.98$.

In order to determine the total polyphenol concentration 30 must samples were measured in the transmission mode threefold and in random order. 90 spectra were divided into 72 calibration and 18 validation spectra. Normalization and performing of the 1st derivative allowed minimizing shifts in the baseline. 4 factors were necessary to obtain a minimum for the PRESS function and to get a maximum agreement of SEE and SEP. Linear regression allowed correlating true and predicted values with a R^2 of 0.97. Compared to the traditionally used Folin - Ciocalteu method in a winery, which is very time-consuming and expensive due to the usage of different chemicals, the NIRS method is very simple, precise and incomparably fast.

Parameter	Unit	SEE		SEP		BIAS	
		a	b	a	b	a	b
Carbohydrates	KMW	0.13	0.21	0.11	0.19	2.30×10^{-15}	3.33×10^{-16}
Total acids	g/l	0.60	0.43	0.61	0.53	7.17×10^{-15}	-1.08×10^{-14}
Tartaric acid	g/l	0.40	0.41	0.54	0.55	-1.08×10^{-14}	-3.43×10^{-15}
Malic acid	g/l	0.43	0.49	0.55	0.65	-4.25×10^{-15}	-2.44×10^{-15}
pH		0.07	0.09	0.06	0.09	-1.26×10^{-15}	-7.15×10^{-15}

Note. a Single analysis; b Simultaneous analysis

Table 1. Prediction results for the determination of the carbohydrate, total acid, tartaric acid, malic acid content and pH

Quality control of coffee ingredients including caffeine, theobromine and theophylline [20] and of food additives deriving from the highly interesting field of Traditional Chinese Medicine (TCM) [21] can be carried out in a similar way. Thereby, emphasis must be put onto the calibration method for which the above mentioned techniques can be applied as a reference. A new analytical method based on near infrared spectroscopy (NIRS) for the quantitation of the three main alkaloids caffeine (Caf), theobromine (Tbr) and theophylline (Tph) in roasted coffee after discrimination of the rough green beans into Arabic and Robusta was established. This validated method was compared to the most commonly used liquid chromatography (LC) connected to UV and mass spectrometric (MS) detection. As analysis time plays an important role in choosing a reference method for the calibration of the NIR-spectrometer, the non-porous silica-C18 phase offers a very fast method. Coupling of the optimised LC method to a mass spectrometer (MS) via an electrospray ionisation (ESI) interface not only allowed to identify Caf, Tbr and Tph by their characteristic fragmentation pattern using collisionally induced dissociation (CID), but also to quantitate the content of the three analytes, which was found to be 6% higher compared to UV-detection. The validated LC–UV method was chosen as a reference method for the calibration of the NIRS system. Analysis of 83 liquid coffee extracts in random order resulted for Caf and Tbr in values for S.E.E. (standard error of estimation) of 0.34, 0.40 g/100 g, S.E.P. (standard error of prediction) of 0.07 and 0.10 g/100 g with correlation coefficients of 0.86 and 0.85 in a concentration range between 0.10 and 4.13 g/100 g. Compared to LC the lower limit of detection (LOD) of the NIRS-method is found at 0.05 g/100 g compared to 0.244–0.60 ng/100 g in LC, which makes it impossible to analyse Tph by NIRS.

The possibility to hyphenate a MIR/NIR spectrometer to a microscope unit allows determining the distribution of active ingredients within a tissue sample down to a resolution of 1.2 μm [22]. A "hyperspectral cube" is recorded with the dimensions of the sample on the x- and y-axis and the absorbance on the z-axis from which the image can be extracted (Figure 9).

Fourier Transform Infrared (FTIR) spectroscopic imaging and mapping techniques have become essential tools for the detection and characterization of the molecular components of biological tissues and the modern analytical techniques enabling molecular imaging of complex samples. These techniques are based on the absorption of IR radiations by vibrational transitions in covalent bonds and their major advantage is the acquisition of local molecular expression profiles, while maintaining the topographic integrity of the tissue by avoiding time-consuming extraction, purification and separation steps. These new techniques enable global analysis of biological samples with high spatial resolution and provide unique chemical-morphological information about the tissue status. With these non-destructive examination methods it is possible to get qualitative and quantitative information of heterogeneous samples.

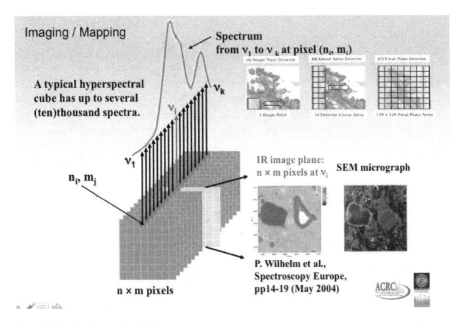

Figure 9. Principle of hyperspectral cube

Additionally, MALDI-TOF/MS imaging can be applied from the same sample of interest to get knowledge concerning the molecular weight distribution. This method is also suitable for studying the effect of nutrition onto different kinds of diseases, e.g. prostate cancer.

3. Conclusions

The techniques described can be applied according to the scheme depicted in Figure 1. This systematic analytical strategy allows getting multifacial knowledge and insights into food and samples derived therefrom.

Acknowledgements

This work was financially supported by the Efre-project "Originalp" (EU) and Agrarmarketing Austria (AMA, Vienna, Austria).

Author details

Christian W. Huck

Institute of Analytical Chemistry and Radiochemistry, CCB – Center for Chemistry and Biomedicine, Innsbruck, Austria

References

[1] Huck C.W., Popp M., Scherz H., Bonn G.K.Development and Evaluation of a New Method for the Determination of the Carotenoid Content in Selected Vegetables by HPLC and HPLC-MS/MS.J. Chromatogr. Sci. (2000). , 38-441.

[2] Stöggl, W. M., Huck, C. W., Scherz, H., Bonn, G. K., Analysis, of., Vitamin, E., in, Food., Phytopharmaceutical, Preparations., by, H. P. L. C., -A, H. P. L. C., -M, P. C. I., & , S. M. S. Chromatographia (2001). , 54-179.

[3] JakschitzT., HuckC.W., LubbadS., Bonn G.K.Monolithic Poly(TMSM-DMSBMS) Stationary Phases for the fast Separation of Oligonucleotides and Proteins.J. Chromatogr. A (2007). , 1147-53.

[4] Huck C.W., Bakry R., Bonn G.K.Progress in capillary electrophoresis of biomarkers and metabolites between 2002 and 2005.Electrophoresis (2006). , 27-111.

[5] Stöggl W.M., Huck C.W., Stecher G., Bonn G.K., Capillary Electrochromatography of Biologically Relevant Flavonoids. (2006). *Electrophoresis*, 27-787.

[6] Huck C.W., Bonn G.K.Review: Polymer based sorbents for solid-phase extraction.J. Chromatogr. A (2000). , 885-51.

[7] Feuerstein I., Najam-ul-Haq M., Rainer M., Trojer L., Bakry R., Hidayat Aprilita N., Stecher G., Huck C.W., Klocker H., Bartsch G., Guttman A., BonnG.K.Material Enhanced Laser Desorption/Ionization (MELDI)- a new protein profiling tool utilizing specific carrier materials for TOF-MS Analysis.J. Am. Soc. Mass Spectrom. (2006). , 17-1203.

[8] Petter C.H., Heigl N., Bachmann S., Huck-Pezzei V.A.C., Najam-ul-Haq M., Bakry R., Bernkop-Schnürch A., Bonn G.K., Huck*C.W.Near Infrared Spectroscopy Compared to Liquid Chromatography Coupled to Mass Spectrometry and Capillary Electrophoresis as a Detection Tool for Peptide Reaction Monitoring.Amino Acids (2008).

[9]   Rainer, M., Sonderegger, H., Bakry, R., Huck, C. W., Morandell, S., Huber, L. A., Gjerde, D. T., & Bonn, G. K. Analysis of protein phosphorylation by monolithic extraction columns based on poly(divinylbenzene) containing embedded titanium dioxide and zirconium dioxide nano-powders. Proteomics (2008). , 8(21), 4593-4602.

[10] Hahn, H., Rainer, M., Ringer, T., Gjerde, D., Huck, C. W., & Bonn, G. K. Ultra-fast Microwave-Assisted In-Tip Digestion of Proteins. J. Proteom. Res. (2009). , 8(9), 4225-4230.

[11] Bonn, G. K., Bakry, R., Huck, C. W., Vallant, R., & Szabo, Z. Analysis of low molecular weight molecules by maldi-ms. Eur. Pat. Appl. ((2008). pp. CODEN: EPXXDW EP 1973142 A1 20080924 AN 2008:1151584

[12] Greiderer A., Clark Ligon S.Jr., Huck C.W., Bonn G.K.Monolithic poly(-bis(p-vinyl-phenyl)ethane capillary columns for simultaneous separation of low- and high-molecular weight compounds.J.Sep. Sci. (2009).

[13] Greiderer A., Trojer L., Huck C.W., Bonn G.K.Influence of the Polymerisation time on the Porous and Chromatographic Properties of Monolithic Poly(1,2-bis(p-vinyl-phenyl)ethane Capillary Columns.J.Chromatogr. A (2009). , 1216(45), 7747-7754.

[14] Heigl, N., Greiderer, A., Petter, C. H., Siesler, H. W., Bonn, G. K., & Huck, C. W. Simultaneous Determination of Physical and Chemical Parameters of Monolithic Porous Polymers with a Combined Use of Fourier-Transform Near Infrared Diffuse Reflection Spectroscopy and Multivariate Techniques. Anal. Chem. (2008). , 80(22), 8493-8500.

[15] Trojer, L., Greiderer, A., Bisjak, C. P., Wieder, W., Heigl, N., Huck, C. W., Bonn, G. K., in, Handbook., of, H. P. L. C., Second, Edition., edited, by., Corradini, D., & Press, . (2010). Print 978-1-57444-554-1eBook ISBN: 978-1-4200-1694-9, 3-45.

[16] Bachmann S., Vallant R., Bakry R., Huck C.W., Corradini D., Bonn G.K.Capillary electrophoresis coupled to matrix assisted laser desorption ionization with novel covalently coated capillaries.Electrophoresis, (2010). , 31, 618-629.

[17] Stöggl W.M., Huck C.W., Stecher G., Bonn G.K.Capillary Electrochromatography of Biologically Relevant Flavonoids.Electrophoresis, (2006). , 27-787.

[18] Petter C.H., Heigl N., Bachmann S., Huck-Pezzei V.A.C., Najam-ul-Haq M., Bakry R., Bernkop-Schnürch A., Bonn G.K., Huck C.W.Near Infrared Spectroscopy Compared to Liquid Chromatography Coupled to Mass Spectrometry and Capillary Electrophoresis as a Detection Tool for Peptide Reaction Monitoring.Amino Acids, (2008). , 34(4), 605-616.

[19] Guggenbichler, W., Huck, C. W., Kobler, A., Bonn, G. K., Near, Infrared., Reflectance, Spectroscopy., Tool, A., for, Quality., Control, In., & Wine, Production. J. Food Agric. Environm., (2006). , 4(2), 98-106.

[20] Huck C.W., Guggenbichler W., Bonn G.K., Analysis of Caffeine, Theobromine and Theophylline in Coffee by Near Infrared Reflectance Spectroscopy (NIRS) Compared

to High Performance Liquid Chromatography (HPLC) Coupled to Mass Spectrometry.Anal. Chim. Acta, (2005). , 538-195.

[21] Mattle, C., Heigl, N., Bonn, G. K., & Huck, C. W. Near Infrared Diffuse Reflection Spectroscopy and Multivariate Calibration Hyphenated to Thin Layer Chromatography for Quality Control and Simultaneous Quantification of Methoxylated Flavones in a Phytomedicine. J. Planar Chromatogr., (2010). , 23(5), 348-352.

[22] Pezzei, C., Pallua, J. D., Schaefer, G., Seifarth, C., Huck-Pezzei, V., Bittner, L. K., Klocker, H., Bartsch, G., Bonn, G. K., Huck, C. W., Prostate, cancer., characterization, by., Fourier, Transform., & infrared, microspectroscopy. Mol. Biosys., (2010). , 6-2287.

Chapter 8

Principle of Meat Aroma Flavors and Future Prospect

Hoa Van Ba, Inho Hwang, Dawoon Jeong and
Amna Touseef

Additional information is available at the end of the chapter

1. Introduction

The population growth fact of the world has been much quickly increasing through the years. As reported by the United Nations Population Fund (UNFPA) the estimated world population of 6.1 billion in the year 2000 and reached to 7 billion in the year 2011, increased 0.9 billion people only after 10 years. The population increases always proportionally accompany to the consumption demands in which including foods. Calculating the global meat consumption only and based on the data collected from IFPRI/ FAO/ILRI by Delgado et al (1999) [1] suggested that global production and consumption of meat will continue to raise from 233 million metric tons in the year 2000 to 300 million metric tons in 2020. On the other hand, income growth of people in most of the countries especially in the developed countries has been significantly increasing in the recent years. Combination of the large populations together with a high-income that will give a big pressure for the food producers in general and meat producers in particular. As a consequence, higher income growth in countries has led to an increase in living standards and changes in consumer diets to include a higher proportion of meat and meat products. While, productivity and provision of meats on the markets has been limited and rising costs of production resulting in not keeping pace with the strong growth in demand, that has caused a rise in meat prices.

Although, a strong demand for meat amounts but consumers are getting quite fastidious to choose meat and meat products since consumer's preference for meat buying is strongly based on quality, freshness and hygiene. Quality factors are very important in the meat purchasing behavior of consumers including marbling (intramuscular fat tissues), texture, color, tenderness and especially flavor characteristics.

Aroma flavor characteristics of cooked meat in particular play the most important level in eating quality of meat, acceptance and preference by consumers. The aroma flavor characteristics of cooked meats are derived from volatile flavor components which derive from thermally induced reactions occurring during heating via the four pathways including (1) Maillard reaction of amino acid or peptides with reducing sugars, (2) Lipid oxidation, (3) interaction between Maillard reaction products with lipid-oxidized products and (4) vitamin degradation during cooking [2]. Aroma flavor is perceived through the nostrils (orthonasal aroma) it gives the first impression of a certain food. When the food is placed in the mouth, the volatile flavor compounds will be transferred through the pharynx to the olfactory receptors (retronasal aroma). It has been reported that flavors together with other sensory attributes such as tenderness and juiciness are specially considered the most important criterion of acceptability and the palatability of meat that affects consumer's purchasing decisions [3,4]. It has been well known that all volatile flavor components are organic and they have low molecular weight [5]. The chemical structures of volatile flavor classes are varied widely including aldehydes, ketones, hydrocarbons, pyrazines, acids, esters, alcohols, nitrogen and sulfur-containing compounds and other heterocyclic compounds as well. Due to the differences in chemical structures therefore their volatility is also quite different.

Many factors have been found to be as influences on the aroma flavors of cooked meat. Rabe et al (2003) [6] found that among all food constituents, lipids generally have the greatest influence on production of aroma flavor components, as they not only reduce the vapour pressure of most flavor compounds. Otherwise, Kinsella (1990) [7] showed that aroma compounds are more lipophilic than hydrophilic therefore fats act as a solvents for aroma compounds reducing their volatility. In addition to these effects, other factors such as diets, breed, sex, chiller ageing, meat pH, cooking conditions which all also affect the flavor [8, 9, 40, 11]

With the crucial importance of aroma flavor of meat for the acceptance and preference of consumers and as well as the factors influencing the generation of aroma flavor compounds as mentioned above, the present chapter aims to highlight the basic information regarding aroma flavor components in terms of mechanisms of formation pathways; current techniques being used for detection; factors that affect aroma flavors; and final ideas and as well as suggestions are also given out to improve flavor quality attributes according to criterion of acceptability, satisfaction and the palatability for consumer.

2. Meat aroma flavor

2.1.The importance of volatile flavor compounds in contributing to the flavor characteristics of cooked meat

Flavor characteristics of cooked meat are directly detected by the nose (i.e., olfactory receptors) before and during chewing. Raw meat has little aroma and only blood-like taste, meat develops its aroma flavor characteristics during cooking as the result of complex interaction of precursors derived from both the lean and fat compositions of meat generating volatile flavor compounds that contribute to meat flavor [12]. To date, approximately thousands of volatile flavor compounds have been detected and identified in cooked meat. There is a large number of these compounds contributing to the flavor characteristics of cooked meat have been identified in previous works [13, 14, 15, 16, 17, 18, 19].

As mentioned above, regarding the chemical structures of volatile flavor classes, among that the heterocyclic compounds especially those containing sulfur are the important flavor compounds produced in the Maillard reaction providing savory, meaty, roasty and boiled flavor characteristics. While, lipid-degraded- compounds which give 'fatty' aromas to cooked meat and compounds which determine some of the aroma flavor differences between meats from different species [20]. The individual volatile compounds have been found to determine distinct aroma flavors of cooked meat represent; dimethylsulfide, 2-butanone, ethyl acetate, 2- and 3-methylbutanal, 2-heptanone, dimethyl trisulphide and nonanal were detected as key flavor compounds of cooked Irish Angus beef, while methional, 2,4-nonadienal and bezothiazole were characterized as meaty, oily notes in cooked Belgian Blue, Limousin and Aberdeen Angus beefs [21]. Kerscher & Grosch, (1997) [22] reported that 2-furfurylthiol, 4-hydroxy-2,5-dimethyl-3(2H)-furanone and 2-methyl-3-furanthiol were the most important odorants of boiled beef. 2-ethyl-3,5-dimethyl pyrazine and 2,3-diethyl-5-methylpyrazine possess roasty, caramel-like, burnt and earthy notes of roasted beef [23]. Other carbonyl compounds such as methional, E-2-undecenal, E-2-dodecenal, decanal, heptanal and 2-methylbutanal also were found to be associated with roasty, sweet, fruity and fatty odor notes of cooked beef [14,17]. Also, a great number of studies considered on the objective volatile flavor components in cooked pork, chicken, lamb, ham and etc… have been documented over the last years [24, 25, 26]. In fact, although thousands of volatile compounds identified but not all of them are important because their high odor detection threshold, only some of them play a significant role in the overall aroma flavor characteristics of cooked meat. An aroma flavor compound with its distinct odor note can be defined as its flavor dilution factor indicating that at the lowest concentration at which the compound still can be detected by the sense of smell. Some represent volatile flavors active-compounds have been detected in cooked meats by using gas chromatography-olfactometry technique (GC-O) are showed in Table 1.

Compound name	Aroma flavor characteristics
Aldehydes	
Methional	Cooked potato, meaty
E,2-nonenal	Fatty
E,E,2,4-decadienal	Fatty
Benzenacetaldehyde	Sweet, honey
E,E,2,4-nonedienal	Fatty
Decanal	Sweet, fruity, like aldehydes, roasty
Heptanal	Fruity, fatty, sweet, oil
Nonanal	Sweet, fatty, green
Undecanal	Sweet, pungent, green
E,2-heptenal	Fatty
E,2-heptenal	Fatty

Hexanal	Green, fatty
E,2-hexenal	Green
E,Z,2,6-nonadienal	Cucumber
Undecanal	Sweet, pungent, green
2-methylbutanal	Pungent, sweet, roasty
E,2-undecenal	Sweet, fruity, fatty
2,E-dodecenal	Sweet, fruity, roasty, pungent
Ethanol	Grilled (weak), acetaldehyde-like
3-methylbutanal	Meaty, fish, rotten, aldehyde,valeric acid, fatty
Octanal	Green, lemon, citrus, aldehyde
E,E,2,4-heptadienal	Aldehyde, green, broth, spicy
Propanal	caramel, sweet, alcoholic, "cooked", broth, spicy
Butanal	smoky, fish, amylic, aldehyde-enal or dienal
Ketones	
2-octanone	Fruity, musty
2-decanone	Fruity, musty
2-dodecanone	Fruity, musty
1-octen-3-one	fresh, mushrooms, pungent, rubbery
3-octanone	Fruity, nutty, moldy, fatty, earthy
2,5-dimethyl-4-hydroxy-3(2H)-furanone	Roasted almonds, sweet
4,5-dihydro-5-propyl-2(3H)-furanone	Fruity, fatty, sweet, pungent, roasty
2,3-butanedione	Sweet, buttery
2-heptanone	Citrus grapefruit, limonene, floral, cheese
2,3-pentanedione	buttery, lemon-like, sweet, fruity
2-nonanone	Hot milk, soap, green, fruity, floral
3-octen-2-one	Nut, crushed bug, earthy, spicy, sweet, mushroom,
6-Methyl 2-heptanone	Cloves, menthol
2-undecanone	Fruity
2,2,6-Trimethylcyclohexanone	Mint, acetone
Alcohols	
1-octen-3-ol	Mushroom
Cyclobutanol	Roasted

1-heptanol	Fragrant, woody, oily, green, fatty, winey, sap
1-hexanol	Woody, cut grass, chemical-winey, fatty, fruity
2-Ethyl 1-hexanol	Resin, flower, green
1-octanol	Penetrating aromatic odor, fatty, waxy, citrus, oily,
2-Octen-1-ol	Green citrus
1-pentanol	Mild odor, fuel oil, fruit, balsamic
Propanol	Alcoholic
Hydrocarbons	
Ethenylbenzene	Pungent, aromatic, fragrant, roasty
1-undecen	Fatty, burnt, nutty, rubbery
Hexane	Faint peculiar odor
(Z)-3-Octene	Fruity, old apples
Pentane	Very slight warmed-over flavor, oxidized
Styrene	Penetrating odor, sweet smell
Tridecane	Alkane
Tetradecane	Alkane
Ethenylbenzene	Aromatic, fragrant, roasty
Pyrazines	
2-ethyl-3,5-dimethylpyrazin	Burnt, fragrant, meaty, green
2-ethenyl-3,6(5)-dimethylpyrazine	Sweet, cooked rice, fatty
2-ethyl-3,6-dimethylpyrazine	Burnt, roasty
2,3-diethyl-5-methylpyrazine	meaty, roasty, fragrant, sweet
2,5-dimethylpyrazine	Fried rice, popcorn, pungent, green
2-ethenyl-5(6)-methylpyrazine	Roasty break-like, cooked rice, coffee-like
2,5-dimethylpyrazine	Fried rice, popcorn, pungent, green
2-ethyl-5-methylpyrazine	Fruity, sweet, pungent
2-ethenyl-5(6)-methylpyrazine	Smoky, roasty, break-like, cooked rice, popcorn
2-ethyl-3,6-dimethylpyrazine	Burnt, pungent, roasty
2-ethenyl-3,6(5)-dimethylpyrazine	Pungent, sweet, cooked rice, fatty
2,3-diethyl-5-methylpyrazine	Meaty, roasty, fragrant, sweet
2-isopentyl-3,6-dimethylpyrazine	Sweet, fragrant, fatty, fruity, pungent
Sulfur & nitrogen containing compounds	
2-fufurylthiol	Roasty

2-acetyl-1-pyrroline	Roasted, sweet
2-formyl-5-methylthiophene	Sulfurous
2-methyl-3-furanthiol	Meaty, sweet, sulfurous
Benzylthiol	Sulphurous
2,4-dimethylthiazole	Rubber y, moldy, fruity, pungent
2-acetylthiazole	Roasted
Dimethyltrisulfide	Fragrant, musty, roasty, rubbery
2-acethylthiophene	Sulphurous, sweet
Bis(2-methyl-3-furyl)disulfide	Meaty-like
Benzothiazole	Metallic
Dimethyldisulfide	Moldy, pungent, rubbery, onion-like
2,4-dimethylthiazole	Rubbery, moldy, fruity, pungent
4,5-dimethylthiazole	Smoky, roasty, fragrant, nutty
2-methylchinoxaline	Aromatic, roasted, nutty, sweet, fruity, fatty
3-mercapto-2-butanone	Fried onion, sulfury, cooked meat
2-mercapto-3-pentanone	Brothy, mashed potatoes meaty, roast meat
2-[(methyldithio)methyl]furan	Brothy, spices, roast, fatty
3-[(2-furanylmethyl)dithio]-2-butanone	onion, burnt rubber, burnt wood

Table 1. The representative volatile flavor compounds with their aroma flavor characteristics found in cooked meat. [References: 13, 14, 20, 15, 27]

2.2. Precursors of meat flavor

Earlier studies on meat flavor, researchers recognized that the low molecular weight, water-soluble compounds and fats in meat constituents are the most important precursor of aroma flavor characteristics of cooked meat [28, 29]. The flavor precursor of meat namely, free sugars, free amino acids, peptides, vitamin, sugar phosphate, nucleotide-bound sugars and nucleotides [30, 31, 32, 33], all of them are able to either participate the Maillard reaction or oxidation/degradation and interaction on heating to generate volatile flavor compounds then create the final aroma flavor characteristics of cooked meat. It is suggested that these precursor components found to contribute to the development of meaty flavor, while the adipose tissues and intramuscular fat not only occupy an important role in development of flavor characteristics of cooked meat but also contribute to the characteristic-specific species flavors. This means that the distinct flavor characteristics between the meats from different species are due to the intramuscular fat content and not from water-soluble precursor compounds. The details on flavor precursors of meat found in the past years are showed in Table 2. However, researchers found that the roles of these flavor precursors in the development of flavor characteristics of cooked meat are not similar. Macey et al (1964) [28] found some sugars present in beef such as glucose, fructose, mannose and ribose, in that ribose was the most heat-labile sugar among these whereas fructose was the most stable. Among the amino acids present in meat, systein and systine are two sulfur-containing amino acids, the reaction of these with other sugars lead to formation of many sulfur-containing flavor compounds [34], while the reaction of other non-sulfur containing amino acids with sugars dominated by the nitrogen-containing products such as pyrazines [72]. In the recent years, researchers have found that the flavor precursor components in meats are influenced by several factors. Koutsidis et al (2008) [31] indicated that diets significantly affected the reducing sugars in beef *longissimus lumborum* muscle, higher total reducing sugars was obtained in beef from concentrate feeding group compared to the grass silage feeding group whereas beef from cattle fed with grass silage had higher level of free amino acids. When the beef was chiller aged for several days at chilling condition resulted in several times increase in free sugars such as ribose, free amino acids also increased with conditioning especially phenylalanine, methionine, lysine, leucine and isoleucine were the amino acids showing the greatest increase with conditioning time [32]. Meinert et al (2009) [35] have found that feeding, fasting and post-mortem ageing factors significantly influenced the concentration of flavor precursors of beef *longissimus dorsi* muscle. Additionally, the recent works also showed that fat-supplemented diets had large effect on the fatty acid compositions, for instance, dietary linseed oil and soybean oil significantly increased the contents of C18:3 and C18:2 in the neutral lipids and phospholipids in both *longissimus* and *biceps brachii* muscles [36], and subsequently influence the volatile flavor compounds of cooked beef [19, 25, 37].

Flavor precursors	Names in detail	Reference
Free amino acids	Systine; systeine; glycine; lysine; alanine; valine; isoleucine; leucine; threonine; serine; proline; asparagines; aspartic acid; methionine; glutamic acid; phenylalanine; glutamine; ornithine; histidine; tyrosine; tryptophan; arginine.	[38,39,40, 31,3232]
Reducing sugars	Ribose; glucose; xylose; starch; mannose; fructose; maltose; mannose 6-phosphate, glucose 6-phosphate; fructose 6-phosphate; ribose 6-phosphate.	[38,39,72, 41,31,32]
Fats/ lipids	Triglycerides and phospholipids Oleic acid (C18:1n-9) Linoleic acid (C18:2n-6) Linolenic acid (C18:3n-3) and etc.	[42,19, 43,34]
Vitamin	Thiamin	[33,44]
Nucleotides and peptides	Glutathione; carnosine inosine; inosine monophosphate; inosine 5'-monophosphate; guanosine 5-monophosphate; creatine; creatinine; Hypoxanthine and etc.	[45,44, 31,32]

Table 2. The representative precursors of meat flavor.

2.3. Pathways for the formation of volatile flavor compounds

2.3.1. Maillard reaction

Maillard reaction, a non-enzymatic browning which plays an important role in generation of volatile flavor compounds and appearances of the cooked foods, it is due to most of important volatile flavor compounds found in cooked foods are originated from this reaction. Otherwise, Maillard reaction also can produce antioxidative components and toxicological implications as well. However, in the present chapter we are focusing on the Maillard reaction in relation to aroma flavor characteristics, particularly the formation of volatile flavor compounds in cooked meat. Maillard reaction was firstly mentioned in the early time, 1912 by Maillard [46] since he wanted to investigate the browning reaction between glucose and glycine. After that many studies focused on determining the fundaments and mechanisms of this reaction [47, 48, 49].

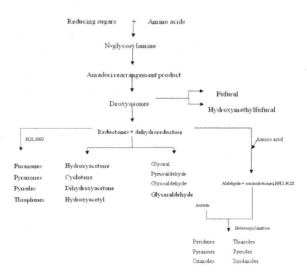

Figure 1. General stages of Maillard reaction showing the formations of flavor compounds (based on van Boekel, 2006) [51].

The Maillard reaction is taken placed with the participation of reducing sugars (e.g., ribose, glucose) and free amino compounds (e.g., amino acids, amines, peptides, proteins, ammonia) at certain heating condition to produce the Maillard products, and usually this reaction is divided into three main stages. In which the firstly initial stage starts with a condensation between a reducing sugar and an amino group, the loss of water from this molecule produces an amine that is able to cyclise resulting in formation of an N-glycosylamine (a sugar attached to NR_2 group) or called Amadori product. The next intermediate stage involves the rearrangement and decomposition of the Amadori product to release amino group and sugar fragmentation. The final stage of Maillard reaction is leading to dehydration, fragmentation, polymeration and cyclization reactions. A general scheme of the Maillard reaction is given in Figure 1.

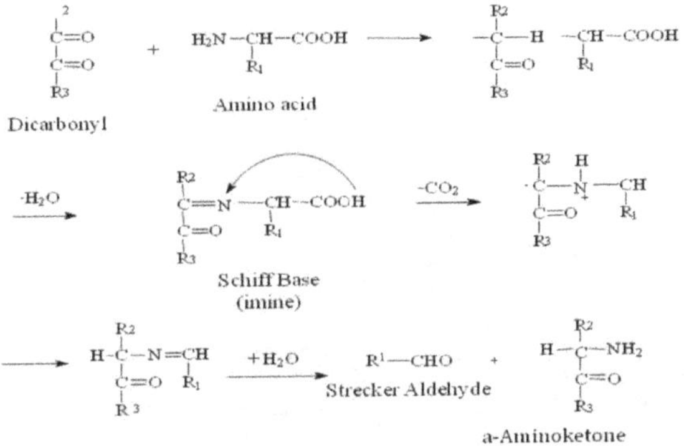

Figure 2. Strecker degradation mechanisms, a part of Maillard reaction

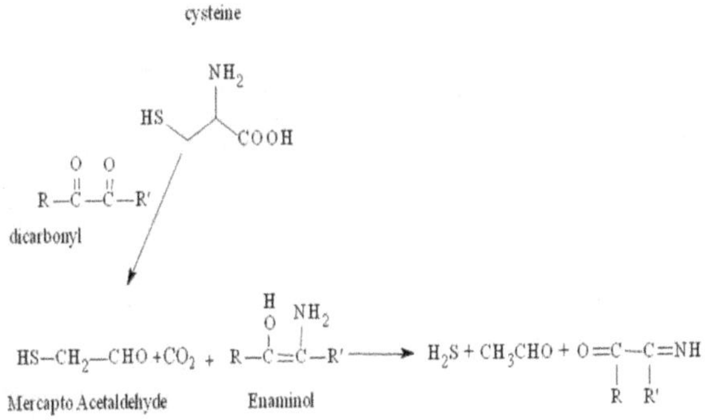

Figure 3. The formation of H_2S from the Strecker degradation of cysteine

Among events occurring in the Maillard reaction, Strecker degradation is one of the quite important events, in which amino acids are undergone degradation processes (oxidative de-amination and decarboxylation) in the presence of a dicarbonyls compound formed from Maillard reaction. The Strecker degradation processes lead to formation of aldehydes (e.g., fufural) and aminoketone (Figure 2). Especially the other important intermediate products such as H_2S, NH_3, etc are also formed from the Strecker degradation by sulphur-containing amino acids such as cystein and systine (Figure 3); all of these intermediate products can further react with other compounds or with each other to produce low and high molecular weight end flavor compounds.

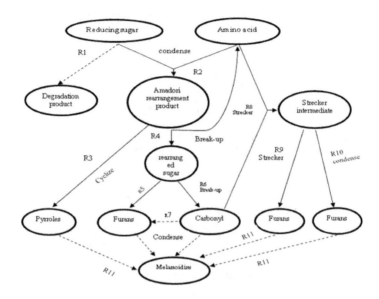

Figure 4. Kinetic scheme of flavor formation by Maillard reaction (Jousse et al., 2002) [50]

Flavor class	Characterized Flavor/aroma notes	Remark
Pyrazines	Cooked, roasted, toasted, baked cereals	
Alkylpyrazines	Nutty, roasted	
Alkylpyridines	Green, bitter, astringent, burnt	Unpleasant flavor
Acetylpyridines	Caracker-like	
Pyrroles	Cereal –like	
Furan, furanones, pyranone	Sweet, burnt, pungent, caramel-like	
Oxazoles	Green, nutty, sweet	
Thiophenes	Meaty	Formed from heated meat by the reaction of systein and ribose

Table 3. Some representative classes of flavor compounds formed from the Maillard reaction (based on van Boekel, 2006) [51].

The formation of volatile flavor compounds in the Maillard reaction largely depend on the reactants (e.g., the nature of reducing sugars and amino acids participated) and also the catalytic condition (e.g., heating temperature, moisture, pH). For the type of reducing sugars and amino acids which determine the kinds of flavor compounds generated for instance, many sulfur-containing flavor compounds are formed from the Maillard reaction between systeine and ribose [34] whereas, the nitrogen-containing compounds (e.g., pyrazines) dominated in the Maillard reaction containing glucose and lysine [72]. Therefore, it should be noted that nature of reactants will require the kinds of Maillard products. For the catalytic condition of Maillard reaction, it usually influences the kinetics of flavor compound generation by Maillard reaction in that depending on each catalytic condition (temperature, pH and etc) will determine the yields and also kinds of Maillard products. The kinetic of flavor compound formation resembles the scheme in Figure 4 with 11 determining steps [50]. Based on the kinetic scheme it shows that there are many chemical classes of flavors are formed via the Maillard reaction, some of the representative classes associated with odor notes are showed in Table 3.

2.3.2 Lipid oxidation and degradation

Lipids and fatty acids play an important role in direct and indirect generating the volatile flavor compounds and some of them contributing to the aroma flavor characteristics of cooked meat. Therefore, the levels of fat contents and as well as fatty acids of meats should be concerned, and it has been reported that the fatty acids of meat are influenced by several factors but almost are the pre-harvest factors such as diets, feed regimes and breeds [52, 53, 54]. Based on our surveillance it seems that the fatty acid profiles significantly vary across the breeds even these breeds are fed with the same diets [55, 56, 57]. Both adipose tissue and intramuscular fat contents are constituted by fatty acids including saturated and unsaturated fatty acids which all are capable to get oxidized and degraded under a certain condition to create a prolific number of volatile flavor compounds [2]. Hundreds of volatile flavor compounds derived from lipid degradation have been found in cooked meat including aliphatic hydrocarbons, aldehydes, ketones, alcohols, carboxylic acids and esters. In general, the odor detection threshold values for the lipid-derived compounds are much higher than those for the sulfur and nitrogen-containing heterocyclic compounds which are formed from the water-soluble precursors via the Maillard reaction. Therefore, the aroma significance of many of these lipid-derived compounds is not as great as that for relatively low concentrations of the heterocyclic compounds. However, certain classes of compounds such as particular aldehydes included saturated and unsaturated aldehydes which containing from 6 to 10 carbons in the structures are major volatile components of all cooked meats and, therefore, they probably play an important part in meat aroma [20]. The oxidation of subcutaneous fat, adipose tissues and intramuscular fat occur in raw meat and continues under the catalysis of many factors such as metals, oxygen, light, heating and etc.

Among the oxidation-induced factors for instance, lights (e.g., ultraviolet) is thought to be thermodynamically capable of production of free radicals directly in lipids, the principles of light-absorbing groups of lipids are double bonds, peroxide bonds and carbonyls which subsequently under the other steps to generate volatiles. And other factors such as oxygen, lypoxygenase, metals and etc which all also affect the lipid oxidation however that is another concern, in the present work we only consider on the heat effect that similar to cooking condition to induce the oxidation and degradation of fatty acids in producing volatile flavor compounds of cooked meat. The degrees of heating temperatures have been reported to affect variously lipid oxidation, in that high heating temperatures (e.g., frying, roasting) can have highly sufficient energies to break the single bonds (e.g., C-C or C-H) in the acyl back bonds to generate a lot of lipid alkyl radicals that participate the radical chain formation of oxidation [58]. Lower heating temperatures have lower energies which can break O-O bonds in traces of ROOH. Mottram (1985) [59] also stated that meat is cooked under boiled and lightly roasted conditions, lipid oxidation products dominated the detected compounds, and many of among them such as aldehydes, alcohols, ketones and lactones which have sufficiently low odor threshold to be contributors of meat aroma flavors.

Early work of Mottram et al (1982) [60] found that lipid has a considerable role in meat flavor, when the adipose tissue is added to lean meat does not affect the lipid-derived flavor compounds. A later study by Mottram and Edwards (1983) [42] found that the removal of intramuscular fats and phospholipids from beef caused marked differences in flavor compounds and sensory characteristics as well. So that the intramuscular fat contents (marbling fats) and membrane lipids are the main source of volatile flavor components and make species-specific flavors. However, it has been demonstrated that high levels of lipids especially polyunsaturated fatty acid contents (PUFA) cause undesirable aroma flavors due to their PUFA-derived products lower or inhibit the formation of some heterocyclic Maillard products [42]. This phenomenon has recently been elucidated by researchers when they used model systems. In the model systems containing systeine, ribose and lipid (e.g., lecithin or individual fatty acids) the concentrations of heterocyclic compounds and especially sulfur-containing compounds were lower several times compared with the model system without lipid content [43, 38, 61, 34]. However, the interaction between the lipid-derived products with Maillard products to form volatile flavor components has been much considered in the previous studies and thought as the important pathway for formation of flavor compounds.

2.3.3. Thiamin degradation

Thiamin is considered as a source of meat flavor generated on heating. Researchers found that the thermal degradation of thiamin produces some ended and intermediate flavor compounds [62,63]. It was assumed that thermal degradation of thiamin is a quite complex reaction including various degradation pathways to produce interesting flavor compounds in which most of them contain one or more sulfur and/or nitrogen atoms, and many of them are heterocyclic structures. The thermal degradation of thiamin under the basic condition to produce several flavor compounds is illustrated in Figure 5.

It was reported that the primary products of thermally-degraded thiamin including 4-methyl-5-(2-hydroxyethyl)thiazole which subsequently responds for formation of thiazoles and other sulfur compounds such as 5-hydroxy-3-mercaptopentan-2-one which then gives some sulfur-containing compounds such as thiophenes and furans as well [62]. Heating temperature and pH conditions have been showed to affect the degradation products of thiamin. At pH 5.0 and 7.0 the 2-methyl-3furanthiol and bis (2-methyl3-furyl) disulfide (meaty aroma) and thiophenes were the dominant aroma volatile compounds. But the levels of these meaty compounds decrease when increasing pH to 9.0 [64]. Similarly, a recent study by Dreher et al (2003) [65] also showed that the most significant thiamin thermal degradation products in the model reaction of orange juice containing 0.024 mM thiamin are 2-methyl-3-furanthiol and bis(2-methyl-3-furyl) disulfide produce intense meaty aromas. Otherwise, some other aroma-active compounds also were found such as 4, 5-dimethylthiazole (skunky, earthy), 3-thiophenethiol (meaty, cooked), 2-methyl-4, 5-dihydro-3(2H)-thiophenone (sour-fruity, musty, green), 2-acethylthiophene (burnt), 2-formyl-5-methylthiophene (meaty), and 2-methyl-3-(methyldithio) furan (meaty).

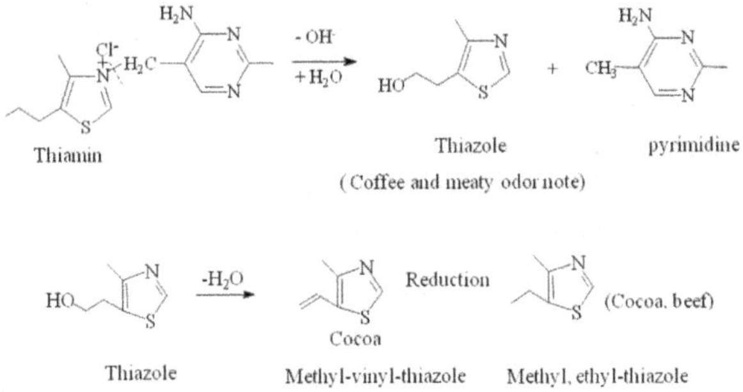

Figure 5. The thermal degradation of thiamin under basic condition

2.3.4. Interaction between lipid-oxidized products with Maillard products

The interaction between oxidized lipids and amino acids or proteins is very complex, in term of a consequence of the contribution of both lipid hydroperoxide and its secondary-oxidized products. This interaction may imply both the formation of physical complexes between the oxidized lipids and the amino acids or protein and the formation of various types of covalent bonds. Protein polymerizarion produced by reaction with peroxy free radicals generated during lipid peroxidation is known to occur during nonenzymatic browning [66, 67, 68]. However, in term of flavor study, the interaction between lipid-oxidized products (secondary products) with amino acids or proteins is the most concerned. Lipid-oxidized products are generic terms used to describe a mixture of aldehydes, alcohols, ketones and other products obtained by the decomposition of lipid hydroperoxides. Although it is not widely recognized, this decomposition does not necessarily imply the breakage of the lipid chain, and the formation of covalent bonds in the reaction between long chain oxidized lipids and amino acids and proteins has been described [69, 70]. This is a consequence of the existence of fatty acids that produce a complex and diverse mixture of lipid oxidation products that are able to react with the different reactive protein residues.

In the Maillard reaction, amino acids can undergo the Strecker degradation process that subsequently generates some reactive radicals such as ammonia, hydrosulfide and etc which also are able to further react with the secondary oxidized products of lipid to produce volatile flavor compounds such as thiols, thiophenes, thiazoles and etc as showed in Figure 6.

The interaction between lipid and Maillard reaction have extensively been studied in a number of studies using model systems containing amino acids and sugars in the presence of lipid [43, 61, 39, 34]. In these studies, systeine and ribose were used for Maillard reaction and in the presence of phospholipids from various sources including egg-yolk and beef. The reaction mixtures produced a lot of aroma volatiles which dominated by sulfur-containing components especially heterocyclics such as thiols and thiophenes. These studies also observed that the presence of phospholipids made a great reduction in amounts of these compounds. Famer and Mottram (1990) [61] also noted that beef-originated triglyceride has much less influence on amounts of heterocyclics than the phospholipids from beef do. The study also found that the addition of beef triglyceride to the Maillard reaction did not influence the sulfurous and rubbery aroma but when beef phospholipids were added resulting in higher meaty aroma note whereas the sulfurous notes were less. However, the Maillard reaction systems containing phospholipids usually had lower level of some meaty compounds especially 2-methyl-3-furanthiol this is due to the lipid limits generation of these compounds and only maintain theme at an optimum level in the reaction mixture.

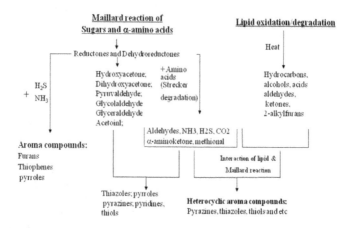

Figure 6. The interaction between lipid-oxidized products with Maillard products.

In general, in Maillard reaction mixtures containing lipids produce a lot of lipids-derived volatile compounds such as aldehydes, furans, hydrocarbons, alcohols and ketones. Furthermore, the reaction mixtures also containing the Maillard products such as H_2S, NH_3, etc. Which all are able to interact with each other to form new heterocyclic aroma volatile compounds as the consequences of the interactions between lipids with Maillard products. The most abundant compounds have been detected as results of the interactions are thiophene class such as 2-pentylthiophene, 2-hexylthiophene and thiol class such as 2-thiophenethiol, 2-furylmethanethiol, 2-methyl-3-furanthiol and etc [38, 61]. A recent study by Elmore and colleagues (2002) [34] concluded that breakdown products of polyunsaturated fatty acids especially are n-3 acids have a shorter chain length have lower odor thresholds will also be present at relatively high concentrations and are more reactive. These breakdown products will affect meat flavor by interacting with the Maillard reaction reducing levels of meaty aroma compounds, such as sulfur-substituted thiophenes and furans. As n-3 PUFAs are readily oxidized, they could initiate the free radical oxidation of more saturated acids, increasing levels of breakdown products of n-6 and n-9 fatty acids, which may also alter the aroma compounds of the cooked meat.

3. The factors affect aroma flavors

3.1 Effect of diets

Diet is as an important indicator to show the growth rate, performance, reproducibility effects and as well as meat quality of cattle. There has been an existed hypothesis of meat flavor changes due to feeding diets in which some works stated a large difference in meat flavor characteristics of the same cattle breed but fed on different diets. Early work by Melton (1983) [71] stated that steers fed with corn-based diets had more intense beef flavor (desirable flavor) than the same age steers fed based pasture or Bermuda pellets. A later study of Melton (1990) [10] found that the less desirable flavor of meat from cattle is mainly caused by several grass species. Conversely, no significant difference in flavors existed between the grass and grain diets-fed animals [73]. The less desirable flavors were also seen on meats from the hay diets-fed animals compared to corn silage diets [74], while Oltjen et al (1971) [75] showed the opposite results. It has been hypothesized that majority of flavor effects due to feeding of forages is mainly due to changes in fatty acid compositions. Fishy off-flavor was significantly higher in meat from grass-finished cattle with increasing unsaturated fatty acids [76]. Recently, researchers have attempted to higher level of PUFA in meat aiming to increase the health benefits by using the fat supplemented-diets (e.g., linseed, sunflower oil and fish oil) to cattle [77, 78], although these works have achieved an increase in several benefit fatty acids however, the detrimental effects on meat flavor characteristics appeared due to higher levels of PUFA [79]. A large number of studies regarding the effect of diets on volatile flavor compounds of cooked meat have been performed. Melton (1983) [71] also noted that the greatest difference in the flavors of meat from cattle fed on grass and grain-based diets is due to fatty acid concentration and type as fatty acids are the primary source of carbonyl. Suzuki and Bailey (1985) [80] indicated that higher concentrations of pentanoic,heptanoic, octanoic, nonanoic, decanoic, and dodecanoic acids were formed in the meat fat from grass-fed animals while heptanal, 2,3-octanedione, 3-hydroxyoctan-2-one, 2-decenal, 2-tridecanone, hexadecane, heptadecane, octodecane, d-dodecalactone, phyt-1-ene, neophytadiene, phyt-2-ene, an isomer of neophytadiene, 2-heptadecanone, dihydrophytol, and phytol with the terpenoids in much higher concentration due to rumen-fermented chlorophyll. Individual volatile flavor compounds like 4-heptanal, 2, 4-heptadienal and 2, 6-nonadienal (derived from C18:3n-3) and hexanal, 2-heptanal and 2, 4-decadienal (derived from C18:2n-6) found to be higher concentration in meats from grass and grain-fed animals, respectively [81]. Elmore et al (1997) [82] also reported that cooked meat from the animals that had been fed fish oil had considerably higher concentrations of saturated and unsaturated aldehydes than meat from the control. While, Descalzo et al (2005) [83] found that some classes of volatile flavor components affected by diets in which aldehydes increased in meat from concentrate diets-fed animals. In general, we can see that diets have a large influence on meat flavors due to directly affect the meat contents especially the intramuscular fat contents which play an important role in interaction and generation of volatile flavor compounds. On the other hand, it is worth noting that the uses of fat –supplemented diets to feed cattle may result in increases of important polyunsaturated fatty acids (e.g., n-3 fatty acids, DHA, EPA) which known to positively affect on consumers health however, a negative effect on meat flavors may appear due to these fatty acids not only produce some unexpected volatile compounds but also inhibit production of other Maillard products.

3.2. Effect of breeds and sex

Researchers have reported that breed also affects volatile flavor components and then influence overall flavor notes of cooked meat. Elmore et al (2000) [25] stated that fifty-four compounds were affected by breed, 75% of which was Maillard reaction products. Over 40 compounds were present at higher levels in the Soay breed than in the Suffolk breed. Other sulfur-containing compounds present at higher levels in the Suffolks than the Soays were bis-(2-furylmethyl) disulfide and 2-methyl-4,5-dihydro-thiophene and the differences in sulfur and nitrogen-containing compounds could contribute to flavor differences between the two breeds. A study on pork flavors as affected by breeds also have found that twenty-three among the detected flavor compounds were significantly affected by breed. Based on sensory analysis indicated that cooked *longissimus* muscle from hybrid breed (Duroc x Landrace x Large White) had the lowest pork flavor intensity and flavor-liking compared with the Chinese indigenous breeds. Laiwu and Dahuabai breeds showed the highest pork flavor intensity and flavor-liking in cooked longissimus muscle [36]. In beef, Insausti and colleagues (2005) [84] also found the differences in volatile flavor compounds among the breeds were considerable and may contributed to the perception of flavor differences in the cooked beef. Particularly, level of dimethyl sulfide probably related to cauliflower notes, was highest for meat from the Pirenaica breed. While, levels of the sulfur-compounds in cooked beef from the Asturiana breed were low-intermediate and potentially related to blood and liver notes and unpleasant flavors.

For the sex effect, it has been reported that meat from bulls has a strong livery and blood flavors while meat from heifers has a strong characteristic flavor. The differences could be associated with the differences in amounts of certain volatile compounds such as hydrocarbons, aldehydes, alcohols and ketones [85]. On the other hand, the differences in meat flavors between bulls and heifers could be explained by the genetic control of animal development and production of sex hormones and their influence the lipid composition which affects the kinds of volatile flavor compounds [86]. Overall, it may be assumed that the differences in meat flavors existing between breeds or sexes are probably due to the differences in the levels of flavor precursors especially the fat contents which large affect the formation of aroma flavor compounds and also interact with other contents in determining flavor characteristics of cooked meat.

3.3. Effect of chiller ageing

Ageing has been become a universal method widely used to improve eating quality of meat (e.g. tenderness, juiciness, flavor). Un-aged beef has a weak, bland odor while aged beef has a strong, savory, roasted odor. Ageing of meat makes an increase in fatty flavor characteristics however; long term ageing (e.g., > 3 weeks) could cause a decrease in positive flavor notes and increase liver-like aroma, bloody, bitter and off-flavor [87, 85, 88]. Ismail et al (2008) [89] stated that ethanol was responsible for the increase in alcohols caused by the microbial growth in beef during storage furthermore, the levels of aldehydes significantly increased after 7 days of storage. Beef from various muscles including gluteus medius, rectus femoris, vastus lateralis, vatsus medialis, teres major, complexus, serratus ventralis, psoas major and longissimus dorsi of heifer carcasses were chiller aged for 7 or 14 days the results showed that flavor-active volatiles included nonanal, 2,3-octanedione, pentanal, 3-hydroxy-2-butanone, 2-pentyl furan, 1-octen-3-ol, butanoic acid, pentanal and hexanoic acid which all often associated with lipid oxidation were affected by enhancement and ageing in the various muscles [90]. Additionally, ageing of beef achieved an increase in characteristic flavor and also aftertaste intensity, making an appreciable improvement of its flavor. After slaughter, loss of circulatory competency results in the accumulation of metabolic by-products, including lactic acid, in the muscle, that induces pH decline. The endogenous enzymes (e.g., cathespins B and L) are activated at near pH 5.4. Spanier and Miller (1993) and Spanier et al (1990) [91, 92] suggested that these thiol proteinases can hydrolyze more peptide bonds than any other group of enzymes, are redistributed during ageing period. Proteolytic enzyme activity is temperature-dependent; some enzymes retain high activity levels even at cooking temperatures. The combined effect of postmortem ageing and cooking, via enzyme redistribution and activity can influence the production of aroma flavor compounds. Toldrá and Flores (2000) [93] stated that enzymes known primarily for textural changes (e.g., μ- and m-calpain) during the postmortem period affect flavors by producing peptides, but it was observed that these enzymes correlate with increases in rancid, sour and salty flavors. The ageing conditions (e.g., oxygen availability, temperature, humidity and aging time) under which beef is aged influences the ultimate flavors of the meat particularly ageing in a higher oxygen environment cause a burnt, toasted off-odor. In addition, dry-ageing increases beef flavor attributes more than ageing in vacuum or in carbon dioxide [94, 95]. Based on the results reported in the previous studies it could be concluded that chiller ageing of meat resulted in increases of most of flavor compounds however a long ageing period (e.g., > 3 weeks) may negatively influences the flavor quality of cooked meat due to increase in amounts of some unexpected compounds which associated with undesirable flavors and decrease in the some important compounds which associated with desirable flavors.

3.4. Effect of cooking temperature and pH conditions

Cooking temperature is one of the important factors impacting the development of flavors through the Maillard reactions and lipid oxidation. Amino acids can undergo Strecker degradation to produce Strecker products. Degradation of sulfur-containing amino acids (e.g., cysteine, cystine and methionine) generates sulfur that contributes to subsequent processes of Maillard reaction. These compounds can react with amines and amino acids to produce a number of flavor-contributing compounds and potent cooked meat odorants such as pyrazines, oxazoles, thiophenes, thiazoles and other heterocyclic sulfur containing compounds [20]. It was well seen that cooking temperatures affect these reactions and then determine flavor characteristics, for instance the stewed meat lacks flavors of the roasted products because of stewed meat has a water activity of approximately 1.0 and not exceed temperature of 100°C while roasted meat has dried surfaces and temperature may exceed 100°C therefore, the conditions like low water activity and high surface temperature will increase production of flavor compounds which give roasted odor notes rather than meat is stewed. Ames et al (2001) [40] concluded that the amounts of most volatile flavor compounds increased with cooking temperature. Cooking at lower temperatures (<165 °C) versus higher temperatures (>180 °C) results in differences in the concentrations of a number of compounds such as 2, 4, 5-trimethyl- 3-oxazoline; 2, 4-dimethyl-5-ethyl-3-oxazoline; 2, 5- dimethyl-4-ethyl-3-oxazoline; 2, 4-dimethyl-3-thiazoline; 2, 4, 5-trimethyl-3-thiazoline [96]. Previous works found that a strong relationship existing between cooking temperature, concentration of free amino acids, carnosine, pyrazines and hexanol, and roasted, burnt and beefy flavor intensity [97, 98]. Cooking beef generates urea content which can also reduce sulfur-containing compounds generating important nitrogen-containing compounds like pyrazines and thiazoles in which pyrazines are formed mostly on the surface of meat and having nutty and roasty odor notes [99]. In general, the higher degree of heating, the higher the concentration of aliphatic aldehydes, benzenoids, polysulfides, heterocyclic compounds and lipid-derived volatiles. Ketones, alcohols sulfur-containing components make smaller contributions.

pH is one of the important factors that influence the kind of volatile flavor compounds formed in the Maillard reaction, and then determine the final flavor characteristics of cooked food. Madruga and Mottram (1995) [8] showed that as pH increases, color and polymeric compounds increase and nitrogen-containing compounds like pyrazines are favored, therefore it was assumed that higher ultimate pH in meat from grass-fed animals may favor the formation of thiazoles and thiophenones due to the availability of amino acid degradation products while decreasing other sulfur volatiles that favor lower pH. A number of early studies have been performed to investigate the effect of pH changes on volatile flavor compounds using model systems (El'Gde et al., 1966; Shu et al., 1985; Meynier and Mottram, 1995) [100, 101, 102]. These studies found that high pH values also favor the formation of many volatile compounds but other compounds are only favored at low pH condition. Meynier and Mottram (1995) [102] used meat-like model systems containing amino acids and ribose on different pH 4.5 and 6.5, results showed that nitrogen-containing compounds such as pyrazines were detected at higher pHs. While, dimethyldisulphide and methional showed decrease as the pH increased, and an increase in the disulphide was observed. It was observed that a large number of sulphur-containing compounds such as 2-methyl-3-furanthiol a strong meaty aroma, whose formation was greatly favored by lower pH condition. Ames et al (2001) [40] used model reactions containing cysteine and reducing sugar at varied pH conditions 5.5, 6.5 and 7.5, results showed that amounts of most of compounds increased with pH especially are pyrazines. Cerny and Biffod (2007) [103] recently found that pH determined strongly which volatile flavors were formed and to what extent. In general, based on the results of the previous studies which all found that pH condition strongly influence the formation of flavor components.

3.5. Effect of irradiation on meat flavors

Irradiation is a food safety technology designed to eliminate disease-causing germs from foods. Depending on the dose levels of irradiation applying on the raw meat and poultry, or ready-to-eat meats that can eliminate bacteria commonly found such as E. coli, Salmonella and Listeria; virus; or parasites. However, irradiation may result in off-odors and flavors. The odors vary with the type of meat, temperature during irradiation, oxygen exposure during and/or after the irradiation process, packaging and presence of antioxidative substances [104]. Most of studies have reported that the aroma flavors of irradiated meat associated with rotten egg, sweet, bloody, cooked meat, barbecued corn, burnt, sulfur, metallic, alcohol, acetic acid, liver-like serumy and bloody [105, 106, 107]. Irradiation can initiate or promote lipid oxidation resulting in undesirable off-odors and flavors [108, 109]. Jo and Ahn, (2000) [110] showed that reactions of sulfur-containing amino acids with radiolytic products of water appear to be the source of hydrogen sulfide and other volatile sulfur-containing compounds which contribute to off-flavor. On the other hand, irradiation may result in the formation of free radicals from unsaturated fatty acids at double bond positions [109]. An increase in lipid peroxidation products such as hexanal and (E)-4,5-epoxy-(E)-2-decenal in combination with a loss of desirable meaty odorants (4-hydroxy-2,5-dimethyl-3(2H)-furanone and 3-hydroxy-4,5-dimethyl-2(5H)-furanone) result in development of warmed over flavor of cooked, refrigerated beef [16]. However, the effects of irradiation on aroma flavors are also depended on: (1) Dose levels of irradiation, it has been demonstrated that the dose levels of irradiation influence variedly on volatile flavor components of cooked meat, as reported by Jo and Ahn (2000) [110] who indicated some of hydrocarbons included 1-heptene and 1-nonene increased with irradiation dose immediately after irradiation of beef. A similar observation also was reported by Yong et al (2000) [111] who indicated that among the 150 flavor compounds indentified in beef the cyclodecene, (E)-2-hexenal, nonene and 2-nonenal showed an increase in a dose-dependent fashion. For the effect of irradiation on chicken flavors, Yong e al (2000) [112] showed that among the 129 identified volatile flavor compounds the cyclotetradecene, 2-methylpentanal and 4-methylcyclohexene were formed specifically in response to irradiation, and level of cyclotetradecene increased in a dose-dependent fashion; (2) Oxygen presence, the presence of oxygen around meats during irradiating can diffuse into the meats, and then results in radiolytic changes which precipitate oxidation and unacceptable secondary breakdown products. As well known, lipid oxidation needs oxygen presence to produce oxidized-products such as aldehydes, Nam and Ahn

(2003) [113] indicated that irradiation of meat in aerobic packaging promoted production of aldehydes such as propanal and hexanal which is assumed as a good indicator of lipid oxidation. The similar observation also was reported by Nam et al (2001) [114] who also showed that irradiation increased TBARS values and off-flavor in aerobically-packaged pork (3) Temperature effect, temperature during irradiating meats has a large effect on aroma flavors of irradiated meat because temperature affects what radiolytic products are formed and what ratios [104]. Using lower temperature during irradiation of meat by freezing meat before irradiation can reduce detrimental effects via retarding autoxidation and extending shelf life; (4) pH effect, it has also been demonstrated that the ultimate pH of meat at the time of irradiation influences lipid oxidation. Nam et al (2001) [114] recently showed that irradiation increased lipid oxidation of normal and pale-soft-exudative (low pH group) muscles, whereas dark-firm-dry (high pH group) muscle was very stable and resistant to oxidative changes. Therefore, to minimize the detrimental effects of irradiation on aroma flavor characteristics we can modify atmosphere packaging by using vacuum packaging (anaerobic packaging) or replacement with inert gases (i.e. nitrogen, helium, hydrogen, carbon dioxide) to eliminate oxygen. Reducing the temperature (freezing) prior to irradiation and addition of antioxidants. Vacuum packaging retains irradiation-generated sulfur-containing compounds, however re-packaging meat in oxygen-permeable materials allows for dissipation of these flavor compounds.

4. Warm-off flavor and liver-like off flavor in cooked meat

Warm-off flavor and liver-like off flavor are undesirable flavors that result from the flavor changes and deterioration in meats that have been pre-cooked, chilled-stored and reheated. The warm-off flavor includes odors and tastes commonly described as stale, cardboard-like, painty, rancid, bitter and sour [115], and together with liver-like off flavor they both are the main factors that negatively affect eating sensory quality, purchase, economic impact of meat industry, and consumer complaint. Researchers have found that warm-off flavor appearing in cooked meat is mainly caused by oxidation of membrane phospholipids [116,115]. A recent report of Byrne et al (2001) [117], which also demonstrated that warm-off flavor associated with the development of lipid oxidation derived nuance off-flavor and odor notes such as rancid-like flavor and linseed oil-like odor, in association with a concurrent decrease in cooked pork meat-like flavor. The development of warm-off flavor usually results in loss of meaty flavor due to mask by lipid-oxidized products. Additionally, processes which involve any action that disrupts the muscle fiber membrane, such as chopping, restructuring, or heating which all can enhance warm-off flavor of meat product [118]. Previous works also suggested that reactions involving sulphydryl–disulfide interchanges in proteins and the degradation of sulfur-containing heteroatomic compounds, leading to a decrease in the "meatiness" of freshly cooked meat may also be an integral part of warm-off flavor [119,120]. For the liver-like off flavor of cooked meat, it was hypothesized that since foodservice preparation traditionally cooked the meat quickly and then held the product in warming ovens until the food was presented to the consumer these conditions might promote the liver-like flavor [27]. James and Calkins, (2005) [121] also hypothesized that the slower cooking and longer hold time allow the undesirable volatile flavor compounds to dissipate.

5. The current techniques used for extraction and detection of aroma flavor components

Up to present time, various techniques have been designed, combined with gas chromatography and mass spectrometry (GC/MS) or Flame ionizing detector (GC/FID) and applied to evaluate volatile flavor components in cooked meat. Of which, simultaneous steam distillation-extraction (SDE), dynamic headspace entrainment on Tenax TA, and solid-phase microextraction (SPME) are the techniques widely used for the extraction of volatile compounds in cooked meat [19, 122, 123, 85, 90, 124, 18,125]. SDE is a simple technique which involves small volumes of solvent, efficient stripping of volatiles and quantitative recovery of many compounds. The sample is dispersed in water which is heated to boiling. The steam that is generated carries volatiles with it into a section of the apparatus where the steam condenses in the presence of extracting solvent vapor. The co-condensation of volatile-laden steam and extracting solvent results in an effective extraction of volatiles [123]. The Dynamic headspace entrainment on Tenax has been used in the studies regarding cooked meat volatile flavor compounds since the 1980s. This technique probably has been used more than any other aroma extraction technique for the analysis of meat aroma and continues to be widely used. The action mechanism of this technique involving purging the headspace of a sample with a purified inert gas (e.g., nitrogen or helium), followed by collection of the volatiles onto a trap containing a suitable adsorbent, which will retain the volatile analytes carried there by the purge gas. Finally, the volatiles of meat samples collected on this trap are desorbed onto a GC or GC-MS column using a modified injection port. In the recent years, SPME technique has been widely adopted and considered as an alternative to isolate volatile flavor components in cooked meat. In SPME, the needle is coated with an absorbent material (e.g. CAR/PDMS), is placed above the cooked meat samples. Volatiles will migrate from the sample matrix to the needle coating and be absorbed. Volatile components will then be desorbed from the needle coating by inserting the needle in GC injection port.

The extraction techniques as mentioned above in combination with GC/MS or GSC/FID can help researchers to tentatively detect the volatile flavor compounds in experimented meat samples but it could not identify the aroma flavors or odor characteristics of detected compounds. It would be advantageous to combine two or more different techniques, such as gas chromatography (GC) and olfactometry, the combination of measuring odor notes is called gas chromatography-olfactometry (GC/O). Gas chromatography-olfactometry (GC-O) is a bioassay that measures human response to odorants separated by gas chromatography. The superior sensitivity and selectivity of human olfaction make GC-O a powerful and meaningful tool for flavor chemistry. In the recent year, GC-O is one of the main techniques which have been used to determine intensity of aroma (odor) characteristics of volatile compounds in cooked meat [15, 21, 125].

6. Conclusion and Implication

In order to have a cooked meat product with its desirable aroma flavors as expectation of consumer, it is important to understand how aroma flavors are derived, the mechanisms by which flavor components are generated, and the factors affect formation of flavor compounds then determine the final aroma flavor characteristics of cooked meat. Regarding the effects of factors on aroma flavors of cooked meat and to minimize the detrimental effects it is suggested if increasing the polyunsaturated fatty acids (e.g. C18:3n-3, DHA, EPA) to increase nutritional benefits to the consumer by using fat-supplemented diets however the undesirable flavors may result. Because the breakdown products of these fatty acids have a shorter chain length therefore are more volatile and they affect meat flavors by interacting with the Maillard reaction results in reducing levels of meaty aroma compounds such as sulfur-substituted thiophenes. Therefore, diets, feeding regimes, welfare and management of animals should be taken into account. Cooking conditions such as temperature, holding time and cooking methods play an important role in determining the formation volatile flavor compounds. In general, it has been demonstrated that cooking meat at high temperature (by roasting, grilling) will produce better aroma flavor characteristics due to the important Maillard products are formed. In addition to the cooking effect, it is suggested that a slow cooking and longer hold time can allow the undesirable volatile flavor compounds to dissipate, thus reduce warm-off flavor. Irradiation of meat can eliminate pathogens however, off-flavor may result therefore, and to minimize the detrimental effect of this method we can lower temperature during irradiation of meat by freezing meat before irradiation. Modifying atmosphere packaging by using vacuum packaging (anaerobic packaging) or replacement with inert gases (i.e. nitrogen, helium, hydrogen, carbon dioxide) to eliminate oxygen in meat during irradiation are also the alternatives. Chiller ageing of meat should be applied to improve eating quality however should not age for a long time (3 week period in maximum is encouraged) because chiller ageing meat for a too long period may result in flavor deterioration and decreasing desirable flavors.

Author details

Hoa Van Ba[1*], Inho Hwang[1], Dawoon Jeong[2] and Amna Touseef[2]

*Address all correspondence to: ba_cnu1981@yahoo.com

1 Department of Animal Science and Biotechnology, Lab of Muscle Biology and Meat Science, Chonbuk National University, South Korea

2 Department of Animal Science and Biotechnology, Lab of Muscle Biology and Meat Science, Chonbuk National University, South Korea

References

[1] Elgado, C., Rosegrant, M., Steinfeld, H., Ehui, S, & Courbois, C. (1999). Paper presented at Livestock to 2020. The Next Food Revolution. Food, Agriculture, and the Environment. Discussion Paper 28. International Food Policy Research Institute, Food and Agriculture Organization of the United Nations and the International Livestock Research Institute., IFPRI, Washington, D.C.

[2] Mac, Leod. G. (1994). The flavor of beef. In Shahidi F (ed) Flavor of meat and meat products. Glasgow Chapman and Hall , 4-37.

[3] Savell, J. W., Branson, R. E., Cross, H. R., Stiffler, D. M., Wise, J. W., Griffin, D. B., & Smith, G. C. (1987). National consumer retail beef study: palatability evaluations of beef loin steaks that differed in marbling. *Journal of Food Science*, 52-517.

[4] Robbins, K., Jensen, J., Ryan, K. J., Homco-Ryan, C., Mc Keith, F. K., & Brewer, M. S. (2003). Consumer attitudes towards beef and acceptability of enhanced beef. *Meat Science*, 65-721.

[5] Landy, P., Courthaudon, J. L., Dubois, C., & Voilley, A. (1996). Effect of interface in model food emulsions on the volatility of aroma compounds. *Journal of Agriculture and Food Chemistry*, 44-526.

[6] Rabe, S., Krings, U., & Berger, R. G. (2003). Influence of oil-in-water emulsion properties on the initial dynamic flavor release. *Journal of the Science of Food and Agriculture*, 83-1124.

[7] Kinsella, J. E. (1990). Flavor perception and binding. *INFORM*, 1(3), 215-226.

[8] Madruga, M. S., & Mottram, D. S. (1995). The effect of pH on the formation of Maillard-derived aroma volatiles using a cooked meat system. *Journal of the Science of Food and Agriculture*, 68-305.

[9] Bredie, W. L. P., Mottram, D. S., & Guy, R. C. E. (1998). Aroma volatiles generated during extrusion cooking of maize flour. *Journal of Agriculture and Food Chemistry*, 46-1497.

[10] Melton, S. L. (1990). Effects of feeds on flavor of red meat: A review. *Journal of Animal Science*, 68-4421.

[11] Mottram, D. S., & Whitefield, F. B. (1994). Aroma volatiles from meat-like Maillard systems. In Thomas H (ed) Thermally generated flavors. ACS Symposium series. American chemical society, Washington, D.C , 543, 180-191.

[12] Mottram, D. S. (1991). Meat: In Hank Maarse (ed) Volatile compounds in foods and Beverages. Marcell Dekker Inc., New York; , 107-177.

[13] Gasser, U., & Grosch, W. (1988). Identification of flavor volatile compounds in high aroma values from cooked beef. *Z. Lebensm. Unters. Forsh*, 186-489.

[14] Specht, K., & Baltes, W. (1994). Identification of volatile flavor compounds with high aroma values from shallow-fried beef. *Journal of Agriculture and Food Chemistry, 42,* 2246-2253.

[15] Rochat, S., & Chaintreau, A. (2005). Carbonyl odorants contributing to the in-oven roast beef top note. *Journal of Agriculture and Food Chemistry, 53-9578.*

[16] Kerler, J., & Grosch, W. (1996). Odorants contributing to warmed-over flavor (WOF) of refrigerated cooked beef. *Journal Food Science, 61*(6), 1271-1274.

[17] Machiels, D., Istasse, L., & van Ruth, S. M. (2004). Gas chromatography-olfactometry analysis of beef meat originating from differently fed Belgian Blue, Limousin and Aberdeen Angus bulls. *Food Chemistry, 86-377.*

[18] , H. V., Oliveros, M. C., Ryu, K. S., & Hwang, I. H. (2010). Development of analysis condition and detection of volatile compounds from cooked Hanwoo beef by SPME-GC/MS analysis. *Journal of Food Science of Animal Resource, 30-73.*

[19] Elmore, J. S., Mottram, D. S., Enser, M., & Wood, J. D. (1999). Effect of the polyunsaturated fatty acid composition of beef muscle on the profile of aroma volatiles. *Journal of Agriculture and Food Chemistry, 47-1619.*

[20] Mottram, D. S. (1998). Flavor formation in meat and meat a review. *Food Chemistry,* 62-415.

[21] Machiels, D., van Ruth, S. M., Posthumus, M. A., & Istasse, L. (2003). Gas chromatography-olfactometry analysis of the volatile compounds of two commercial Irish beef meats. *Talanta, 60-755.*

[22] Kerscher, R., & Grosch, W. (1997). Comparative evaluation of potent odorants of boiled beef by aroma extracts dilution and concentration analysis. *Zeitschrift für Lebensmitteluntersuchung und Forschung A, 204,* 3-6.

[23] Cerny, C., & Grosch, W. (1992). Evaluations of potent odorants in roasted beef by aroma extract dilution analysis. *Zeitschrift für Lebensmitteluntersuchung und Forschung A,* 194, 323-325.

[24] Cañedo, A. R., Juez-Ojeda, C., Nuñez, M., & Fernández-García, E. (2011). Effects of high-pressure processing on the volatile compounds of sliced cooked pork shoulder during refrigerated storage. *Food chemistry, 124,* 749-758.

[25] Elmore, J. D., Mottram, D. S., Enser, M., & Wood, J. D. (2000). The effects of diet and breed on the volatile compounds of cooked lamb. *Meat Science, 55,* 149-159.

[26] Wettasinghe, M., Vasanthan, T., Temelli, F., & Swallow, K. (2001). Volatile flavor composition of cooked by-product blends of chicken, beef and pork: a quantitative GC-MS investigation. *Food research international, 34,* 149-158.

[27] Calkins, C. R., & Hodgen, J. M. (2007). A fresh look at meat flavor. *Meat Science, 77,* 63-80.

[28] Macey, R. L., Naumann, H. D., & Bailey, M. E. (1964). Water-soluble flavor and odor precursors of meat. (II) Effects of heating on amino nitrogen constituents and carbohydrates in lyophilized diffusates from aqueous extracts of beef, pork and lamb. *Journal of Food Science*, 29, 142-148.

[29] Macey, R. L., Naumann, H. D., & Bailey, M. E. (1970). Water-soluble flavor and odor precursors of meat. 5. Influence of heating on acidextractable non-nucleotide chemical constituents of beef, lamb and pork. *Journal of Food Science*, 35, 83-87.

[30] Mottram, D. S. (1994). Some aspects of the chemistry of meat flavor. In Shahidi, F (ed) the flavor of meat and meat products: Blackie Glasgow , 210-230.

[31] Koutsidis, G., Elmore, J. S., Oruna-Concha, M. J., Campo, M. M., Wood, J. D., & Mottram, D. S. (2008). Water-soluble precursors of beef flavor: I. Effect of diet and breed. *Meat Science*, 79, 124-130.

[32] Koutsidis, G., Elmore, J. S., Oruna-Concha, M. J., Campo, M. M., Wood, J. D., & Mottram, D. S. (2008). Water-soluble precursors of beef flavor: part II. Effect of diet post-mortem conditioning. *Meat Science*, 79, 270-277.

[33] Dwivedi, B. K., & Arnold, R. G. (1973). Chemistry of thiamine degradation in food products and model systems: a review. *Journal of Agriculture and Food Chemistry*, 21, 54-60.

[34] Elmore, J. S., Campo, M. M., Enser, M., & Mottram, D. S. (2002). Effect of Lipid composition on Meat-like model systems containing cystein, ribose and polyunsaturated fatty acids. *Journal of Food chemistry*, 50, 1126-1132.

[35] Meinert, L., Tikk, K., Tikk, M., Brockhoff, P. B., Bredie, W. L. P., Bjergegaard, C., & Aaslyng, M. D. (2009). Flavor development in pork. Influence of flavor precursor concentrations in longissimus dorsi from pigs with different raw meat qualities. *Meat Science*, 81, 255-262.

[36] Lu, P., Zhang, L. Y., Yin, J. D., Everts, A. K. R., & Li, D. F. (2008). Effects of soybean oil and linseed oil on fatty acid compositions of muscle lipids and cooked pork flavor. *Meat Science*, 80, 910-918.

[37] Elmore, J. S., Cooper, S. L., Enser, M., Mottram, D. S., Sinclair, L. A., & Wilkinson, R. G. (2005). Dietary manipulation of fatty acid composition in lamb meat and its effect on the volatile aroma compounds of grilled lamb. *Meat Science*, 69, 233-242.

[38] Farmer, L. J., Mottram, D. S., & Whitfield, F. B. (1989). Volatile compounds produced in Maillard reaction involving systeine, ribose and phospholipids. *Journal of the Science of Food and Agriculture*, 49, 347-369.

[39] Salter, L. J., Mottram, D. S., & Whitfield, F. B. (1988). Volatile compounds produced in the Maillard reaction involving glycine, ribose and phospholipids. *Journal of the Science of Food and Agriculture*, 46, 227-242.

[40] Ames, J. M., Guy, R. C. E., & Kipping, G. J. (2001). Effect of pH and temperature on the formation of volatile compounds in cysteine/reducing sugar/starch mixtures during extrusion cooking. *Journal of Agriculture and Food Chemistry*, 49, 1885-1894.

[41] Tai, C. Y., & Ho, C. T. (1997). Influence of cysteine oxidation on thermal formation of Maillard aromas. *Journal of Agricultural and Food Chemistry*, 45, 3586-3589.

[42] Mottram, D. S., & Edwards, R. A. (1983). The role of triglycerides and phospholipids in the aroma of cooked beef. *Journal of the Science of Food and Agriculture*, 34, 517-522.

[43] Whitfield, F. B., Mottram, D. S., Brock, S., Puckey, D. J., & Salter, L. J. (1988). Effect of phospholipid on the formation of volatile heterocyclic compounds in heated aqueous solutions of amino acids and ribose. *Journal of the Science of Food and Agriculture*, 42, 261-272.

[44] Huang, T. C., & Ho, C. T. (2001). Flavors of meat products. In Hui. Y. H., Nip, W. K., Roger, R. W and Young, O. A (eds) Meat Science and Application Marcel Dekker, Inc , 71-102.

[45] Tai, C. C., & Ho, C. T. (1998). Influence of glutathione oxidation and pH on thermal formation of Maillard-type volatile compounds. *Journal of Agriculture and Food Chemistry*, 46, 2260-2265.

[46] Maillard, L. C. (1912). Action des acides amines sur les sucres: formation des melanoidines par voie methodique. *Compte-rendu de l'Academie des Sciences, tome*, 154, 66-68.

[47] van den, Ouweland. G. A. M., Peer, H. G., & Tjan, S. B. (1978). Occurrence of Amadori and Heyns rearrangement products in processed foods and their role in flavor formation. In Charalambous, G and Inglett, G. E (eds) flavor in foods and Beverages Academic press New York , 131-143.

[48] Mouron, J. (1981). The Maillard reaction in food: a critical review from the nutritional standpoint. In Erickson, C (ed) Maillard reaction in food Pergamon Press Oxford , 3-35.

[49] Hurrent, R. F. (1982). Maillard reaction in flavor. In Morton, I. D and Macleod, A. J (eds) food flavor Elsevier Amsterdam , 399-437.

[50] Jousse, F., Jongen, W., Agterof, W., Russell, S., & Braat, P. (2002). Simplified kinetic scheme of flavor formation by the Maillard reaction. *Journal of Food Science*, 7, 2534-42.

[51] van Boekel, M. A. J. S. (2006). Formation of flavor compounds in the Maillard reaction. *Biotechnology Advances*, 24, 230-233.

[52] Realini, C. E., Duckett, S. K., Brito, B. M., Dalla, Rizza. M., & De Mattos, D. (2004). Effect of pasture vs. concentrate feeding with or without antioxidants on carcass characteristics, fatty acid composition, and quality of Uruguayan beef. *Meat Science*, 66, 567-577.

[53] Warren, H. E., Scollan, N. D., Enser, M., Hughes, S. I., Richardson, R. I., & Wood, J. D. (2008). Effects of breed and a concentrate or grass silage diet on beef quality in cattle of 3 ages. I: Animal performance, carcass quality and muscle fatty acid composition. *Meat Science*, 78, 256-269.

[54] Cristina, P. M. A., Susana, P. A., Susana, I. V. M., Ana, S. H. C., Carlos, M. G. A. F., Jose, P. C. L., Rui, J. B. B., & Jose, A. M. P. (2009). Effect of the feeding system on in-tramuscular fatty acids and conjugated linoleic acid isomers of beef cattle, with em-phasis on their nutritional value and discriminatory ability. Food Chemistry; , 114, 939-946.

[55] Cuvelier, C., Clinquart, A., Hocquette, J. F., Cabaraux, J. F., Dufrasne, I., Istasse, L., & Hornick, J. L. (2006). Comparison of composition and quality traits of meat from young finishing bulls from Belgian Blue, Limousin and Aberdeen Angus breeds. *Meat Science*, 74, 522-531.

[56] Muchenje, V., Hugo, A., Dzama, K., Chimonyo, M., Strydom, P. E., & Raats, J. G. (2009). Cholesterol levels and fatty acid profiles of beef from three cattle breeds raised on natural pasture. *Journal of Food Composition and Analysis*, 22, 354-358.

[57] Moreno, T., Keane, M. G., Noci, F., & Moloney, A. P. (2008). Fatty acid composition of M. Longissimus dorsi from Holstein-Friesian steers of New Zealand and European/American descent and from Belgian Blue Holstein-Friesian steers, slaughtered at two weights/ages. *Meat Science*, 78, 157-169.

[58] Nawar, W. W. (1969). Thermal degradation of lipids-a review. *Journal of Agriculture and Food Chemistry*, 17, 1-9.

[59] Mottram, D. S. (1985). Effect of cooking conditions on the formation of volatile heter-ocyclic compounds in pork. *Journal of Science and Food Agriculture*, 36, 377-382.

[60] Mottram, D. S., Edwards, R. A., & Macfie, H. J. H. (1982). A comparison of flavor vol-atiles from cooked beef and pork meat systems. *Journal of the Science of Food and Agri-culture*, 33, 934-944.

[61] Farmer, J. J., & Mottram, D. S. (1990). Recent study on the formation of meat-like aro-ma compounds. In Bessere, Y and Thomas, A. F (eds) Flavor Science and technology Wiley, Chichester, UK , 113-116.

[62] van der Lide, L. M., van Dort, J. M., de valois, P., Boelens, H., & de Rijike, D. (1979). Volatile components from thermally degraded thiamin. In Land, D. G and Nursten, H. E (eds) progress in flavor research. Applied science London , 219-224.

[63] Guntert, M., Bruning, J., Emberger, R., Kopsel, M., Kuhn, W., Thielmann, T., & Werkhoff, P. (1990). Identification of formation of some selected sulfur-containing flavor compounds in various food model systems. *Journal of Agriculture and Food Chemistry*, 38, 2027-2041.

[64] Reineccius, G. A., & Liardon, R. (1985). The use of charcoal traps and microwave de-sorption for the analysis of headspace volatiles above heated thiamin solutions. In R.

G, Berger, S. Nitz and P, Schreier (eds)Topics in flavor research Eichhorn, Marzling-Hangenhan , 125-136.

[65] Dreher, J. G., Rouseff, R. L., & Naim, M. (2003). GC-Olfactometric Characterization of Aroma Volatiles from the Thermal Degradation of Thiamin in Model Orange Juice. *Journal of Agriculture and Food Chemistry*, 51, 3097-3102.

[66] Karel, M., Schaich, K., & Roy, R. B. (1975). Interaction of Peroxidizing Methyl Linoleate with Some Proteins and Amino Acids. *Journal of Agriculture and Food Chemistry*, 23, 159-163.

[67] Kikugawa, K., Kato, T., Beppu, M., & Hayasaka, A. (1990). Fluorescent and Cross-linked Proteins Formed by Free Radical and Aldehyde Species Generated During Lipid Oxidation in Lipofuscin and Ceroid Pigments. E. A. Porta, Plenum Press New York., 345-357.

[68] Neukom, H. (1980). Oxidative Crosslinking of Proteins and Other Biopolymers. In Simic, M. G. and Karel, M (eds.) Autoxidation in Food and Biological Systems Plenum Press New York , 249-259.

[69] Gardner, H. W., Kleiman, R., Weisleder, D., & Inglett, G. E. (1977). Cysteine adds to lipid hydroperoxide. *Lipids*, 12, 655-660.

[70] Hidalgo, F. J., & Zamora, R. (1995). In Vitro Production of Long Chain Pyrrole Fatty Esters from Carbonyl-Amine Reactions. *Journal of Lipid Research*, 36, 725-735.

[71] Melton, S. L. (1983). Effect of forage feeding on beef flavor. *Food Technology*, 37, 239-248.

[72] Ames, J. M., Defaye, A. B., & Bates, L. (1997). The effect of pH on the volatiles formed in an extruded starch-glucose-lysine model system. *Food chemistry*, 58, 323-327.

[73] French, P., O'Riordan, E. G., Monahan, F. J., Caffrey, P. J., Mooney, M. T., & Troy, D. J. (2001). The eating quality of meat of steers fed grass and/or concentrates. *Meat Science*, 57, 379-386.

[74] Dube, G., Bramblett, V. D., Howard, R. D., Homler, B. E., Johnson, H. R., & Harrington, R. B. (1979). Dietary effects on beef composition.4. Processing and palatability attributes. *Journal of Food Science*, 36, 147-154.

[75] Oltjen, R. R., Rumsey, T. S., & Putnam, P. A. (1971). All-forage diets for finishing beef cattle. *Journal of Animal Science*, 32(2), 327-333.

[76] Nuernberg, K., Wood, J. D., Scollan, N. D., Richardson, R. I., Nute, G. R., & Nuernberg, G. (2005). Effect of a grass-based and a concentrate feeding system on meat quality characteristics and fatty acid composition of longissimus muscle in different cattle breeds. *Livestock Production Science*, 94, 137-147.

[77] Mandell, I. B., Buchanan-Smith, J. G., Holub, B. J., & Campbell, C. P. (1997). Effects of fish meal in beef cattle diets on growth performance, carcass characteristics, and fatty acid composition of longissimus muscle. *Journal of Animal Science*, 75(4), 910-919.

[78] Scollan, N., Richardson, I., Moloney, A., Dannenberger, D., Hocquette, J. F., & Nuern-
      berg, K. (2006). Innovations in beef production systems that enhance the nutritional
      and health value of beef lipids and their relationship with meat quality. *Meat science*,
      74(1), 17-33.

[79] Miller, R. K. (2001). Beef flavor: A white paper. Centennial, CO, National Cattlemens'
      Beef Association.

[80] Suzuki, J., & Bailey, M. E. (1985). Direct sampling capillary GLC analysis of flavor
      volatiles from ovine. *Food Chemistry*, 33(3), 343-347.

[81] Larick, D. K., Hedrick, H. B., Bailey, M. E., Williams, J. E., Hancock, D. L., & Garner,
      G. B. (1987). Flavor constituents of beef as influenced by forage- and grain-feeding.
      Journal of Food Science, 52(2), 245-251.

[82] Elmore, J. S., Mottram, D. S., Enser, M., & Wood, J. D. (1997). Novel if thiazoles and
      3-thiazolines in cooked beef aroma. *Journal of Agriculture and Food Chemistry*, 45,
      3603-3607.

[83] Descalzo, A. M., Garcia, P. T., Pensel, N. A., Josifovich, J. A., Insani, E. M., & Biolatto,
      A. (2005). Influence of pasture or grain-based diets supplemented with vitamin E on
      antioxidant/oxidative balance of Argentine beef. *Meat Science*, 70(1), 35-44.

[84] Insausti, K., Goni, V., Petri, E., Gorraiz, C., & Beriain, M. J. (2005). Effect of weight at
      slaughter on the volatile compounds of cooked beef from Spanish cattle breeds. *Meat
      Science*, 70, 83-90.

[85] Gorraiz, C., Beriain, M. J., Chasco, J., & Insausti, K. (2002). Effect of aging time on vol-
      atile compounds, odor, and flavor of cooked beef from Pirenaica and Friesian bulls
      and heifers. *Journal of Food Science*, 67, 916-922.

[86] Sink, J. D. (1979). Symposium on meat flavor factors influencing the flavor of muscle
      foods. *Journal of Food Science*, 44, 1-5.

[87] Spanier, A. M., Flores, M., Mc Millin, K. W., & Bidner, T. D. (1997). The effect of post
      mortem aging on meat flavor quality in Brangus beef. Correlation of treatments, sen-
      sory, instrumental and chemical descriptors. *Food Chemistry*, 59, 531-538.

[88] Yancey, E. J., Grobbel, J. P., Dikeman, M. E., Smith, J. S., Hachmeister, K. A., & Cham-
      bers, E. C. (2006). Effects of total iron, myoglobin, hemoglobin, and lipid oxidation of
      uncooked muscles on livery flavor development and volatiles of cooked beef steaks.
      Meat Science, 73, 680-686.

[89] Ismail, H. A., Lee, E. J., Ko, K. Y., & Ahn, D. U. (2008). Effects of aging time and natu-
      ral antioxidants on the color, lipid oxidation and volatiles of irradiated ground beef.
      Meat Science, 80, 582-591.

[90] Stetzer, A. J., Cadwallader, K., Singh, T. K., Mckeith, F. K., & Brewer, M. S. (2008).
      Effect of enhancement and ageing on flavor and volatile compounds in various beef
      muscles. *Meat Science*, 79, 13-19.

[91] Spanier, A. M., & Miller, J. A. (1993). Role of Proteins and Peptides in Meat Flavor. In Spanier, A.M., Okai, H. and Tamura, M (eds) Food Flavor and Safety. ACS Symposium Series Am. Chem. Soc. Washington, D.C (528), 78-97.

[92] Spanier, A. M., Mc Millin, K. W., & Miller, J. A. (1990). Enzyme activity levels in beef: effect of postmortem aging and end point cooking temperature. *Journal of Food Science*, 55, 318-322.

[93] Toldrá, F., & Flores, M. (2000). The use of muscle enzymes as predictors of pork meat quality. *Food Chemistry*, 69, 387-395.

[94] Campbell, R. E., Hunt, M. C., Levis, P., & Chambers, E. I. V. (2001). Dry-aging effects on palatability of beef longissimus muscle. *Journal of Food Science*, 66, 196-199.

[95] Jeremiah, L. E., & Gibson, L. L. (2003). The effects of postmortem product handling and aging time on beef palatability. *Food Research International*, 36, 929-941.

[96] Mussinan, C. J., Wilson, R. A., Katz, I., Sanderson, A., & Vock, M. H. (1975). Identification and flavor properties of some 3oxazolines and 3-thiazolines isolated from cooked beef. Abstract, Journal of American Chemical Society AGFD , 170, 22.

[97] Lorenzen, C. L., Davuluri, V. K., Adhikari, K., & Grün, I. U. (2005). Effect of end point temperature and degree of doneness on sensory and instrumental flavor profile of beefsteaks. *Journal of Food Science*, 70, 113-118.

[98] Cambero, M. I., Seuss, I., & Honikel, K. O. (1992). Flavor compounds of beef broth as affected by cooking temperature. *Journal of Food Science*, 57, 1285-1290.

[99] Hogan, B. (2002, July). Putting punch in meat flavor profiles. *Food Product Design*.

[100] El'Ode, K. E., Domseifer, T. P., Keith, K. S., & Powers, J. J. (1966). Effect of pH and temperature on the carbonyls and aromas produced in heated amino acid-sugar mixtures. *Journal of Food Science*, 31, 351-8.

[101] Shu, C. K., Hagedom, M. L., Mookherjee, B. D., & Ho, C. T. (1985). pH effect on the volatile components in the thermal degradation of cysteine. *Journal of Agriculture and Food Chemistry*, 33, 442-6.

[102] Meynier, A., & Mottram, D. S. (1995). The effect of pH on the formation of volatile compounds in meat-related model systems. *Food Chemistry*, 52, 361-366.

[103] Cerny, C., & Briffod, M. (2007). Effect of pH on the Maillard Reaction of [13C5] Xylose, Cysteine and Thiamin. *Journal of Agriculture and Food Chemistry*, 55, 1552-1556.

[104] Brewer, M. S. (2009). Irradiation effects on meat flavor: A review. *Meat Science*, 81, 1-14.

[105] Hampson, J. W., Fox, J. B., Lakritz, L., & Thayer, D. W. (1996). Effect of low dose gamma radiation on lipids in five different meats. *Meat Science*, 42, 271-276.

[106] Jo, C., Lee, J. I., & Ahn, D. U. (1999). Lipid oxidation, color changes and volatile production in irradiated pork sausage with different fat content and packaging during storage. *Meat Science*, 51(4), 355-361.

[107] Lee, M., Sebranek, J. G., Olson, D. G., & Dickson, J. S. (1996). Irradiation and packaging of fresh meat and poultry. *Journal of Food Protection*, 59(1), 62-72.

[108] Lescano, G., Narvaiz, P., Kairiyama, E., & Kaupert, N. (1991). Effect of chicken breast irradiation on microbiological, chemical and organoleptic quality. *Lebensmittal Wissenund Technology*, 24, 130-134.

[109] Thakur, B. R., & Singh, R. K. (1994). Food irradiation Chemistry and applications. *Food Reviews International*, 10(4), 437-473.

[110] Jo, C., & Ahn, D. U. (2000). Volatiles and oxidative changes in irradiated pork sausage with different fatty acid composition and tocopherol content. *Journal of Food Science*, 65(2), 270-275.

[111] Yong, J., Hun, K., Sung, Y. P., So, J. K., & Young, J. Y. (2000). Identification of irradiation- induced volatile flavor compounds in beef. *Journal of Korean Society of Food Science and Nutrition*, 29(6), 1042-1049.

[112] Yong, J., Hun, K., Sung, Y. P., Wo, J. C., Seong, S. Y., & Young, J. Y. (2000). Identification of irradiation-induced volatile flavor compounds in chicken. *Journal of Korean Society of Food Science and Nutrition*, 29(6), 1050-1056.

[113] Nam, K. C., & Ahn, D. U. (2003). Double-packaging is effective in reducing lipid oxidation and off-odor volatiles of irradiated raw turkey meat. *Poultry Science*, 82(9), 1468-1474.

[114] Nam, K. C., Ahn, D. U., Du, M., & Jo, C. (2001). Lipid oxidation, color, volatiles, and sensory characteristics of aerobically packaged and irradiated pork with different ultimate pH. *Journal of Food Science*, 66, 1220-1225.

[115] St, Angelo. A. J., Vercellotti, J. R., Legendre, M. G., Vinnett, C. H., Kuan, J. W., James Jr, C., Jr, & Dupuy, H. P. (1987). Chemical and instrumental analysis of warmed-over flavor in beef. *Journal of Food Science*, 52, 1163-1168.

[116] Ingene, J. O., & Pearson, A. M. (1979). Role of phospholipids and triglycerides in warmed-over flavor development in meat model systems. *Journal of Food Science*, 44, 1285-1290.

[117] Byrne, D. V., Bredie, W. L. P., Bak, V., Bertelsen, G., Martens, H., & Martens, M. (2001). Sensory and chemical analysis of cooked porcine meat patties in relation to warmed-over flavor and pre-slaughter stress. *Meat Science*, 59, 229-249.

[118] St Angelo, A. J. (1996). Lipid oxidation in foods. *Critical Reviews in Food Science and Nutrition*, 36(3), 175-224.

[119] St, Angelo. A. J., Vercellotti, J. R., Dupuy, H. P., & Spanier, A. M. (1988). Assessment of beef flavor quality: a multidisciplinary approach. *Food Technology*, 42, 133-138.

[120] St, Angelo. A. J., Crippen, K. L., Dupuy, H. P., & James Jr, C., Jr. (1990). Chemical and sensory studies of antioxidant-treated beef. *Journal of Food Science*, 55, 1501-1539.

[121] James, J. M., & Calkins, C. R. (2005). Cooking rate and holding time effect on the flavor of muscles from the beef chuck and the round. In Proceedings of the international congress of meat science and technology Baltimore, MD.

[122] Elmore, J. S. (2008). Aroma. In Nollet L. M. L and Toldra. F (eds.) Handbook of muscle foods analysis Boca Raton CRC , 242-262.

[123] Madruga, M. S., Elmore, J. S., Dodson, A. T., & Mottram, D. S. (2009). Volatile flavor profile of goat meat extracted by three widely used techniques. *Food Chemistry*, 115, 1081-1087.

[124] Moon, S. Y., Cliff, M. A., & Li-Chan, E. C. Y. (2006). Odour-active components of simulated beef flavor analyzed by solid phase microextraction and gas chromatography-mass spectrometry and-olfactometry. *Food Research International*, 39, 294-308.

[125] Xie, J. C., Sun, B. G., & Wang, S. B. (2008). Aromatic constituents from Chinese traditional smoke-cured bacon of mini-pig. *Food science and technology international*, 14, 329-340.

Quality Control in Pharmaceutics

Chapter 9

New Approaches in Drug Quality Control: Matrices and Chemometrics

Sigrid Mennickent, M. de Diego, B. Schulz, M. Vega
and C. G. Godoy

Additional information is available at the end of the chapter

1. Quality control

Quality control refers to the process of quality evaluation that focuses on the internal measurement of the quality of a process, institution, product, service, or other. Often used interchangeably with *quality management* and *quality assurance* [1-3].

2. Drug quality control

Quality Assurance plays a very important role in making sure that the GMP standards are met and products comply with the international quality standards. The main functions carried out by drug quality control are:

• Approval of raw materials

• Monitoring of manufacturing processes

• Approval of finished products

• Documentation of technical information

• Implementation of cGMP

Manufacturing processes are monitored and controlled by testing of raw materials, in-process parameters. Final active pharmaceutical ingredients and dosage forms are tested for specified parameters before release. Analytical testing is carried out with highly sophisticated instruments: viz. HPLC, GC, IR, UV spectrophotometer mettler titrators, particle size analyzer etc.

All the analytical test procedures and manufacturing procedures are well documented and revision is undertaken as per specified protocol. Analytical methods are validated to give the reproducible results. Stability study as per stability protocol is considered to be very important area of Quality Assurance.

Automated systems are becoming increasingly important tools for appropriate monitoring and controlling of the pharmaceutical packaging process. Solutions for comprehensive quality assurance or production data acquisition and evaluation are just as important as applications that meet the legislative requirements of different countries in terms of serial numbering and the unique marking of products.

Quality control involves many phases, such as sample collection, measuring, analysis of results, and the approval/rejection of the batch. Nonetheless, the most important thing is the continuity and systematization of the quality control.

Effective process validation contributes significantly to assuring drug quality. The basic principle of quality assurance is that a drug should be produced that is fit for its intended use. This principle incorporates the understanding that the following conditions exist: Quality, safety, and efficacy are designed or built into the product.

Quality cannot be adequately assured merely by in-process and finished-product inspection or testing.

Process validation is defined as the collection and evaluation of data, from the process design stage through commercial production, which establishes scientific evidence that a process is capable of consistently delivering quality product. Process validation involves a series of activities taking place over the lifecycle of the product and process. Usually, process validation includes three stages:

- Process Design: The commercial manufacturing process is defined during this stage based on knowledge gained through development and scale-up activities.

- Process Qualification: During this stage, the process design is evaluated to determine if the process is capable of reproducible commercial manufacturing.

- Process Verification: Ongoing assurance is gained during routine production that the process remains in a state of control [1-3].

3. New approaches in drug quality control

3.1. Matrices

3.1.1. Residue analysis of pharmaceuticals in the aquatic environment

Residue analysis of pharmaceuticals in the aquatic environment has attracted considerable interest during the last few years.

Traces of such compounds have been detected in surface water samples from all countries where pharmaceuticals are widely in use.

Pharmaceutically active compounds have captured the attention of the scientific community because such pollutants result not primarily from manufacturing but from widespread, continual use in human and veterinary clinical practice. The biological activity of these compounds can lead to adverse effects in aquatic ecosystems and potentially have an impact on drinking-water supplies [4].

In the human body, pharmaceuticals can be transformed to one or more metabolites and excreted as a mixture of parent compound and metabolites, in which the parent compound is often the minor component. However, some drugs are poorly metabolized and are excreted unchanged. The degree of metabolism depends on a number of parameters, including age, gender and ethnicity, the constitution of the patient and the time of administration. Drug-drug interactions caused by enzyme induction or inhibition, as well as enhanced metabolism due to previous exposure, can also influence the pharmacokinetics of drugs [5].

Both the parent compound and the metabolites enter the aquatic environment once they are excreted from the human body. Monitoring studies in the environment have demonstrated the discharge of pharmaceuticals and their metabolites through municipal wastewater-treatment plants (WWTPs). Although unchanged drugs can undergo biochemical transformations during sewage treatment, some studies indicate that the absence of pharmaceutical compounds in treated water does not necessarily imply their complete removal. In most instances, human drugs are metabolized in the body to more polar compounds that are more likely to pass through the WWTP. In some cases, pharmaceuticals and their human metabolites can be microbially degraded in the activated sludge treatment.

Knowledge of the formation of stable metabolites in WWTPs is also important in order to understand the environmental fate of the parent compound. Once in the environment, these compounds can be transported and distributed in rivers, streams, and possibly further biodegraded. For most pharmaceuticals and their biotransformation products, these pathways in the aquatic environment are largely unknown, and investigations into their occurrence in environmental compartments are still rare.

Studies have been carried out to investigate their fate not only in surface waters, but also in sediment and soil environments. By nature, most pharmaceuticals are designed to be at least moderately water-soluble and to possess half-lives in the human body in the range of hours. Because human and microbial degradates will generally coexist with their parent compounds in the environment, indicators that summarize all the information on parent substances and degradates would be important instruments for decision-making and assessment [6].

Progress in instrumental analytical chemistry has resulted in the availability of methods that allow a monitoring of these pollutants at ng levels.

Improvements in detection limits over the past years have mainly been due to sophisticated mass spectrometric detection techniques. Furthermore, robust sample preparation and preconcentration protocols have contributed significantly to the achievements observed so far.

Nowadays it is a well-established fact that pharmaceutical drugs used during medical treatment may partly be excreted in an un-metabolized form, enter municipal sewage systems, and can even survive the passage through the sewage treatment plant. Therefore, sewage treatment plant effluents are the major source for introduction of pharmaceuticals into the aquatic environment. Furthermore, pharmaceuticals employed in veterinary medicine may be introduced into soil (and eventually into water) via manure, or may find a direct way into the aquatic system when used in fish farms.

Unfortunately, the consequences of continuous presence of low concentrations of pharmaceuticals for the ecosystem are still not fully known.

In many cases, the analytical procedures for residue analysis of pharmaceutical drugs nowadays available includes a pre-concentration and clean-up step by solid-phase extraction or related techniques, followed by chromatography in combination with mass spectrometry (MS) as detector.

Although GC–MS may still be the perfect technique for certain classes of pharmaceuticals, high-performance liquid chromatography (HPLC) hyphenated with atmospheric pressure ionization-MS has established itself as the better choice for simultaneous determination of pharmaceuticals of widely differing structures.

The concentration levels of pharmaceuticals found in environmental water samples are generally too low to allow a direct injection into a chromatographic system. Therefore, efficient pre-concentration steps are necessary which should also result in some sample clean-up. One of the most widely used sample treatment technique for residue analysis of pharmaceuticals in water is the extraction of the analytes by means of a solid sorbent.

This extraction procedure can be based on multiple equilibria between the liquid phase and the sorbent filled into a small cartridge (solid-phase extraction, SPE), or on a single equilibrium (sorptive extraction) [7-23].

3.1.1.1. Solid-phase extraction

Pharmaceuticals of adequate hydrophobicity can easily be pre-concentrated using any reversed-phase material such as alkyl-modified silica or polymer-based materials. Deprotonation of acidic compounds and protonation of basic compounds should be suppressed to ensure sufficient hydrophobicity of the analytes. Therefore, acidic pharmaceuticals should be pre-concentrated under acidic conditions, whereas basic analytes should be pre-concentrated at an alkaline pH. Alternatively, mixed-mode SPE materials can be used which exhibit both reversed-phase and cation-exchange properties due to the presence of sulfonic acid groups on the hydrophobic surface of the particles. Using acidified sample solutions, acidic and neutral analytes would be extracted by hydrophobic interactions, whereas protonated basic analytes would interact via ion exchange mechanisms.

A recent review has summarized new SPE materials that can improve the recoveries for polar analytes. These materials are mainly polymeric sorbents that improve the retention of polar compounds either by novel functional groups in the polymeric structure (resulting in a hydrophilic–hydrophobic balance material) or by considerably increased surface area. Some of these new materials have turned out to be well suited for multi-class analysis of pharmaceuticals in water samples. Nowadays, one of the most widely used sorbent is a copolymer of divinylbenzene and vinylpyrrolidone [7-23].

3.1.1.2. Sorptive extraction

Sorptive extraction based on a single partitioning equilibrium of analytes between the aqueous sample and a solid sorbent includes solid-phase microextraction (SPME), stir-bar sorptive extraction (SBSE), and several related variants. Originally, these techniques were based on polydimethylsiloxane (PDMS) as material for trapping trace analytes from a water sample due to partitioning between the aqueous matrix and the PDMS phase. Besides PDMS, some alternative sorptive materials have become commercially available recently, such as polyacrylates, copolymers of PDMS with divinylbenzene, copolymers of polyethylene glycol with divinylbenzene, and mixtures of carboxen (an inorganic adsorbent) with PDMS or divinylbenzene [7-23].

3.1.1.3. Sample pre-concentration procedures for sediment and sludge samples

Extraction of pharmaceuticals from sediment and sludge is generally done by blending the sample with an organic solvent or with mixtures of aqueous buffers and organic solvents.

Ultrasonication is frequently applied to assist the extraction process.

Additional clean-up steps for the extract may be necessary employing SPE or liquid–liquid extraction. Somewhat more advanced procedures are based on pressurized liquid extraction (accelerated solvent extraction) which may need less time and less solvent consumption [7-23].

3.1.1.4. Derivatization of the compounds

Various groups of pharmaceuticals can be derivatized to make them suited for GC analysis. Typical derivatization reagents for acidic pharmaceuticals include pentafluorobenzylbromide, methyl chloromethanoate, methanol/BF3, or tetrabutylammonium salts (for derivatization during injection). Phenazone-type drugs have been derivatized by silylation using N-tert-butyldimethylsilyl-N-methyltrifluoroacetamide (MTBSTFA). Silylation procedures are also commonly used for synthetic estrogens [7-23].

3.2.1.Some latest researches in this area

3.2.1.1. Pharmaceuticals in the aquatic environment: a critical review of the evidence for health effects in fish

The authors review the current data on the presence and reported biological effects in fish of some of the most commonly detected pharmaceuticals in the aquatic environment; namely nonsteroidal anti-inflammatory drugs (NSAIDs), fibrates, beta-blockers, selective serotonin reuptake inhibitors (SSRIs), azoles, and antibiotics. Reported biological effects in fish in the laboratory have often been shown to be in accordance with known effects of pharmaceuticals in mammals. Water concentrations at which such effects have been reported, however, are generally, between microg L(-1) and mg L(-1), typically at least 1 order of magnitude higher than concentrations normally found in surface waters (ng L(-1)). There are exceptions to this, however, as for the case of synthetic oestrogens, which can induce biological effects in the low ng L(-1) range. Although generally effect levels for pharmaceuticals are higher than those found in the environment, the risks to wild fish populations have not been thoroughly characterised, and there has been a lack of consideration given to the likely chronic nature of the exposures, or the potential for mixture effects. As global consumption of pharmaceuticals rises, an inevitable consequence is an increased level of contamination of surface and ground waters with these biologically active drugs, and thus in turn a greater potential for adverse effects in aquatic wildlife [24].

3.1.1.2. Human Pharmaceuticals, Hormones and Fragrances: The Challenge of Micropollutants in Urban Water Management

The observed concentrations of pharmaceuticals and personal care products (PPCPs) in raw wastewater confirm that municipal wastewater represents the main disposal pathway for the PPCPs consumed in households, hospitals and industry. In sewage treatment plant effluents most PPCPs are still present, since many of these polar and persistent compounds are being removed only partially or, in some cases, not at all. Treated wastewater therefore represents an important point source for PPCPs into the environment. After passing a sewage treatment plant the treated wastewater is mostly discharged into rivers and streams or sometimes used to irrigate fields. If drinking water is produced using resources containing a substantial proportion of treated wastewater (e.g. from river water downstream of communities) the water cycle is closed and indirect potable reuse occurs. Human Pharmaceuticals, Hormones and Fragrances provides an overview of the occurrence, analytics, removal and environmental risk of pharmaceuticals and personal care products in wastewater, surface water and drinking water. [25].

3.2.1.2. Factors affecting the concentrations of pharmaceuticals released to the aquatic environment

Although recent research has demonstrated that pharmaceuticals are widely distributed in the aquatic environment, it is difficult to assess the threat that they

pose to drinking water supplies or their rate of attenuation in natural systems without an adequate understanding of the sources of contamination. To identify pharmaceutical compounds of significance to water supplies in the United States, the authors have reviewed available data on the use of prescription drugs. Results of our analysis indicate that approximately 40 compounds could be present in municipal wastewater effluent at concentrations above 1,000 ng/L and at least 120 compounds could be present at concentrations above 1 ng/L. Important classes of prescription drugs include analgesics, beta-blockers, and antibiotics. Analysis of a group of the most commonly used pharmaceuticals in the United States indicates that they are ubiquitous in wastewater effluents. Authors have detected concentrations ranging from approximately 10- 3,000 ng/L for high use pharmaceuticals such as beta-blockers (*e.g.,* metoprolol, propranolol) and acidic drugs (*e.g.,* gemfibrozil, ibuprofen). The concentration of pharmaceuticals in effluent from conventional wastewater treatment plants is similar. Advanced wastewater treatment plants equipped with reverse osmosis systems reduce concentrations of pharmaceuticals below detection limits. In addition to removal during biological wastewater treatment, pharmaceuticals also are attenuated in engineered natural systems (*i.e.,* treatment wetlands, ground water infiltration basins). Preliminary evidence suggests limited removal of pharmaceuticals in engineered treatment wetlands and nearly complete removal of pharmaceuticals during ground water infiltration [26].

3.2.1.3. A preliminary ecotoxicity study of pharmaceuticals in the marine environment

Environmental fates and effects of pharmaceuticals in the aquatic environment have been the focus of recent research in environmental ecotoxicology. Worldwide studies of common over-the-counter pharmaceuticals have reported detectable levels in the aquatic environment, but there are few studies examining impacts on marine habitats. These drugs can affect the functions of various vertebrates and invertebrates. The stability of two pharmaceuticals, cyclizine (CYC) and prochlorperazine (PCZ), in seawater was examined under light and dark conditions, as well as the toxicity of these compounds to larvae of the barnacle Balanus amphitrite, which is a cosmopolitan marine organism found in most of the world's oceans. CYC was very stable under all the tested conditions. On the other hand, PCZ degraded in light but not in the dark, and was more stable in seawater than fresh water. For the barnacle larvae, the LC50 of prochlorperazine was 0.93 microg/mL and the LC50 for CYC was approximately 0.04 microg/mL [27].

3.2.1.4. Estrogenic activity of pharmaceuticals in the aquatic environment

In the last years pharmaceuticals have aroused great interest as environmental pollutants for their toxic effects towards non target organisms. This study wants to draw attention to a further adverse effect of drugs, the endocrine interference. The most representative drugs of the widespread classes in environment were investigated. The YES-test and the E-screen assay were performed to detect the capability of these substances to bind the human estrogenic receptor alpha (hER alpha) in comparison with 17beta-estradiol. Out of 14 tested pharmaceuticals, 9 were positive to YES-assay and 11 were positive to E-screen assay; in particular, Furosemide and the fibrates (Bezafibrate, Fenofibrate and Gemfibrozil) gave the maximal estrogenic response. Tamoxifen showed its dual activity as agonist and antagonist of hER alpha [28].

3.2.1.5. Colloids as a sink for certain pharmaceuticals in the aquatic environment

The occurrence and fate of pharmaceuticals in the aquatic environment is recognized as one of the emerging issues in environmental chemistry and as a matter of public concern. Existing data tend to focus on the concentrations of pharmaceuticals in the aqueous phase, with limited studies on their concentrations in particulate phase such as sediments. Furthermore, current water quality monitoring does not differentiate between soluble and colloidal phases in water samples, hindering our understanding of the bioavailability and bioaccumulation of pharmaceuticals in aquatic organisms. In this study, an investigation was conducted into the concentrations and phase association (soluble, colloidal, suspended particulate matter or SPM) of selected pharmaceuticals (propranolol, sulfamethoxazole, meberverine, thioridazine, carbamazepine, tamoxifen, indomethacine, diclofenac, and meclofenamic acid) in river water, effluents from sewage treatment works (STW), and groundwater in the UK. Colloids were isolated by cross-flow ultrafiltration (CFUF). Water samples were extracted by solid-phase extraction (SPE), while SPM was extracted by microwave. All sample extracts were analyzed by liquid chromatography-tandem mass spectrometry (LC-MS/MS) in the multiple reaction monitoring.

Five compounds propranolol, sulfamethoxazole, carbamazepine, indomethacine, and diclofenac were detected in all samples, with carbamazepine showing the highest concentrations in all phases. The highest concentrations of these compounds were detected in STW effluents, confirming STW as a key source of these compounds in the aquatic environments. The calculation of partition coefficients of pharmaceuticals between SPM and filtrate, between SPM and soluble phase, and between colloids and soluble phase showed that intrinsic partition coefficients are between 25% and 96%, and between 18% and 82% higher than relevant observed partition coefficients values, and are much less variable. Secondly, K_{coc} values are 3–4 orders of magnitude greater than Kocint values, indicating that aquatic colloids are substantially more powerful sorbents for accumulating pharmaceuticals than sediments. Furthermore, mass balance calculations of pharmaceutical concentrations demonstrate that between 23% and 70% of propranolol, 17–62% of sulfamethoxazole, 7–58% of carbamazepine, 19–84% of indomethacine, and 9–74% of diclofenac are present in the colloidal phase.

The results provide direct evidence that sorption to colloids provides an important sink for the pharmaceuticals in the aquatic environment. Such strong pharmaceutical/colloid interactions may provide a long-term storage of pharmaceuticals, hence, increasing their persistence while reducing their bioavailability in the environment.

Recommendations and perspectives from this study:

Pharmaceutical compounds have been detected not only in the aqueous phase but also in suspended particles; it is important, therefore, to have a holistic approach in future environmental fate investigation of pharmaceuticals. For example, more research is needed to assess the storage and long-term record of pharmaceutical residues in aquatic sediments by which benthic organisms will be most affected. Aquatic colloids have been shown to account for the accumulation of major fractions of total pharmaceutical concentrations in the aquatic environment, demonstrating unequivocally the importance of aquatic colloids as a sink for such residues in the aquatic systems. As aquatic colloids are abundant, ubiquitous, and highly powerful sorbents, they are expected to influence the bioavailability and bioaccumulation of such chemicals by aquatic organisms. It is therefore critical for colloids to be incorporated into water quality models for prediction and risk assessment purposes [29].

4. Chemometrics

Chemometrics is the science of extracting information from chemical systems by data-driven means. It is a highly interfacial discipline, using methods frequently employed in core data-analytic disciplines such as multivariate statistics, applied mathematics, and computer science, in order to address problems in chemistry, biochemistry, medicine, biology and chemical engineering.

Chemometrics is applied to solve both descriptive and predictive problems in experimental life sciences, especially in chemistry. In descriptive applications, properties of chemical systems are modeled with the intent of learning the underlying relationships and structure of the system (i.e., model understanding and identification). In predictive applications, properties of chemical systems are modeled with the intent of predicting new properties or behavior of interest. In both cases, the datasets can be small but are often very large and highly complex, involving hundreds to thousands of variables, and hundreds to thousands of cases or observations.

Chemometric techniques are particularly heavily used in analytical chemistry and metabolomics, and the development of improved chemometric methods of analysis also continues to advance the state of the art in analytical instrumentation and methodology. It is an application driven discipline, and thus while the standard chemometric methodologies are very widely used industrially, academic groups are dedicated to the continued development of chemometric theory, method and application development [30-33].

Author details

Sigrid Mennickent[1*], M. de Diego[1], B. Schulz[1], M. Vega[2] and C. G. Godoy[1]

*Address all correspondence to: smennick@udec.cl

1 Department of Pharmacy, Faculty of Pharmacy, University of Concepción, Concepción,, Chile

2 Department of Bromatology, Nutrition and Dietetic, Faculty of Pharmacy, University of Concepción, Concepción, , Chile

References

[1] USP (1999). The United States Pharmacopeia/ The National Formulary (USP 24/NF 19), United States Pharmacopeial Convection, Inc., Rockville

[2] ICH. (2003). *The Sixth ICH International Conference on Armonization of Technical Requirements for Registration of Pharmaceuticals for Human Use, Osaka,*.

[3] Buchberger, W. W. (2007). *Analytica Chimica Acta*, 593, 129-139.

[4] Jones, O., Lester, J. N., & Voulvoulis, N. (2005). *Trends in Biotechonology*, 23(4), 163-167.

[5] Lemmer, B. (1996). Chronopharmacology- Cellular and Biochemical Interactions. Birkhäuser,, New York, USA.

[6] Boxall, A., Fenner, K., Kolpin, D. W., & Maund, S. (2004). *Environ. Sci. Technol.*, 38, 369A.

[7] Moldovan, Z. (2006). *Chemosphere*, 64, 1808.

[8] Cunningham, V. L., Buzby, M., Hutchinson, T., Mastrocco, F., Parke, N., & Roden, N. (2006). *Env. Sci. Technol*, 40, 3457.

[9] Fent, K., Weston, A. A., & Caminada, D. (2006). *Aquatic Toxicol*, 76, 122.

[10] Crane, M., Watts, C., & Boucard, T. (2006). *Sci. Tot. Environ*, 367, 23.

[11] Hernando, M. D., Mezcua, M., Fernandez-Alba, A. R., & Barcelo, D. (2006). *Talanta*, 69, 334.

[12] Benito-Peña, E., Partal-Rodera, A. I., Leon-Gonzalez, M. E., & Moreno-Bondi, M. C. (2006). *Anal. Chim. Acta*, 556, 415.

[13] Fontanals, N., Marce, R. M., & Borrull, F. (2005). Trends Anal. Chem ., 24, 394.

[14] Gomez, M. J., Petrovic, M., Fernandez-Alba, A. R., & Barcelo, D. (2006). *J. Chromatogr. A*, 1114, 224.

[15] Gros, M., Petrovic, M., & Barcelo, D. (2006). *Talanta*, 70, 678.

[16] Petrovic, M., Gros, M., & Barcelo, D. (2006). *J. Chromatogr. A*, 1124, 68.

[17] Trenholm, R. A., Vanderford, B. J., Holady, J. C., Rexing, D. J., & Snyder, S. A. (2006). *Chemosphere*, 65, 1990.

[18] Roberts, P. H., & Bersuder, P. (2006). *J. Chromatogr. A*, 1134, 143.

[19] Himmelsbach, M., Buchberger, W., & Klampfl, C. (2006). *Electrophoresis*, 27, 1220.

[20] Seitz, W., Weber, W. H., Jiang, J. Q., Lloyd, B. J., Maier, M., Maier, D., & Schulz, W. (2006). *Chemosphere*, 64, 1318.

[21] Pozo, O. J., Guerrero, C., Sancho, J. V., Ibañez, M., Pitarch, E., Hogendoorn, E., & Hernandez, F. (2006). *J. Chromatogr. A*, 1103, 83.

[22] Rodriguez-Mozaz, S., Lopez de Alda, D., & Barcelo, D. (2007). *J. Chromatogr. A*, 1152, 97.

[23] Quintana, J. B., Miro, M., Estela, J. M., & Cerda, V. (2006). *Anal. Chem.*, 78, 2832.

[24] Corcoran, J., Winter, M. J., & Tyler, C. R. (2010). *Crit, Rev. Toxicol*, 40(4), 287-304.

[25] Ternes, T. (2006). Human Pharmaceuticals, Hormones and Fragrances: The Challenge of Micropollutants in Urban Water Management. Iwa Publishing.

[26] Sedlak, D., & Pinkston, K. (2011). *Factors affecting the concentrations of pharmaceuticals released to the aquatic environment*, University of California.

[27] Choong, A. M., Teo, S. L., Leow, J. L., & Ho, P. C. (2006). *J. Toxicol. Environ. Health A.*, 69(21), 1959-1970.

[28] Isidori, M., Bellota, M., Cangiano, M., & Parrella, A. (2009). *Environ. Int*, 35(5), 826-829.

[29] Maskaoui, K., & Zhou, J. (2010). *Environmental Science and Pollution Research*, 17(4), 898-907.

[30] Verenitch, S. S., Lowe, C. J., & Mazumder, A. (2006). *J. Chromatogr. A*, 1116.

[31] Gemperline, P. J. (2006). Practical guide to chemometrics. 2nd Edition, CRC Press 10.1201/9781420018301

[32] Mark, H., & Workman, J. (2007). Chemometrics in spectroscopy. Academic Press-Elsevier.

[33] Maeder, M., & Neuhold, Y. M. (2007). Practical Data Analysis in Chemistry. Elsevier.

Chapter 10

Microbial Quality
Concerns for Biopharmaceuticals

Farzaneh Lotfipour and Somayeh Hallaj-Nezhadi

Additional information is available at the end of the chapter

1. Introduction

Finding an appropriate definition or a clear classification for biologically occurring pharmaceutical products is a complicated task because of overlapping borders and consequent misconceptions in this area. Indeed, numerous definitions and classifications for this category of products have been proposed so far, and different points of view for this concept can be found in research literature, business, industry, and even the general public [1, 2].

To obtain a better view of biopharmaceutical concept, first, it is necessary to know the present definitions for the main constituents of the word, that is, pharmaceutical product and biological product.

According to the WHO, a finished pharmaceutical product (FPP) is "A finished dosage form of a pharmaceutical product, which has undergone all stages of manufacture, including packaging in its final container and labeling." [3]

An active pharmaceutical ingredient can be defined as "A substance used in a finished pharmaceutical product (FPP), intended to furnish pharmacological activity or to otherwise have direct effect in the diagnosis, cure, mitigation, treatment or prevention of disease, or to have direct effect in restoring, correcting or modifying physiological functions in human beings." [3] Hence, in brief, it can be said that any material, regardless of its origin or structure, with treatment, diagnosis, or prevention applications and passing regulatory requirements, is a pharmaceutical product.

On the other hand, the FDA definition for biological products is as follows: "Biological products or biologics are medical products made from a variety of natural sources (human, animal or microorganism). Like drugs, some biologics are intended to treat diseases and medical conditions or to prevent or diagnose diseases." [4] Consequently, any product of biological origin with treatment, diagnosis, or prevention applications is a biological product.

A biotechnology-derived product is another concept that should be taken into consideration. It is defined by Walsh as "any pharmaceutical product used for a therapeutic or in vivo diagnostic purpose, which is produced in full or in part by either traditional or modern biotechnological means." [5]

On comparing the definitions for a biotechnology-derived product and a biological product, both of which should be of biological origin, it is obvious that the key element in the former definition is the application of biotechnological means for production.

In practice, the regulatory requirements needed for a biotechnology-derived product and a biological product are methodologically different from the pharmaceutical product due to their biological essence. For example, the determination of adventitious agents such as viruses, transmitting spongiform encephalopathy (TSE), and mycoplasma are included in most of the related guidelines and pharmacopeias for a biotechnology-derived product and a biological product.

Finally, a biopharmaceutical is defined by Walsh as "A protein or nucleic acid based pharmaceutical substance used for therapeutic or in vivo diagnostic purposes, which is produced by means other than direct extraction from a native (non-engineered) biological source." This definition that will be used in the present chapter for biopharmaceuticals includes all pharmaceutical products produced by modern biotechnology techniques as well as nucleic acid (DNA or RNA) based pharmaceutical products for gene therapy. Hence, the overlapping area between biotechnology-derived products and biopharmaceuticals is the application of modern biotechnological means in their production. However, the differentiating area can be the application of traditional biotechnological means for the production of biotechnology-derived products. In addition, nucleic acid-based pharmaceutical products that are categorized as biopharmaceuticals are not biotechnology-derived products [6]. Figure 1 illustrates these overlapping and differentiating areas. Moreover, some examples of products in these categories are shown in Table1.

Biological products	Biotechnology-derived product by:		Biopharmaceuticals
	Traditional technology	Modern technology	
Blood and blood products	Therapeutic proteins from natural sources	Recombinant proteins	Recombinant proteins
Human cells and tissues	Antibiotics fully or partially from microorganisms	Monoclonal antibody produced by hybridoma technology	Nucleic acid-based pharmaceutical products for gene therapy

Table 1. Some examples of products related to biological, biotechnology-derived, and biopharmaceutical products.

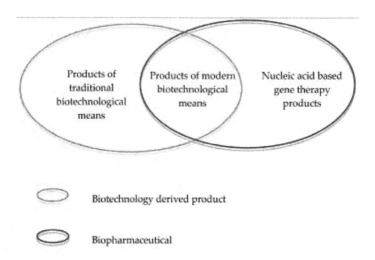

Figure 1. The schematic representation for biotechnology-derived products and biopharmaceutical categories and the overlapping areas between them.

2. Methods for biopharmaceutical production

2.1. Production of an original recombinant system

2.1.1. Recombinant DNA technology

The main category of biopharmaceuticals is manufactured via recombinant DNA technology. Indeed, recombinant DNA technologies are enabling techniques that manipulate and engineer different gene fragments and which have been introduced less than 50 years ago by the revolutionary invention of Polymerase Chain Reaction (PCR) by Kary Mullis [7].

DNA and RNA extraction from different cell types, cutting DNA fragments using restriction endonucleases, joining DNA fragments by DNA ligases, PCR to amplify gene fragments, cloning of the gene fragments into different vectors, introduction of recombinant constructs into proper hosts, protein expression, extraction, and purification are some of the most widely used means in recombinant protein production.

Figure 2 schematically represents the summarized process of production of a recombinant protein. As can be seen from the chart, first, the gene of interest should be isolated and amplified from the original cell. According to the type of the cell, it can be done through direct total DNA extraction followed by a PCR using proper primers to obtain the gene in prokaryotes. On the other hand, in eukaryotes, due to the existence of introns and some modifications that occur in the transcribed mRNA, the process is considerably complicated. Introns are non-coding sequences which are removed after transcription versus coding sequences that are called *exons*. In addition, mRNA is more modified by the addition of a methylated guanine (CAP) on its 5′end and a poly-adenine tail on its 3′end. After these modifications, mature mRNA is exported to the cytoplasm in order to start the translation process. Consequently, to obtain a gene of interest in eukaryotes, the mature mRNA should be extracted from the cell, and the complementary DNA should be synthesized followed by amplification of the gene by PCR using proper primers. However, in both cases (prokaryotes and eukaryotes), the short genes can be obtained by a solid-phase synthesis process.

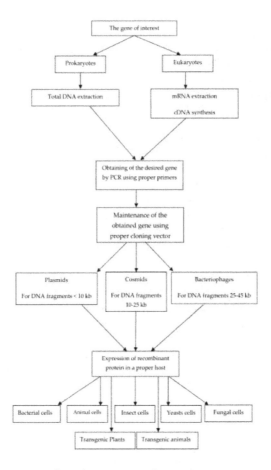

Figure 2. Schematic representation of recombinant protein production process

Based on their sizes, the obtained genes can now be introduced into a proper vector for maintenance, replication, or expression purposes. Plasmids, cosmids, and bacteriophages are the most important cloning vectors that are classified according to the size of the DNA fragment that can be inserted into them. Ultimately, the new recombinant construct should be introduced into an expression system for production. Different classes of expression systems with their certain merits and disadvantages are available and range from cell systems such as bacterial, animal, fungal, and yeast cells to transgenic systems such as transgenic plants and animals [7, 8].

2.1.2. Monoclonal antibody production

2.1.2.1. Classical hybridoma technology

Each specific antibody is secreted by a specific B cell and could recognize a specific region on the antigen that is called *epitope*. Each antibody-secreting B cell could be used as a source of an antibody of interest if it is isolated and cultured in vitro. Nevertheless, B cells are not considered a satisfactory source, as they are not immortalized and cannot survive for a long time. The main approach for overcoming this problem is cell hybridization, which includes the fusion of antibody-secreting B cells with tumor cells (such as mouse myeloma cells) proliferating ever more. The classical hybridoma technology was first introduced by Georges Kohler and Cesar Milstein in the mid 1970s for the generation of immortalized hybridoma cells that could grow in cell culture for a long time and produce the desired monoclonal antibodies [9, 10]. The basic process (Figure 3) includes the immunization of a mouse with the desired antigen. The mouse was then sacrificed, and B lymphocytes secreting antibodies that were selective for the specific epitope on the antigen were isolated from the spleen. The spleen is considered the most ready source for antigen-specific lymphocytes that provides access to a large number of antibody-secreting cells [1]. The isolated B cells were subsequently fused with immortal mouse myeloma cells. The resultant hybridoma cells were then separated from the unfused cells by culturing in specific cell culture media. The cell culture media for the hybridoma growth and production of monoclonal antibodies have been reviewed in detail by Bols et al. [11].

In general, for the successful fusion of hybridomas, the cells are grown in HAT selection medium. The selection medium is called *HAT*, as it has Hypoxanthine, Aminopterin, and Thymidine. This is because a mutation in either the hypoxanthine-guanine phosphoribosyltransferase (HGPRT) or the thymidine kinase (TK) gene of the cells would cause their death in the HAT medium. Generally, a TK-deficient cell (TK-negative mutant) is resistant to bromodeoxyuridine (BrdU), and an HGPRT-deficient cell (HGPRT-negative mutant) is resistant to 6-thioguanine (6-TG) and 8-azaguanine. Hence, in order to make myeloma cells sensitive to HAT (unable to grow in HAT media), they are treated with one of these drugs before their passage to HAT media.

Normal cells can synthesize the required nucleotides in two pathways: (1) the main one or de novo biosynthetic pathway, and (2) the alternative one or the salvage pathway (when the main pathway is blocked).

Aminopterin (a folic acid analog that inhibits dihydrofolate reductase) blocks the activation of tetrahydrofolate, which is required for the synthesis of nucleotides via the de novo synthetic pathway, and, therefore, the main pathway is blocked. Thus, in aminopterin-treated

cells (HGPRT⁺ and TK⁺), the synthesis of nucleotides shifts to the salvage pathway only if hypoxanthine and thymidine are supplied in the medium. HGPRT and TK, the two enzymes, are required for the salvage pathway, and they catalyze the synthesis of purine and thymidylate from hypoxanthine and thymidine substrates, respectively.

Since unfused myeloma cells lack HGPRT or TK, they cannot use the salvage pathway. Thus, the unfused myeloma cells get killed in the HAT medium, as both biosynthetic pathways are blocked. Normal unfused B cells die in the HAT medium, as they are not immortalized and cannot grow for a long time. Nevertheless, the fusion of normal B cells with the HGPRT⁻or TK⁻myeloma cells allows the hybridoma cells to grow in HAT medium, as the B cells provide the necessary enzymes for growth of the hybridoma cells.

Hence, the HAT selection medium offers an ideal environment for the isolation of fused myeloma and B cells (hybridoma cells) from unfused myeloma cells and unfused B cells, as this medium allows only the hybridoma cells to survive in the culture.

The production of monoclonal antibodies could be accomplished by ascites (ascitic fluid) production (in vivo) or by cell culture (in vitro) methods. In the in vivo method, hybridoma cells are injected intraperitoneally into mice. The peritoneum serves as a growth chamber for the injected cells. These cells could secrete a high-titered solution of desired antibodies as they grow in the cavity. Finally, the produced antibodies are extracted from the ascitic fluid accumulated in the peritoneal cavity [6]. The antibody concentrations typically range between 1 and 15 mg/ml. The in vivo method offers a very high concentration of monoclonal antibody that often does not need more concentration procedures. Nevertheless, monoclonal antibodies produced by this technique may be contaminated by considerable levels of mouse proteins and other contaminants that might require more complicated, subsequent downstream purifications. The other disadvantage of the ascites production is related to animal welfare issues, as these could cause distress in mice.

Currently, more than 90% of monoclonal antibodies are produced by in vitro techniques [12] that use large-scale manufacturing plants containing several 10,000-L or larger culture bioreactors [13]. The in vitro method of monoclonal antibody production decreases the use of mice and also avoids the need for experienced personnel for animal handling. Regardless of the privileges and importance of the in vitro methods of antibody production, there are some situations in which this method is not applicable; for instance:

1. Hybridoma cells do not adapt well to in vitro conditions.

2. Downstream purification methods cause protein denaturation or decreased antibody activity.

3. The cell line cannot maintain the production of monoclonal antibodies.

4. When hybridoma cells are contaminated with infectious agents (such as yeasts or fungi), the cells must often be passed through mice. Since removal of the organisms cannot be accomplished by current antimicrobial drugs, thus the in vivo method may save a valuable hybridoma.

5. When in vitro methods result in monoclonal antibodies that are glycosylated at positions different from those harvested from mouse ascites, they affect antigen-binding capacity as well as biological functions [12].

Taken together, the cell culture technique is a method of choice for large-scale monoclonal antibody production due to the simplicity of the cell culture and financial considerations without ethical concerns that are related to animal use.

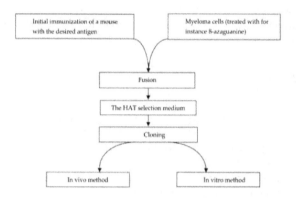

Figure 3. The diagram of the monoclonal antibody production via classical hybridoma technology

2.1.2.2. Chimeric and humanized antibodies

In 1986, about 10 years after the conception of monoclonal antibody technology, Orthoclone OKT3 was approved by the FDA for use in patients with acute rejection of a transplanted kidney [14]. Unfortunately, early clinical applications of murine monoclonal antibodies were disappointing. This was due to the fact that monoclonal antibodies produced via the classical method are of murine origin and are, therefore, immunogenic to human subjects. In general, patients receiving an antibody exhibit HAMA responses (human anti-mouse antibodies) within two weeks. Multiple infusions of murine monoclonal antibodies significantly enhance the HAMA reactions [6]. In addition, the immune system eliminates the murine monoclonal antibody molecule. Thus, murine monoclonal antibodies demonstrate short serum half lives after administration to humans. Furthermore, the other main difficulty related to murine monoclonal antibodies is the poor recognition of the Fc region by human effector systems of complement and Fc receptors.

Thus, new strategies that are used for producing humanized mouse antibodies that are less immunogenic have been discovered. The first strategy includes the production of functional specific recombinant IgG molecules consisting of mouse variable regions and human constant regions; these are known as chimeric antibodies. Taken together, in the chimeric antibody, 8 out of 12 domains are of human origin (constant regions of the heavy and light chains) (C_H and C_L) [15]. Chimeric antibodies exhibit reduced HAMA responses compared with mouse antibodies, but the affinity and the selectivity are the same. Furthermore, since the Fc region contains human sequences, the activation of Fc-mediated immune effector functions is allowed.

To further minimize the antigenicity of murine antibodies, humanized antibodies were developed. For their generation, hyper-variable complementarity-determining regions (CDRs) of the specific murine antibody are transferred to a fully human framework. In comparison with the mouse antibodies, humanized antibodies suggest a lower occurrence of HAMA responses.

Further efforts have been invested in the development of technologies that generate fully human monoclonal antibodies. One of the approaches entails the development of transgenic mice, in which a repertoire of human immunoglobulin germline gene segments is inserted into the mouse genome. After the immunization of these mice, they produce fully human antibodies, which can subsequently be separated with the classical hybridoma technology [15].

Figure 4 illustrates the schematic structures of mouse, chimeric, humanized, and human antibodies.

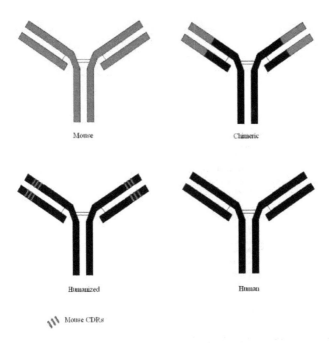

Mouse

Chimeric

Humanized

Human

111 Mouse CDRs

Figure 4. The structure of mouse (shown in red color), chimeric, humanized (shown in black color), and human antibodies. Chimeric antibodies comprise mouse variable regions and human constant regions. Humanized antibodies consist of murine hyper-variable complementarity-determining regions (CDRs) that are grafted to fully human framework.

2.2. Mass production of a recombinant product

Mass production of recombinant products can be achieved in a process that is divided into two main sections called *upstream* and *downstream* processing, as schematically depicted in Figure 5.

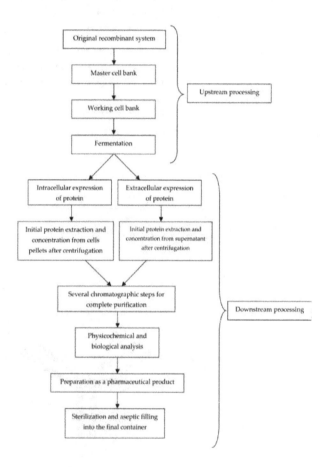

Figure 5. Mass production of a recombinant product.

The first step, the upstream processing step, is the mass production of a recombinant protein via the fermentation process. The original recombinant system that is used for the expression of the recombinant protein (i.e. in the form of a recombinant plasmid maintained in a suitable host cell) forms the cell deposit in a cell banking system. There are two levels of cell deposits in the cell banking system: The first line is called *master cell bank*, which is prepared directly from a culture of the original recombinant system that includes several hundred stored ampoules.

The second line that is referred to as the *working cell bank* is produced from a single master cell bank ampoule. Each ampoule from the working cell bank is thawed and used to seed the fermentor for the production of a batch. Obviously, the fermentation process for various recombinant systems, such as bacterial fermenting systems or animal cell systems, is quite different and needs its own certain requirements.

On the other hand, *downstream processing*, which is the next step, refers to the purification of the mass produced protein. The first step in downstream processing is the initial extraction and concentration of the product, which depends on the situation of the expressed protein; that is, it should be extracted from the pellet cells for intracellular proteins or from the supernatant for extracellular proteins after centrifugation.

The second stage entails (1) several chromatographic steps that complete the purification of the product; (2) the potency test; (3) the addition of suitable excipients; (4) sterilization; (5) filling of the product in its final form (liquid or solid) into the final container before sealing; and labeling [6].

3. Sources of biological contamination of biopharmaceuticals

In line with conventional pharmaceutical products, the main sources of biological contamination in biopharmaceuticals can be related to raw materials and the production environment. Indeed, the biological contaminant content of any pharmaceutical product is a representative of their starting materials and the production environment flora.

3.1. Raw materials

Animal origin materials, such as cell culture media, sera, and supplements that are extensively used in biopharmaceutical production, are of high contamination risk. These materials can be considered the main source for the contamination of biopharmaceuticals with adventitious agents such as TSEs, viruses, and mycoplasmas. Therefore, they should be supplied from reliable resources, and special attention should be paid to their quality control procedure. It should be ensured that all raw materials, especially those of high risk, gain quality specifications for current good manufacturing practice.

Standard methods for sterilization of cell culture media, sera, and supplements should be established according to the properties of the materials. Due to the heat-labile nature of the majority of materials used in biopharmaceutical production, autoclaving is usually replaced with alternative strategies such as filter-sterilization or less frequently high-temperature, short-time treatment strategies. In spite of the routine filter-sterilization procedure that uses 0.22 μm, it is usually performed with 0.1-μm membrane filters due to the risk of contamination with adventitious agents.

Furthermore, high-temperature, short-time treatment strategies are sometimes employed for the elimination of biological contaminants from small solutes such as vitamins and amino acids [16].

Another important raw material that is used in the production of any pharmaceutical product, including biopharmaceuticals, is water, which can be considered an important source for contamination, with water-borne bacteria such as Pseudomonas spp., Alcaligenes spp., Flavobacterium spp., Chromobacter spp., and Serratia spp. Water for pharmaceutical purposes is discussed in detail in the USP [17]. Due to the fact that the intended administration of biopharmaceuticals in the majority of cases is via injection, Water for Injection (WFI) which is sterile and apyrogen is routinely used in this area.

3.2. Production environment

Pharmaceutical products' contamination may occur from the transformation of microorganisms from the production environment to the product. The production environment includes air, surfaces, instruments, equipments, and personnel.

The main groups of microorganisms that are isolated from air are the spore-forming bacteria (Bacillus spp. and Clostridium spp., the non-sporing bacteria Staphylococcus spp., Streptococcus spp., and Corynebacterium spp.), the molds (Penicillium spp., Cladosporium spp., Aspergillus spp., and Mucor spp.), and the yeast (Rhodotorula spp.). These contaminants may be air borne or can be initiated from process equipment or personnel [16]. Consequently, environmental monitoring programs in a production environment are essential actions. Furthermore, the critical operations in biopharmaceutical production should be performed in controlled environments or clean rooms. A clean room is a place with high control of the entrance of particles via the establishment of some air filters called *high-efficiency particulate air (HEPA) filters*. HEPA filters made from a microglass material with a pleated construction system provide a large surface area that efficiently filters the incoming air and generates a constant air motion. Based on the permitted quantity of viable microorganisms and particulates, various classes of clean rooms can be established using HEPA filters with required efficiencies.

According to the *EC Guide to Good Manufacturing Practice for Medicinal Products* (EC GGMP), four grades for clean rooms are available, such as grade A, B, C, or D, based on the number of viable microorganisms and particulates (Table 2).

Clean room grade	Maximum permitted number of particles/m$_3$	Maximum permitted CFU of viable microorganisms/m$_3$ in air sample
A	3500	<1
B	3500	10
C	350000	100
D	3500000	200

Table 2. Clean room grades according to the number of viable microorganisms and the number of particulates

Critical operations such as inoculum preparation and aseptic filling are generally performed in the highest air grade (A); however, less critical operations can be performed in lower grades or even non-classified air.

In addition to the establishment of suitable filters in the clean rooms, special attention should be paid to the position, type, and texture of surfaces, floors, and fixtures. They should be made from smooth and chemically stable materials. In addition, a distinct transfer lock area should exist before entry to the clean room for sanitization of materials and personnel or garment changing. Furthermore, all doors should be interlocking [6].

4. Hazards of biological contamination of biopharmaceuticals

Similar to other pharmaceuticals, biological contamination of biopharmaceuticals may perhaps cause product spoilage. It may result in product metabolization by microorganisms, and, therefore, lead to a decrease in biopharmaceutical potency. The product spoilage may also provide a potential health hazard to patients and lead to outbreaks of infections that may cause additional complications. In addition, microbial-derived agents secreted in products such as endotoxins can be hazardous to a patient's health.

5. Determination of biological contaminants

5.1. Bacteria and fungi

Bacteria and fungi can be considered important contamination sources for all kinds ofpharmaceutical products, including biopharmaceuticals; hence, the control of them is of critical importance. The control of both bacteria and fungi is considered to be worthy of mandatory tests for nearly all kinds of pharmaceuticals in pharmacopoeias. All the related tests and procedures are covered in detail in the major pharmacopoeias such as USP and EP [17, 18].

Since almost all the biopharmaceuticals are administered intravenously, general sterility testing must be carried out for these products. Basically, sterility testing can be defined as "a test that evaluates whether a sterilized pharmaceutical product is free of contaminating microorganisms." The European Pharmacopoeia (2002) proposes two media for sterility testing:

(1) fluid mercaptoacetate medium (also known as *fluid thioglycollate medium*), which is mainly appropriate for the culture of anaerobic organisms at 30–35°C; and (2) soyabean casein digest medium, which is used for the culture of both aerobic bacteria at 30–35°C and fungi at 20–25°C.

Two main methods are used for sterility tests: (1) direct inoculation of the test samples in the media mentioned earlier; or (2) filtration of the test material through a sterile membrane filter with a pore size of 0.45 μm; then, the filter containing any microorganism present in the fluids is divided aseptically, and portions are transferred to the media.

The eradication of bacteria and fungi from the products is generally carried out via inactiva-tion and sterile filtration.

5.2. Endotoxins

Since most of the biopharmaceuticals are administered intravenously, finished-product bio-pharmaceuticals must be sterile and free from pyrogenic substances. The endotoxin limit for the intravenous administration of pharmaceutical and biological products is 5 endotoxin units (EU)/kg of body weight/hour by all pharmacopoeias [19]. Hence, the detection and re-moval of pyrogenic substances, especially endotoxins (lipopolysaccharides in the cell wall of gram-negative bacteria), are necessary to ensure safety of biopharmaceutical products. Cur-rently available methods for endotoxin detection include the U.S. Pharmacopeia rabbit test and the Limulus amebocyte lysate (LAL) test [7].

The rabbit pyrogen test entails measurements of the rise in body temperature of rabbits after an intravenous injection of a test substance. The presence of pyrogens of all kinds can be tested using this method. However, this method suffers from a number of disadvantages and limitations: (1) Endotoxin tolerance occurs after repeated use of rabbits; (2) variations in the response depending on sex, age, and species; (3) differences between the responses of rabbits and humans to various pyrogen types; and (4) the rabbit pyrogen test is inadequate for sera, radiopharmaceuticals, chemotherapeutics, analgesics, cytokines, immunosuppres-sive agents, and others [20].

Accordingly, the use of the rabbit pyrogen test has been reduced. Nowadays, the most wide-ly used endotoxin detection systems are based on the highly sensitive LAL test. It is based on the coagulation cascade of the blood of a horseshoe crab, Limulus polyphemus, which is induced by lipopolysaccharide. The currently known methods for lipopolysaccharide detec-tion entail (1) gel-clot assay, (2) turbidimetric LAL technique, and (3) the chromogenic LAL technique.

The gel-clot assay is a limit test that provides simple positive or negative results. The LAL reagent is introduced to a sample, and the test material is considered endotoxin positive if a gel is formed via a clotting reaction.

The turbidimetric and the chromogenic LAL techniques are quantitative tests. The former is based on the fact that turbidity increases as a result of the precipitation of the clottable pro-tein that is related to endotoxin concentration in the sample. The optical density is read by a spectrophotometer at either a fixed time (for the end-point method) or progressively (for the kinetic assay) as turbidity develops.

The chromogenic LAL technique makes use of a synthetic substrate which contains an amino acid sequence similar to that of the clottable protein, coagulogen, in order to detect endotoxin. The enzyme cleaves a yellow-colored substance from the chromogenic sub-strate, and the color intensity produced is proportional to the amount of endotoxin present in the sample.

Endotoxins are temperature and pH stable, and, therefore, their removal is one of the most challenging issues. Numerous techniques are used to reduce endotoxin contamination of biopharmaceuticals, including ion-exchange chromatography, sucrose gradient centrifugation, gel filtration chromatography [19], affinity adsorption [21], charged membrane/depth filtration, and ultrafiltration [22].

5.3. Viruses

Owing to the risks of transmission of adventitious agents to patients, the different cell levels should be studied for the absence of these agents. Among the adventitious agents, special attention should be paid to viruses that are capable of contaminating the original species. Generally, the virological safety of biopharmaceuticals includes several levels of control at various manufacturing stages, including 1 - rigorous screening of cell banks (both master cell bank and working cell bank) for viruses; 2 - screening of each cell culture harvest for adventitious agents; and 3 - a demonstration that the purification process can clear potential adventitious agents [15].

The detection of viruses in cell lines can be carried out via various techniques. The commonly used methods of detecting viral infections include

- co-cultivation assays (specific in vitro tests),

- in vivo assays,

- antibody production in animals (MAPs, RAPs, or HAPs),

- immunoassays for viral specific proteins,

- Transmission Electron Microscopy (TEM),

- Polymerase Chain Reaction (PCR).

For the co-cultivation assays (specific in vitro tests), the cells used for production, or culture supernatant, or the final product are incubated with the detector cells. The detector cell lines are susceptible to different viruses and are used to detect desired viruses via monitoring subsequent cytopathic effects, hemadsorption, morphological changes, or other signs of viral infection. The detector cells usually contain humans, primates, and cells from the same species.

The in vivo assay can be performed by the inoculation of cells or cell lysates into animals, including newborn and adult mice, guinea pigs, rabbits, or embryonated chicken eggs to detect viruses. The animals are consequently monitored for any abnormality.

Species-specific viruses potentially present in rodent cell lines can be examined using assays for antibody production in the animals. The MAP, RAP, and HAP (mouse, rat, and hamster antibody production assays, respectively) tests involve an injection of the test article into the animals. The inoculated animals are bled after four weeks, and the sera are tested for the presence of the antibodies against the specific viral antigens. For instance, Hantaan virus, Lactic Dehydrogenase virus, and Sendai virus have been screened using MAP.

An immunoassay for viral-specific proteins can be undertaken through production of the relevant antibodies after an injection of a virus of interest into animals. Currently commercially available immunoassays are able to detect various viruses.

Another method that is used for virus detection is TEM (Transmission Electron Microscopy). TEM is a quantitative assay that is based on the visualization and morphological identification of virus particles in samples [23].

Nevertheless, more sensitive methods, such as the PCR identification methods, can be employed for the detection of sequences of the viruses [16].

Since the biopharmaceuticals can be originated from mammalian cell lines with a high risk of endogenous retroviruses, on one hand, and these products may be infected with adventitious viruses through processing, on the other hand, virus inactivation and removal steps in the purification process are required [24]. These entail gamma irradiation, low pH treatment, or virus filtration.

Indeed, ensuring the absence of virus contamination in biopharmaceuticals is challenging. For instance, a limited number of commercial poultry vaccines were contaminated by avian leukosis virus even after routine quality assurance procedures. In addition, reovirus was found as a contaminant in urokinase. On the whole, sourcing and testing alone cannot guarantee the virological safety of biopharmaceuticals owing to some limitations: the limit of sensitivity for cell culture and PCR tests and also due to the fact that cell culture or in vivo tests are not able to detect all known kinds of potential contaminants [25]. Thus, practical methods are required for the virological safety of biopharmaceuticals, which involve the inclusion of risk assessment as well as management policies.

5.4. Mycoplasma

Mycoplasmas are the smallest free-living and self-replicating organisms in nature that are sized between 50 and 500nm. They lack a rigid cell wall and, consequently, are highly pleomorphic from round to filamentous. They are filterable and penicillin-resistant forms. Furthermore, their membrane contains sterol and due to this, mycoplasmas require the addition of serum or cholesterol to the growth medium. They grow on special media in aerobic or anaerobic conditions with optimum growth at 37°C and pH 7.0 and form with a "fried egg" morphology on agar media (Figure 6).

Mycoplasma contamination of cell culture systems for the production of mycoplasmas is a critical problem due to its effect on various parameters within the cell culture system. Mycoplasma contaminates cell cultures approximately without any sign, and it persists for a long time. Indeed, mycoplasma-positive cell cultures can be considered the major source of biopharmaceutical infection, and they should be discarded or effectively decontaminated. Taken together, mycoplasma-positive cell cultures pose a serious problem and should be effectively detected and eradicated [26].

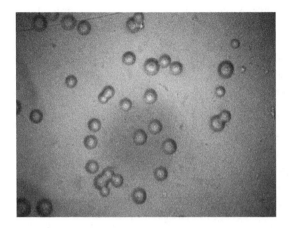

Figure 6. Mycoplasma colonies with fried egg morphology on mycoplasma agar medium. Picture was taken at Myco-plasma Reference laboratory, Razi vaccine and serum research institute, Iran

Different methods are used in international pharmacopoeias and guidance for detecting my-coplasma in biological test samples, mainly categorizing them as direct assay by microbio-logical culture, indirect assay by indicator mammalian cell culture, and PCR.

Direct assay by microbiological culture: The principle of detection is based on the growth of mycoplasma on supporting agar and liquid media (broth). First, the test sample is intro-duced into a special broth culture, is incubated for an appropriate time, and, consequently, it is sub-passaged to plate agar. After the required incubation period, the presence of myco-plasma colonies is observed microscopically in the agar plates (Figure 6).

Indirect assay by indicator mammalian cell culture: The indirect method requires the co-cul-tivation of the test sample with an indicator cell line for two to three days. Typically, VERO cells with a large cytoplasm area around the nucleus were used. Consequently, the cells were stained using a DNA binding stain (such as Hoechst stain) that binds specifically to DNA and is observed via fluorescent microscopy. Due to the affinity of mycoplasmas for the mammalian cell membrane, mycoplasmas appear as granules surrounding the nucleus.

Mycoplasma PCR: In this method, detection is carried out using specific oligonucleotide pri-mers for the amplification of mycoplasma DNA. This method is specially recommended for detecting contamination with the non-cultivable strains of *M. hyorhinis* [27].

On the whole, it is advisable to use two different methods in the detection of mycoplasmas in order to allow for the differentiation between false-positive and false-negative results.

5.5. DNA

The importance of DNA contamination detection in biopharmaceuticals is related to the fact that the DNA from some sources such as hybridoma cell lines in monoclonal antibody pro-duction may act as active oncogenes. These kinds of DNA contaminants can be introduced and expressed in human cells and result in the initiation of cancer cells. According to guidelines, the acceptable level of residual DNA in recombinant products is 10 pg per therapeutic dose. DNA hybridization studies that use radiolabeled DNA probes with a specific nucleic acid sequence constitute one of the most widely used methods for the detection of DNA contaminants in the product to a nanogram (ng) range [6]. The important steps involved in DNA hybridization are shown in Figure 7.

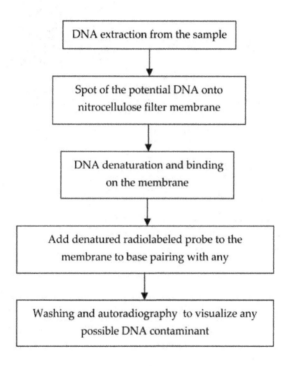

Figure 7. The main steps of the DNA hybridization procedure

5.6. Cross-contamination

Cell cultures may be infected with other cell types due to the use of contaminated items or operator mistakes. Also fail of the sterilization process can be another reason. The detection of cross-contamination is very challenging due to the fact that macroscopic and microscopic properties of the original and contaminant cells are commonly the same. Cross-contamination in the production of biopharmaceuticals would prove to be disastrous and terrible.

Various tests for detecting cross-contaminations can be applied; however, a product-specific identity test will be the best choice [16].

6. Summary

Microbial quality control plays a prominent role in the manufacture of safe and effective bio-pharmaceuticals. The main sources of microbial contamination can be related to raw materials and the production environment. The main categories of raw materials that are involved in the manufacturing of biopharmaceuticals with a high risk of contamination are those of animal origin such as cell culture media, sera, and supplements. The production environment includes air, surfaces, instruments, equipments, and personnel. All these can be considered the main source for the contamination of biopharmaceuticals with adventitious agents such as viruses, bacteria, fungi, transmitting spongiform encephalopathy, and mycoplasma. The use of contaminated biopharmaceuticals causes product spoilage, which may lead to (i) metabolization of the therapeutic agents by microorganisms, thus bringing about a decrease in the potency of the therapeutic agent; (ii) a potential health hazard to patients as a result of either infectious diseases or microbial-derived agents such as endotoxins that are secreted into products.

Various methods are used for detecting and eliminating different biological contaminants that are used in the manufacturing of biopharmaceuticals. Generally, bacteria and fungi can be detected by standard sterility testing or macroscopic and microscopic characteristics, as well as biochemical tests. In addition, viruses can be detected via a number of methods such as co-cultivation assays (specific in vitro tests), in vivo assays, antibody production in animals (MAPs, RAPs, or HAPs), immunoassays for viral specific proteins, TEM, or PCR. The detection of endotoxin can be carried out using the pharmacopeial rabbit test or LAL test. The available approaches for the detection of mycoplasma include direct assay using special culture media, indirect assay by mammalian cells, and DNA staining, as well as PCR. Furthermore, DNA hybridization is a widely used approach for the detection of DNA contaminants in biopharmaceuticals. The best method for cross-contamination detection includes a product-specific identity test.

With regard to the collection of tests for biological quality control of biopharmaceuticals summarized in this chapter, it is obvious that various sets of methods are available in different guidelines and pharmacopeias which are complicated and problematic. The development and compilation of harmonized guidelines for biological quality control of biopharmaceuticals is a critical necessity that can facilitate the control of the safety of these ever-increasing products.

Author details

Farzaneh Lotfipour and Somayeh Hallaj-Nezhadi

Faculty of Pharmacy, Immunology Research Center, Tabriz University of Medical Sciences, Tabriz, Iran

References

[1] Rader, R. A. (2005). What is a Biopharmaceutical, Part 1: (Bio)Technology-Based Definitions BioExecutive. March and May

[2] Rader, R. A. (2005). What is a Biopharmaceutical, Part 2: Company and Industry Definitions. BioExecutive. March and May

[3] WHO. Definition of active pharmaceutical ingredient.(2011). July Available from: http://www.who.int/medicines/areas/quality_safety/quality_assurance/DefinitionAPI-QAS Rev1-08082011.pdf.

[4] FDA. What is a biological product? ; Available from: http://www.fda.gov/AboutFDA/Transparency/Basics/ucm194516.htm.

[5] Walsh, G. (2002). Biopharmaceuticals and biotechnology medicines: an issue of nomenclature. Eur J Pharm Sci. 15(2):, 135-138.

[6] Walsh, G. (2003). Biopharmaceuticals Biochemistry And Biotechnology. Second ed, England: John Wiley & Sons, Ltd.

[7] Denyer, S. P., Hodges, N. A., & Gorman, S. P. (2004). Hugo and Russell's Pharmaceutical Microbiology. SEVENTH ed: Blackwell Science.

[8] Brown, T.A., Gene Cloning and DNA Analysis: An Introduction.th ed(2010). Wiley Blackwell.

[9] Kohler, G., & Milstein, C. (2005). Continuous cultures of fused cells secreting antibody of predefined specificity. 1975. J Immunol. 174(5):, 2453-2455.

[10] Kohler, G., & Milstein, C. (1975). Continuous cultures of fused cells secreting antibody of predefined specificity. Nature. 256(5517):, 495-497.

[11] Bols, N. C., et al. (1988). Media for hybridoma growth and monoclonal antibody production. Biotechnol Adv. 6(2):, 169-182.

[12] ANTIBODIES, C.O.M.O.P.M., *Monoclonal Antibody Production A Report of the Committee on Methods of Producing Monoclonal Antibodies Institute for Laboratory Animal Research National Research Council.*, (1999). : Washington, DC.

[13] Li, F., et al. (2010). Cell culture processes for monoclonal antibody production. MAbs. 2(5):, 466-479.

[14] Ho, R. J. Y., & Gibaldi, M. (2003). Biotechnology and Biopharmaceuticals: Transforming Proteins and Genes into Drugs, New Jersey.: A John Wiley & Sons, Inc.

[15] Knäblein, J. (2005). Modern Biopharmaceuticals: Design, Development and Optimization: WILEY-VCH Verlag GmbH & Co. KGaA, Weinheim.

[16] Denyer, S. P., & Baird, R. M. (2007). Guide to Microbiological Control in Pharmaceuticals and Medical Devices. second ed: CRC Press.

[17]   United States Pharmacopocia 29, National Formulary 24. USP Convention,Rockville (2006).

[18]   European Pharmacopoeia, 4th ed. EPSecretariat, Strasbourg.(2002).

[19]   Magalhaes, P. O., et al. (2007). Methods of endotoxin removal from biological preparations: a review. J Pharm Pharm Sci. 10(3):, 388-404.

[20]   Daneshian, M., et al. (2006). In vitro pyrogen test for toxic or immunomodulatory drugs. J Immunol Methods. 313(1-2):, 169-175.

[21]   Petsch, D., & Anspach, F. B. (2000). Endotoxin removal from protein solutions. J Biotechnol. 76(2-3):, 97-119.

[22]   Salema, V., Saxena, L., & Pattnaik, P. (2009). Removing endotoxin from biopharmaceutical solutions. Pharmaceutical Technology Europe. 21(10):, 36.

[23]   Vale, F. F., et al. (2010). Applications of transmission electron microscopy to virus detection and identification Microscopy: Science, Technology, Applications and Education.

[24]   Liu, H. F., et al. (2010). Recovery and purification process development for monoclonal antibody production. MAbs,. 2(5):, 480-499.

[25]   Bailey, A. (2011). Learning from Experience European Biopharmaceutical Review, Spring.

[26]   Fleckenstein, E., & Drexler, H.G. Iochemica n 1996 1.

[27]   Edition, T. J. P. F. Mycoplasma Testing for Cell Substrates used for the Production of Biotechnological/Biological Products. Available from: http://db.yaozh.com/foreign/JP15/jp5/F5_14.pdf.

Chapter 11

Quality Control of Formulated Medicines

Alexandre S. Leal, Maria Ângela de B. C. Menezes,
Ilza Dalmázio, Fernanda P. Sepe,
Tatiana C. B. Gomes, Amalia S. Santana,
Luzia H. da Cunha and Radojko Jaćimović

Additional information is available at the end of the chapter

1. Introduction

A pharmaceutical drug is technically obtained or prepared for prophylactic, curative, palliative or diagnostic purposes. The final product must meet quality standard, be safe and effective. In Brazil, there is a high demand for formulated drugs. This is mainly due to their lower price compared to manufactured drugs, evidenced by the rapid growth – an increase of 350% from 1998 to 2010.

Even after the ANVISA's (Agency National Health Surveillance) establishment of the new handling standards to be followed by the magistral pharmacies, several serious cases, including death reports, caused by the consumption of formulated drugs have recently become public [1-5].

Other problems related to this subject occurred in 2004, when deaths caused by manipulated medicines of low therapeutic index (clonidine and levotiroxine) led ANVISA to modify the regulation for manipulated medicines. The concentration of each compound was not totally assured and the contamination by impurities, not included in the original formula, were present in the final product.

In a previous work, we have also observed the presence of impurities – such as metals - in different kinds of medicines. The ingestion of metals, even at low levels, can be very harmful to humans. Besides this, the long-term uptake of some drugs is also risky. This should require attention and surveillance from the public health-related agencies [6-10].

The quality and safety of drugs must follow the specifications described in the official compendia - among them, the pharmacopoeias. Medicines cannot contain impurities or other substances that endanger the patient's health. According to the second edition of the Brazilian Pharmacopoeia National Formulary [1], to ensure safety, efficacy and quality of the handled products it is necessary correct calculations, exact measurements, and adequate conditions and procedures of preparation. The prudent judgment of the pharmacist, who must be a qualified professional for this purpose, is another fundamental aspect. Additionally, an appropriate profile with a proven stability must be sought in the literature [11-14].

The requirements of sanitary legislation and quality control of raw materials for magistral solid preparations are:

- raw material: character sensory, solubility, pH determination, melting point, density, weight and volume; analysis report of manufacturer/supplier;

- raw material of vegetal origin: organoleptic characters, solubility, pH determination, melting point, density, weight and volume, evaluation of vendor analysis report;

- manipulated product: solid dosage forms: description, appearance and organoleptic characteristics, determination of average weight

The legislation also determines that all pharmacies must perform analyzes every two months of at least one of the formulas containing drug(s) ≤ 25 mg of drugs. The priority is to those that contain ≤ 5 mg of drugs. The legislation establishes special quality control requirements for preparations of substances with low therapeutic index, like hormones, antibiotics and cytotoxic drugs, homeopathic products, and sterile products. The raw materials used in sterile preparations must also be analyzed [15-17].

The Legislation on Good Practices for Handling does not require impurity tests for the raw materials received by the pharmacies. It is only necessary to check the certificate of a qualified supplier – issued in accordance with methods described in the pharmacopoeia, which are only suitable for the detection of some elements (Ag, As, Bi, Cd, Hg, Mo, Pb, Sb, and Sn) [18].

Quality control tests for the products handled do not include detection and quantification of impurities. Moreover, the analysis required for formulated preparations allow limited conclusions about the quality of the process, since they do not testify the homogeneity of the active principle directly, but only as to the uniformity of filling of the capsules. So, a particular formulation can have the acceptance criteria for average mass, standard deviation and coefficient of variation but not the uniformity of this active content in the capsules [19].

Periodic reviews performed every two months for formulated drugs do not statistically have significant value, so that a reliable conclusion about the quality of formulated drugs can not be reached [20]. The analysis of thirty batches of 20 mg of Sinvastatin medicine manipulated in pharmacies of Belo Horizonte, showed that only fourteen of them, met the quality standard required by pharmacopeia. Thus, the therapeutic efficacy of 53% of the analyzed products can not be totally dependable [21].

In this study, the quality of medicines Omeprazole and Enalapril Maleate from five (5) different magistral pharmacies was evaluated according to the methodology described in pharmacopoeia. The analyses for mass determination, identification of active principle, content, content uniformity and related compounds were performed.

The target drugs, Omeprazole and Enalapril Maleate, were chosen because of their representativeness of consumption and availability of related reference data in the pharmacopoeias.

In order to evaluate the presence and concentration of chemical elements, the technique used in this study was neutron activation analysis (NAA), applying the k_0-standardization method [23-25]. The neutron activation analysis is a very sensitive and reliable multielemental technique, suitable for determination of the elements such as: As, Ba, Br, Ca, Ce, Cl, Co, Cr, Eu, Fe, Hf, Mg, Mn, Na, Sb, Sc, Sm, Ti and Zn, in different drugs [14]. The technique is based on the principle that when the material is irradiated by neutrons, some elements with suitable nuclear characteristics become radioactive isotopes. Thus, the concentration of each element can be determined by counting the respective radiation emitted by the corresponding radionuclide [26].

The results described here are part of a wider project which also includes the analyses of Fluoxetin and Sinvastatin medicines and will be published briefly.

2. Quality control of formulated drugs

2.1. The pharmacopeia

The 5th edition of the Brazilian Pharmacopoeia [27] defines quality control as: "The set of measures to ensure, at any time, the batch production of medicines and other products that meet the standards of identity, activity, content, purity, efficacy and safety." According to Resolution RDC Nº. 67, October 8, 2007 [15], which provides the Technical Regulation establishing the Good Handling Practices in Pharmacies (Good Compounding Practices) quality control of magistral and officinal preparations, is given by the completion of at minimum, the tests described in Table 1, according to the Brazilian Pharmacopoeia or other Official Compendium recognized by the National Health Surveillance Agency (ANVISA).

Results of tests must be recorded in the same order of handling, in addition to other relevant information. The pharmacist must evaluate the results to approve or not the preparation for dispensing. Each pharmacy is responsible for the quality of magistral preparations that handles, keeps, transports and dispenses. Raw materials should be checked in its receipt and moved to quarantine soon after, until the release of the reports of quality control. In the absence of pharmacopoeia monograph, the scientific literature should be used as a reference, and only with the lack of literature, the specification provided by the supplier may be used. All results must be written and stored [15].

Preparation	Test
Solid	Description, appearance, organoleptic characteristics, average mass
Semi-solid	Description, appearance, organoleptic characteristics, pH (where applicable), mass
Non-sterile liquid	Description, appearance, organoleptic characteristics, pH, mass or volume before filling

Table 1. Tests for quality control of magistral drugs

However, some studies also show that the rule of Good Practices on Handling does not answer and does not guarantee the quality of compounded drugs [20].

2.2. Analyses performed

The analyses of quality control were performed at the Laboratory for Quality Control of Chemical Physics Drug, and Cosmetic Sanitizing of the Ezequiel Dias Foundation (FUNED). The following tests were performed [15,27,28]:

- Aspect;

- Identification ;

- Labeling;

- Content;

- Related compounds;

- Dosage uniformity;

- Unit Change in mass;

The test of aspect is just a visual description of the product to be analyzed, coloration of the capsule and its content.

The test of identification allows determining the presence of the active principle in the product analyzed. It is performed through the high performance liquid chromatography (HPLC) [28].

The analysis of content aims to verify whether the drug has a dose of active ingredient on the label provided and used to quantify the active ingredient in the product analyzed. This test is performed according to the pharmacopoeia for each product, and may be performed in the ultraviolet and visible spectrophotometry, by high performance liquid chromatography, among other methods. The test uses usually ten to twenty capsules and each capsule analyzed separately, but the "pool" of these. There are limits specified in the monograph, which should be within the active drug, usually 90 to 110%. Results below the limit can result in ineffective therapy and above, intoxication, depending on the drug analized [28].

The analysis of related compounds determines the amount of by-products of synthesis of the substance and / or its degradation products and / or contaminants from the process of obtaining the substance which can be normally found within a specified limit. This test is done only when specified in the pharmacopoeia.

The variation of the mass allows checking the uniformity of mass between units within a batch. For products in hard capsules should be weighed individually, twenty units, the contents of each one should be removed, properly cleaned and reweighed. The mass content of each capsule is determined by mass difference between the full and the empty capsule. Then the average mass of the contents can be determined. For hard capsules, the limit of variation is ± 10% of the mass corresponding to less than 300 mg. If the mass corresponds to 300 mg or more, the maximum range is ± 7.5%. It cannot be tolerated more than two units outside the limits specified in the official compendia, but none can be above or below twice the percentages indicated [27].

The uniformity of dosage units evaluate the uniformity of distribution of active component units in a single batch can be determined by two methods: mass variation and content uniformity. The mass variation test is only applicable in specific cases. The test for content uniformity is based on the content of each active ingredients in a number of unit doses in order to determine whether the content is within specified limits, being applicable in all cases [28].

3. Methodology

3.1. High performance liquid chromatography

In this study the identification tests, content, related compounds and content uniformity was performed by high performance liquid chromatography (HPLC) according to the specifications of literature [28]. The chromatograph Shimadzu detector was coupled to molecular absorption spectrophotometry in the ultraviolet-visible Perkin Elmer Lambda 25 model, Class-VP software. All chemical reference substances (SQR) were purchased from USP (The United States Pharmacopeia).

To analyze the Enalapril Maleate, L7 C_8 column (4.6 mm x 25 cm x 5 mm) was used. Isocratic elution was performed with a buffer monobasic sodium phosphate pH 2.2 /acetonitrile at a ratio of 75:25. Solvents and solutions were degassed in ultrasonic bath (Elma Transsonic Digitals) and filtered through a Millipore membrane of 0.45 micrometers. Chromatography was performed at 50°C, flow rate of 2 mL.min⁻¹, with injections of 50 µL, detection at 215 nm and running time of 30 min. The calculations were based on the content of the samples obtained areas of the areas of the SQR of Enalapril Maleate. For related compounds the content of diketopiperazine compounds and enalaprilat was also calculated.

For omeprazole, L7 C_8 column (4.6 mm x 15 cm x 5 mm) was used. Elution was performed by mixing two solutions – solution A (6 g of glycine in 1500 mL water, pH 9) and solution B (acetonitrile and methanol, 85:15 ratio) – as shown in Table 3. Solvents and solutions were degassed in ultrasonic bath (Elma Transsonic Digitals) and filtered through a Millipore membrane of 0.45 micrometers. Chromatography was performed with a flow of 1,2 mL.min⁻¹, with injections of 10 µL, detection at 305 nm and running time of 30 min. The calculations were based on the content of the samples obtained areas of the areas of the SQR of omeprazole.

Time (minutes)	Solution A (%)	Solution B (%)	Elution
0 – 20	88 → 40	12 → 60	Linear gradient
20 – 21	40 → 88	60 → 12	Linear gradient
21 – 25	88	12	Isocratic

Table 2. Parameters of elution of the HPLC analysis of Omeprazole

3.1.1. Results and discussion

a.   Appearance, Identification and Labeling

Both, Omeprazole and Enalapril Maleate samples, showed similar aspects as their samples: hard capsule containing white pellets for Omeprazole, and hard capsule containing white powder varying only the color of the hard capsule used by each pharmacy. All samples, Omeprazole and Enalapril Maleate, were satisfactory for labeling and identification, confirming that the identity of the material was in accordance with the label from its packaging. In addition, all labels contain information provided by RDC Resolution Nº 67, October 8, 2007 [15]:

1.   Name of the prescriber;

2.   Name of the patient;

3.   Registration Number of the formulation;

4.   Data handling and shelf life;

5.   Formulation components and their quantities;

6.   Number of units;

7.   Dosage;

8.   Identification of pharmacy, full address and federal registration;

9.   Name and professional register of the responsible person.

b.   Related substances (Enalapril Maleate)

The test for related substances is performed only when described in the pharmacopeia of the compound to be analyzed, or another official compendium regulated by ANVISA [28]. For the Enalapril Maleate it is specified that no more than 5% of diketopiperazine and enalaprilat can be found in the final product. All samples of Enalapril Maleate were satisfactory for this analysis and the results are shown in Table 5.

Pharmacy	Enalaprilat (%)	Diketopiperazine (%)	Enalaprilat + Diketopiperazine (%)
A	0.66	0.82	1.48
B	0.16	0.07	0.23
C	0.53	0.87	1.40
D	0.05	0.001	0.055
E	1.18	2.77	3.95

Table 3. Content of related compounds of Enalapril Maleate

c. Content

The reference values for the content of both drugs should not be less than 90% nor exceed 110% of the declared value, 10 mg and 20 mg for omeprazole and enalapril, respectively. The results for content of active ingredient are described in Table 6.

It can be observed that four from the five samples of omeprazole were unsatisfactory; two of them with content above the permissible and the other two with the content below. For the samples of enalapril, two were unsatisfactory, one exceeding the limit and the other with recommended content lower than expected, as showed in Table 6.

Pharmacy	Omeprazole (10 mg/caps)	Enalapril Maleate (20 mg/caps)
A	(11.3 ± 0.4) mg/caps or 112.7% declared	(18.5 ± 0.2) mg/caps or 92.6% of declared
B	(8.4 ± 2.2) mg/caps or 84.4% declared	(20.5 ± 0.1) mg/caps or 102.7% declared
C	(6.9 ± 2.6) mg/caps or 68.7% declared	(18.5 ± 0.1) mg/caps or 92.5% declared
D	(11.2 ± 0.1) mg/caps or 111.5% declared	(11.2 ± 4.3) mg/caps or 56.0% declared
E	(11.0 ± 0.2) mg/caps or 109.6% declared	(16.9 ± 1.2) mg/caps or 84.7% do declared

Table 4. Final content of Omeprazole and Enalapril Maleate

d. Uniformity of the dosage unit

All Omeprazole samples were considered unsatisfactory for uniformity of the dosage unit. Three samples were satisfactory for Enalapril Maleate. The results for uniformity of dosage unit are described in Table 7 as contained in the final analysis report issued by FUNED. Variations in dose uniformity should not exceed 15% [28].

e. Mass Variation

The acceptable limit for the analysis of variation in mass of capsules, weighing less than 300 mg is ± 10% above the average mass, and it is tolerable no more than two units outside the specified limit and any unit may be above or below twice the percentages indicated. Thus, only a sample of Omeprazole was considered unsatisfactory. The results for the samples of Omeprazole and Enalapril Maleate are presented in Tables 8 and 9, respectively [27].

Pharmacy	Omeprazole (10 mg/caps)	Enalapril Maleate (20 mg/caps)
A	18.7%	7.8%
B	24.0%	14.2%
C	47.9%	10.6%
D	15.6%	14.0%
E	15.8%	46.5%

Table 5. Dose uniformity of the capsules of Omeprazole and Enalapril Maleate

Pharmacy	average weight (mg/caps.)	Lower	Higher
*A	220.4 ± 1.2	2.4	1.6
B	226.8 ± 5.8	9.5	8.7
C	210.0 ± 4.9	9.7	7.5
*D	119.0 ± 2.1	6.5	10.9
**E	120.7 ± 2.9	10.9	7.9

*One unit above the limit. ** Two units above the limit. Caps, capsules

Table 6. Variation (%) in mass of the capsules of Enalapril Maleate (20 mg/caps)

Pharmacy	average mass (mg/caps.)	Lower	Higher
*A	108.3 ± 3.0	7.1	15.1
B	195.4 ± 1.8	4.6	3.0
C	175.9 ± 3.0	9.1	4.7
**D	107.0 ± 7.0	15.3	40.8
***E	105.0 ± 2.1	10.6	7.2

*Two units above the limit. ** Four units above the limit. Unsatisfactory. *** One unit above the limit.

Table 7. Variation (%) in mass of the capsules of Enalapril Maleate (20 mg/caps)

From the ten samples analyzed, seven were rated as *unsatisfactory*, considering the analysis of aspect, mass variation, identification, related substances, uniformity of dosage units, content and labeling.

It was observed that, if only the official established procedures (description, appearance, organoleptic characteristics and average mass) were considered from the seven samples rated as unsatisfactory, just one would be classified in this status. The remaining six samples would erroneously be rated satisfactory, meaning that would be approved for human consumption [18].

Some factors may cause deviations, inherent to the handling process of drugs in capsules, such as the loss of substance during the grinding, mixing and filling the capsules. Miscalculations and weight of the formulation components, errors inherent to the operator and the use of damaged equipment may also compromise the process and therefore the quality of the final product [29].

The results of Omerazole and Enalapril Maleate were analyzed by ANOVA followed by Tukey's test for uniformity of content and unit dose. Results were considered significantly different at $p < 0.05$.

3.2. Neutron activation analysis

3.2.1. Material and methods

All samples of Omeprazole and Enalapril Maleate were purchased in the market of the Belo Horizonte, state of Minas Gerais, Brazil from five (5) different magistral pharmacies.

Due to operational reasons, Jožef Stefan Institute (JSI) performed analyses only from three (3) different pharmacies from the sampling group. Due to same operational reasons, the JSI did not analyze the short half-lives radionuclides of elements like Al, Cl, Mg, Mn and Ti.

The samples of Omeprazole and Enalapril Maleate performed by the JSI were packed in polyethylene capsules in plastic bottle containing 20 capsules each. Whole powder mass from 20 capsules was taken to prepare homogenized samples, which was transferred in clean polyethylene bottle. In the samples of Omeprazole performed by CDTN, just one the mass of one capsule taken randomly was considered by each sample. The difference of procedures carried out by both Institutes was due to operational reasons.

Both institutes CDTN/CNEN and JSI followed the same procedure to prepare the samples. The aliquots of each sample were manually crushed or ground using an agate mortar with pestle, whenever necessary, to avoid any contamination. In most cases, unless the amount of material did not allow it, two replicates were taken and weighed in polyethylene vials. It is relevant to emphasize that no additional chemical sample preparation was performed. At CDTN/CNEN and IJS, the samples were irradiated together with several Al–0.1% Au disks as neutron flux monitors, according to the k_0-standardisation method procedure [23,24,30].

Table 10 shows the characteristics of the applied technique such as the parameters f (thermal to epithermal fluxes ratio) and the α (parameter which measures the epithermal flux deviation from the ideal (1/E) distribution), needed for the k_0-method, the irradiation times and gamma spectrometry systems at each Institute.

3.2.2. Results and discussion

The obtained results of NAA from the medicines Omeprazole and Enalapril Maleate are showed in the Tables 11 to 13.

The technique applied was suitable for determining 20 chemical elements – Al, Br, Ca, Cl, Co, Cr, Fe, Mg, Mn, Na, Sb, Sc, Sm, Sr, Ta, Th, Ti, U and Zn – in a large range of concentration, without any chemical process. The elements Cl, Fe, K, Mg, Mn, Na, and Zn could be expected in this kind of samples. Other elements, not considered essential, for the human being such as As and Sr, found in lower concentration compared to Cl, Fe, K, Mg, Mn, Na, and Zn can also represent a health problem in a long term consumption. Even essential elements were determined but in high concentrations, like Fe may be toxic.

High concentration of elements such as Cl, Ca, Mg, Na and Ti are expected because they are frequently components of excipients in the preparation of pellets. The presence of Mg is due to the excipients usually used: magnesium is a component of magnesium estearate $(Mg[C_{18}H_{35}O_2])$, a lubricant for tablets and capsules and opadry, coloring agent, respectively [26]. Mg also is present in magnesium silicate $(Mg_3SiO_4(OH)_2]$ Na is a component of sodium laurilsulfate, $([CH_3(CH_2)_{10}(CH_2O)(SO_3)Na]$ and sodium bicarbonate $NaHCO_3$. Ca is added as excipient as calcium phosphate and Ti as titanium dioxide, TiO_2. Fe comes from red iron oxide, used as excipient as well [10,13]. The impurities such as Br, Co, Cr, Hf, La, Sb, Sc, Sm, Sr, Ta, Th and U, are probably original from the raw material and/or from the process of production and manipulation of the medicine. All elements determined not foreseen in the original formula can be considered as impurities.

	INSTITUTE	
	CDTN/CNEN	JSI
Thermal Flux (neutrons cm^{-2} s^{-1})	6.4×10^{11}	1.1×10^{12}
k_0-standardisation parameters		
f	20.4	28.6
α	0.197	- 0.011
Irradiation time (h)	8	13
Detector nominal efficiency (%)	50	40
Software used for:	Genie 2000	Genie 2000
Acquisition spectra	(CANBERRA)	(CANBERRA)
Spectra Analysis	HyperLab	HyperLab
Concentration calculation	Kayzero for Windows, V.2.42	Kayzero for Windows, V.2.42
Sample mass (mg)	200-250	240-250

Table 8. Experimental information of neutron activation analysis

The data presented in Tables 12, 13 and 14 cannot be compared directly because the samples analyzed are not from the batch, but the results are, in general, very similar. Most results determined by the CDTN in one capsule of Omeprazole taken randomly were also determined by the JSI in the homogenized samples, except for the elements Br, Cr and La. The concentrations of the elements determined by both institutes have, in general, the same magnitude.

The discussion about toxicity levels and possible consequences for humans being is very difficult, due to the low concentration of the elements and limitations on the studies available in the literature. For most trace elements, there are just some available data on acute and chronic toxicity in experimental animals, not sufficient data to assess the risks to the human health on a long term daily intake [22].

4. Conclusion

The obtained results of samples of omeprazole and enalapril from five different magistral pharmacies of Belo Horizonte, Brazil, confirm the concern about the quality and safety for consumption of formulated medicines. They represent a preliminary part of a more complete investigation, still under way.

From the ten samples analyzed, seven were considered unsatisfactory. Most of the problems found through analyses Omeprazole and Enalapril Maleate medicines, like the variation of active principle mass, mass variation and dosage unit, come from the inadequacy of procedures for handling the ingredients in the pharmacy.

Problems can also be caused by the quality of the raw material used and inefficient or inexistence of test for checking the material. Diversified impurities reinforce the hypothesis that these elements are not controlled by the quality system. It also suggests that quality control over the purity of medicines in general should be established, as well as the concentration limits for the impurities, at least for some elements like As, Cd, Cu, Hg, Pb and Sn, already foreseen for food in the Brazilian legislation.

The possible harmful and/or toxicological effects for the human health as a consequence of long term use of the formulated medicines represent an important concern for the authorities of the public health system. Recent cases of contamination and death in Brazil due to the consumption of inadequate formulated medicines has been enhancing the debate about the quality of the magistral pharmacy.

In conclusion, the results point out the necessity of prompt and efficient actions by the authorities of the health public system to assure the quality of formulated medicines. The aim of this work is just to provide evidences in order to contribute with this initiative.

	Pharmacy													
Element	A			B			C			D			E		
Al	532	±	20	260	±	10	305	±	11	452	±	17	335	±	12
Br	DL			0.60	±	0.03	DL			DL			DL		
Ca	17740	±	793	9379	±	446	11230	±	512	19600	±	880	14260	±	190
Cl	806	±	48	313	±	18	262	±	18	490	±	30	514	±	31
Co	0.5	±	0.1	0.3	±	0.1	0.3	±	0.1	DL	±		0.10	±	0.01
Cr	11.7	±	0.5	7.9	±	0.3	6.7	±	0.3	11.6	±	0.5	13	±	1
Fe	65	±	5	64	±	11	47	±	10	49	±	11	51	±	5
Mg	4643	±	192	449	±	28	390	±	28	998	±	57	697	±	47
Mn	2.8	±	0.3	1.4	±	0.1	DL			1.8		0.2	2.2		0.2
Na	8134	±	326	4003	±	144	3918	±	140	6838	±	241	6718	±	247
Sb	0.09	±	0.01	0.41	±	0.02	0.04	±	0.01	0.06	±	0.01	0.13	±	0.01

Table 9. Elemental concentration (mg.kg^{-1}) for Omeprazole (CDTN/CNEN)

	Pharmacy													
Element	A			B			C			D			E		
Sc	0.03	±	0.01	0.03	±	0.01	0.01	±	0.01	0.02	±	0.01	0.02	±	0.01
Sm	DL			0.02	±		DL			0.02		0.01	DL		
Sr	DL			DL			DL			21	±	4	DL		
Ta	0.02	±	0.01	0.14	±	0.01	DL			0.15	±	0.01	0.09	±	0.01
Ti	2748	±	105	1483	±	55	897	±	34	2124	±	79	1907	±	71
U	DL			0.22	±	0.01	DL			DL			0.4	±	0.1
Zn	3.4	±	0.4	1.8	±	0.3	DL			2.9	±	0.4	2.5	±	0.3

* DL – Lower than the Detection Limit

Table 10. Elemental concentration (mg.kg^{-1}) for Omeprazole (CDTN/CNEN)

	Pharmacy								
Element	A			B			C		
Br	0.19	±	0.01	0.17	±	0.01	0.22	±	0.01
Ca	16453	±	592	14908	±	540	12817	±	467
Ce	DL			DL	±		0.09	±	0.01

	Pharmacy							
Element	**A**			**B**			**C**	
Co	0.18	±	0.01	0.016	±	0.001	0.51	±	0.02
Cr	0.52	±	0.03	0.26	±	0.02	0.59	±	0.04
Fe	102	±	4	53	±	2	265	±	9
Hf	0.020	±	0.001	0.009	±	0.001	0.021	±	0.002
La	0.019	±	0.002	0.030	±	0.004	0.040	±	0.002
Mo	0.34	±	0.05	DL	±		DL		
Na	6616	±	232	5988	±	210	4836	±	169
Sb	0.014	±	0.001	0.012	±	0.001	0.011	±	0.001
Sc	0.013	±	0.005	0.010	±	0.001	0.022	±	0.001
Sm	DL			DL			0.0052	±	0.0003
Sr	22.3	±	1.1	17.4	±	1.0	9.0	±	1.0
Ta	0.34	±	0.01	0.076	±	0.003	0.42	±	0.02
Th	0.012	±	0.002	DL			0.027	±	0.002
U	0.09	±	0.01	0.14	±	0.01	0.053	±	0.004
Zn	0.60	±	0.1	0.4	±	0.1	0.7	±	0.1

* DL – Lower than the Detection Limit

Table 11. Elemental concentration (mg.kg⁻¹) for Omeprazole (JSI)

	Pharmacy							
Element	**A**			**B**			**C**	
Br	0.13	±	0.01	0.47	±	0.02	0.24	±	0.02
Cr	0.07	±	0.01	0.15	±	0.01	0.10	±	0.01
Na	12540	±	439	271	±	10	72480	±	2538
Sc	0.0009	±	0.0001	0.0007	±	0.0001	0.0054	±	0.0002
Sb	0.09	±	0.01	0.41	±	0.02	0.04	±	0.01
Th	DL			DL			0.015	±	0.001
Zn	0.49	±	0.04	DL			0.015	±	0.001

* DL – Lower than the Detection Limit

Table 12. Elemental concentration (mg.kg⁻¹) for Enalapril Maleate (JSI)

Acknowledgements

The authors would like to thank Dr. Adailton Pereira de Paiva and Dr. Marco Antonio Franzero for their kind and helpful collaboration.

Author details

Alexandre S. Leal[1*], Maria Ângela de B. C. Menezes[1], Ilza Dalmázio[1], Fernanda P. Sepe[1], Tatiana C. B. Gomes[1], Amalia S. Santana[2], Luzia H. da Cunha[2] and Radojko Jaćimović[3]

*Address all correspondence to: asleal@cdtn.br

1 Centro de Desenvolvimento da Tecnologia Nuclear/Comissão Nacional de Energia Nuclear (CDTN/CNEN), Belo Horizonte, Brazil

2 Fundação Estadual Ezequiel Dias (FUNED), Belo Horizonte, Brazil

3 Jožef Stefan Institute (JSI), Ljubljana, Slovenia

References

[1] Formulário Nacional Da Farmacopeia BrasileiraEd. 2. (2011). http://www.anvisa.gov.br/farmacopeiabrasileira/arquivos/FNFB%202%20Vers%C3%A3o%20DICOL%2009%20Dez%202012.pdfAccessed 23 May 2012)., 37.

[2] BrasilLei nº 5991, de 17 de dezembro de (1973). Dispõe sobre o controle sanitário do comércio de drogas, medicamentos, insumos farmacêuticos e correlatos, e dá outras providências. Diário Oficial da República Federativa do Brasil, Brasília, 19 Dec. 1973.

[3] Szatkowski, L. T. D, & Oliveira, C. L. O uso de medicamentos manipulados no município de Toledo. Infarma, Brasília, DF, n. 1-2, (2004). , 16, 77-80.

[4] Conselho Federal De FarmáciaHttp://Www.Cff.Org.Br/Accessed 01 Oct. (2011).

[5] Agência Nacional De Vigilância Sanitária (ANVISA)Boletim Informativo. Ed. 56. Jun. 2005. http://www.anvisa.gov.br/divulga/public/boletim/56_05.pdfAccessed (26 Sep. 2011).

[6] Gisele, H. Comunicação na Oficina: "Medicamentos Manipulados: um Desafio para o Sistema Nacional de Vigilância Sanitária". Rio de Janeiro, 08 and 09 May (2006).

[7] UOLFarmácia assume culpa por contaminação que causou doping de Cielo. http://esporte.uol.com.br/natacao/ultimas-noticias/2011/07/01/farmacia-assume-culpa-por-contaminacao-que-causou-doping-de-cesar-cielo.htmAccessed (10 Oct. 2011).

[8]   Notícia, A. Remédio pode ter matado duas pessoas em Corupá, Norte de SC. http://
      www.clicrbs.com.br/anoticia/jsp/default.jsp?uf=2&local=18&section=Geral&news-
      ID=a3497429.xmlAcessed 10 Oct. (2011).

[9]   G1MG. Análise parcial comprova erro em produção de remédio, diz secretaria.
      http://g1.globo.com/minas-gerais/noticia/2011/12/analise-parcial-comprova-erro-em-
      producao-de-remedio-diz-secretaria.html (Acessed 23 Dec. 2011).

[10] Remington, J. P, & Gennaro, A. R. The Science and Practice of Pharmacy. Philadel-
      phia College of Pharmacy and Science, Philadelphia, ed. 20, (2000). , 2077.

[11] Fergusson, J. E. The Heavy Elements: Chemistry, Environmental Impact and Health
      Effects. Pergamon, Oxford, (1990). , 614.

[12] World Health Organization (WHO)www.who.intAcessed 03 Mar. (2010).

[13] Leal, A. S, Menezes, M. Â. B. C, Vermaercke, R. R, & Rodrigues, O. Andonie; Sneyers,
      L. Investigation of chemical impurities in formulations, phytotherapics and polyvita-
      minic medicines by k0-instrumental neutron activation analysis. Nucl. Instrum.
      Methods Phys. Res. A 564, (2006). , 729-732.

[14] Leal, A. S, Menezes, M. Â. B. C, Vermaercke, P, Sneyers, L, & Jensen, C. A compara-
      tive neutron activation analysis study of common generic manipulated and reference
      medicines commercialized in Brazil. App. Rad. Isotop. 66, (2008). , 1307-1312.

[15] BrasilResolução RDC n° 67, de 8 de outubro de (2007). Diário Oficial da União, Poder
      Executivo, Brasília, DF, 09 Oct. 2007. Seção I, , 29-58.

[16] BrasilResolução RDC n° 87, de 21 de novembro de (2008). Diário Oficial da União,
      Poder Executivo, Brasília, DF, 24 Nov. 2008, Seção I, , 58-59.

[17] BrasilResolução RDC n° 21, de 20 de maio de (2009). Diário Oficial da União, Poder
      Executivo, Brasília, DF, 21 May 2009, Seção I, , 53.

[18] Wang, T, Wu, J, Hartman, R, Jia, X, & Egan, R. S. A multi-element ICP-MS survey
      method as an alternative to the heavy metals limit test for pharmaceutical materials.
      Journal of Pharmaceutical and Biomedical Analysis. 23, (2000). , 867-890.

[19] Buurma, H, Smet, P. A. G. M, Hoff, O. P, Sysling, H, Storimans, M, & Egberts, A. C.
      G. Frequency, nature and determinants of pharmacy compounded medicines in
      Dutch community pharmacies. Pharmacy World & Science, Netherlands, n. 6,
      (2003). , 25, 280-287.

[20] Almeida, M. L, & Filho, A. P. N. Análise das cápsulas manipuladas segundo a RDC
      67/2007 da ANVISA/MS para a garantia da qualidade. Rev. Bras. Farm., n. 3, (2010). ,
      91, 119-125.

[21] Marinho, F. D. M. Zanon, J.C.C; Sakurai, E. Reis, I.A.; Lima, A.A.; Soares, C.D.V.
      Quality evaluation of simvastatin compounded capsules. Brazilian Journal of Phar-
      maceutical Sciences, n. 3, (2011). , 47, 495-502.

[22] Oskarsson, A, & Sandstrom, B. A Nordic Project-risk evaluation of essencial trace elements: esencial versus toxic levels of intake. Analyst., (1995). , 120, 911-912.

[23] De Corte, F, & The, k. standardisation method; a move to the optimisation of neutron activation analysis. Ed. Ryksuniversiteit Gent, Faculteit Van de Wetenschappen, (1986). , 464.

[24] De Wispelaere, F, De Corte, F, Bossus, D. A. W, Swagten, J. J. M. G, & Vermaercke, P. Re-determination and re-evaluation of the f and α parameters in channels Y4 and S84 of the BR1 reactor for use in K0- NAA at DSM research. Nuclear Instruments and Methods in Physics Research Section A, (2005). , 564, 636-640.

[25] Vermaercke, P, Robouch, P, Eguskiza, M, De Corte, F, Kennedy, G, Smodis, B, Yonezawa, C, Matsue, H, Lin, X, Blaauw, M, & Kučêra, J. Characterization of synthetic multi-element standards SMELS used for validation of K0- NAA. Nuclear Instruments and Methods in Physics Research Section A, (2006). , 564, 675-682.

[26] Nordberg, G. F, et al. Handbook on the Toxicology of Metals. (2007). http://pt.scribd.com/doc/59673422/Toxic-Metals-HandbookAcessed 01 Oct. 2011).

[27] Farmacopéia BrasileiraAgência Nacional de Vigilância Sanitária, Ed. 5, Brasília, (2010).

[28] USP 32 (The United States Pharmacopeia 32)United States Pharmacopeial Convention, (2009).

[29] Futuro, D. O, & Silva, R. F. Uso de ferramentas de controle estatístico para o entendimento do processo de produção de cápsulas em farmácias magistrais. XXVIII Encontro Nacional de Engenharia de Produção Foz do Iguaçu, Paraná, Brasil, Oct. (2007). , 09-11.

[30] Menezes, M. Â. B. C, Jacimovic, R, & Optimised, k. instrumental neutron activation method using the TRIGA MARK I IPR-R1 reactor at CDTN/CNEN, Belo Horizonte, Brazil. Nuclear Instruments and Methods in Physics Research Section A, (2006). , 564, 707-715.

Permissions

The contributors of this book come from diverse backgrounds, making this book a truly international effort. This book will bring forth new frontiers with its revolutionizing research information and detailed analysis of the nascent developments around the world.

We would like to thank Dr. Isin Akyar, for lending her expertise to make the book truly unique. She has played a crucial role in the development of this book. Without her invaluable contribution this book wouldn't have been possible. She has made vital efforts to compile up to date information on the varied aspects of this subject to make this book a valuable addition to the collection of many professionals and students.

This book was conceptualized with the vision of imparting up-to-date information and advanced data in this field. To ensure the same, a matchless editorial board was set up. Every individual on the board went through rigorous rounds of assessment to prove their worth. After which they invested a large part of their time researching and compiling the most relevant data for our readers. Conferences and sessions were held from time to time between the editorial board and the contributing authors to present the data in the most comprehensible form. The editorial team has worked tirelessly to provide valuable and valid information to help people across the globe.

Every chapter published in this book has been scrutinized by our experts. Their significance has been extensively debated. The topics covered herein carry significant findings which will fuel the growth of the discipline. They may even be implemented as practical applications or may be referred to as a beginning point for another development. Chapters in this book were first published by InTech; hereby published with permission under the Creative Commons Attribution License or equivalent.

The editorial board has been involved in producing this book since its inception. They have spent rigorous hours researching and exploring the diverse topics which have resulted in the successful publishing of this book. They have passed on their knowledge of decades through this book. To expedite this challenging task, the publisher supported the team at every step. A small team of assistant editors was also appointed to further simplify the editing procedure and attain best results for the readers.

Our editorial team has been hand-picked from every corner of the world. Their multi-ethnicity adds dynamic inputs to the discussions which result in innovative outcomes. These outcomes are then further discussed with the researchers and contributors who give their valuable feedback and opinion regarding the same. The feedback is then collaborated with the researches and they are edited in a comprehensive manner to aid the understanding of the subject.

Apart from the editorial board, the designing team has also invested a significant amount of their time in understanding the subject and creating the most relevant covers. They scrutinized every image to scout for the most suitable representation of the subject and create an appropriate cover for the book.

The publishing team has been involved in this book since its early stages. They were actively engaged in every process, be it collecting the data, connecting with the contributors or procuring relevant information. The team has been an ardent support to the editorial, designing and production team. Their endless efforts to recruit the best for this project, has resulted in the accomplishment of this book. They are a veteran in the field of academics and their pool of knowledge is as vast as their experience in printing. Their expertise and guidance has proved useful at every step. Their uncompromising quality standards have made this book an exceptional effort. Their encouragement from time to time has been an inspiration for everyone.

The publisher and the editorial board hope that this book will prove to be a valuable piece of knowledge for researchers, students, practitioners and scholars across the globe.

List of Contributors

Osamu Morinaga and Yukihiro Shoyama
Department of Pharmacognosy, Faculty of Pharmaceutical Sciences, Nagasaki International University, Sasebo, Japan

Marcelo Gonzaga de Freitas Araújo and Taís Maria Bauab
Biological Sciences Department, Faculty of Pharmaceutical Sciences, São Paulo State University – UNESP, Araraquara, Brazil

Takuhiro Uto, Nguyen Huu Tung and Yukihiro Shoyama
Faculty of Pharmaceutical Sciences, Nagasaki International University, Japan

Hiroyuki Tanaka
Faculty of Pharmaceutical Sciences, Kyushu University, Japan

Elba Lúcia Cavalcanti de Amorim, Valérium Thijan Nobre de Almeida de Castro, Allan Jonathan Chernichiarro Corrêa
Department of Pharmacy, Federal University Pernambuco, Recife/PE, Brazil

Joabe Gomes de Melo
Department of Biology, Federal Rural University of Pernambuco, Brazil

Tadeu José da Silva Peixoto Sobrinho
School of Medicine, Federal University of Tocantins, Palmas/TO, Brazil

Sunday Ameh and Florence Tarfa
Department of Medicinal Chemistry & Quality Control, National Institute for Pharmaceutical Research and Development (NIPRD), Idu Indusrial Area, Nigeria

Magaji Garba
Department of Pharmaceutical & Medicinal Chemistry, Ahmadu Bello University, Nigeria

Karniyus Gamaniel
Office of the Director General, NIPRD, Idu Indusrial Area, Nigeria

Edoardo Capuano and Saskia M. van Ruth
RIKILT – Institute of Food Safety, Wageningen University and Research Centre, The Netherlands

Christian W. Huck
Institute of Analytical Chemistry and Radiochemistry, CCB – Center for Chemistry and Biomedicine, Innsbruck, Austria

Hoa Van Ba and Inho Hwang
Department of Animal Science and Biotechnology, Lab of Muscle Biology and Meat Science, Chonbuk National University, South Korea

Dawoon Jeong and Amna Touseef
Department of Animal Science and Biotechnology, Lab of Muscle Biology and Meat Science, Chonbuk National University, South Korea

Sigrid Mennickent, M. de Diego, B. Schulz and C. G. Godoy
Department of Pharmacy, Faculty of Pharmacy, University of Concepción, Concepción, Chile

M. Vega
Department of Bromatology, Nutrition and Dietetic, Faculty of Pharmacy, University of Concepción, Concepción, Chile

Farzaneh Lotfipour and Somayeh Hallaj-Nezhadi
Faculty of Pharmacy, Immunology Research Center, Tabriz University of Medical Sciences, Tabriz, Iran

Alexandre S. Leal, Maria Ângela de B. C. Menezes, Ilza Dalmázio, Fernanda P. Sepe and Tatiana C. B. Gomes
Centro de Desenvolvimento da Tecnologia Nuclear/Comissão Nacional de Energia Nuclear (CDTN/CNEN), Belo Horizonte, Brazil

Amalia S. Santana and Luzia H. da Cunha
Fundação Estadual Ezequiel Dias (FUNED), Belo Horizonte, Brazil

Radojko Jaćimović
Jožef Stefan Institute (JSI), Ljubljana, Slovenia